Concise Review of Veterinary Microbiology

Concise Review of Veterinary Microbiology

Second Edition

P.J. Quinn   MVB, PhD, MRCVS

Professor Emeritus
Former Professor of Veterinary Microbiology and Parasitology
School of Veterinary Medicine
University College Dublin

B.K. Markey   MVB, PhD, MRCVS, Dip. Stat

Senior Lecturer in Veterinary Microbiology
School of Veterinary Medicine
University College Dublin

F.C. Leonard   MVB, PhD, MRCVS

Senior Lecturer in Veterinary Microbiology
School of Veterinary Medicine
University College Dublin

E.S. FitzPatrick   FIBMS, FRMS

Former Chief Technical Officer
School of Veterinary Medicine
University College Dublin

S. Fanning   BSc, PhD

Professor of Food Safety and Zoonoses
Director of UCD Centre for Food Safety
School of Public Health, Physiotherapy and Sports Science
University College Dublin

WILEY Blackwell

Contents

Preface

The first edition of this book provided undergraduate veterinary students with a brief introduction to veterinary microbiology and diseases caused by pathogenic microorganisms. Since its publication in 2003, there have been many changes in veterinary microbiology, some related to the classification of pathogenic microorganisms and others associated with the increased understanding of the pathogenesis of infectious diseases. Developments in molecular aspects of microbiology have broadened the scope of diagnostic methods and have improved our understanding of the epidemiological characteristics of many infectious diseases. New developments relating to the emergence of antibacterial resistance are of particular importance in veterinary therapeutics and in public health.

The second edition of this book includes new chapters on bacterial genetics, antibacterial resistance, immunology, antifungal chemotherapy, biosecurity and vaccination. Topics of particular importance in veterinary medicine are given extended coverage. Important changes which have occurred in veterinary microbiology in recent years are presented in relevant chapters. There are five sections in this book and the Appendix includes a list of relevant websites to facilitate readers requiring additional information on topics referred to in the book. Colour has been used to enhance the quality of the illustrations and to facilitate interpretation of complex diagrams.

Acknowledgements

We wish to acknowledge the assistance provided by colleagues who reviewed chapters, provided scientific, technical and editorial advice or who assisted in other ways: James Buckley, Rory Breathnach, Louise Britton, Jill Bryan, Marguerite Clyne, Hubert Fuller, James Gibbons, Stephen Gordon, Laura Luque-Sastre, Aidan Kelly, Pamela Kelly, Dores Maguire, Marta Martins, Kerri Malone, Jarlath Nally, David Quinn, Michael Quinn, Eoin Ryan, John Ryan, Patrick Raleigh, Shabarinath Srikumar, Graham Tynan, Patrick Wall and Annetta Zintl.

The facilities and support provided by the librarian, Carmel Norris and staff at the Veterinary Library are acknowledged with gratitude. We are grateful to Justinia Wood, Catriona Cooper and their colleagues at Wiley for the help and advice provided during the preparation of the book.

Dublin, January 2015

Abbreviations and definitions

AGID	agar gel immunodiffusion
ATP	adenosine triphosphate
BCG	bacille Calmette–Guérin
bp	base pairs
cAMP	cyclic adenosine monophosphate
CD	cluster of differentiation
CFT	complement fixation test
CNS	central nervous system
cELISA	competitive enzyme-linked immunosorbent assay
DNA	deoxyribonucleic acid
ELISA	enzyme-linked immunosorbent assay
EU	European Union
FA	fluorescent antibody
Fc	crystallizable fragment, portion of an immunoglobulin without an antigen combining site
IFA	indirect fluorescent antibody
IFN	interferon
Ig	immunoglobulin
LPS	lipopolysaccharide
KOH	potassium hydroxide
MBC	minimal bactericidal concentration
MHC	major histocompatibility complex
MIC	minimal inhibitory concentration
MLST	multi-locus sequence typing
mRNA	messenger RNA
MRSA	methicillin-resistant *Staphylococcus aureus*
MZN	modified Ziehl–Neelsen
nm	nanometre, 10^{-9} metre
NK cells	natural killer cells
OIE	Office International des Épizooties (World Organization for Animal Health)
ORF	open reading frame
PAS	periodic acid–Schiff
PCR	polymerase chain reaction
PFGE	pulsed-field gel electrophoresis
RFLP	restriction fragment length polymorphism
RNA	ribonucleic acid
rRNA	ribosomal RNA
RT-PCR	reverse transcriptase-polymerase chain reaction
RTX	repeats-in-toxin
SMEDI	stillbirth, mummification, embryonic death, infertility
V factor	nicotinamide adenine dinucleotide
VP	viral protein
UK	United Kingdom
μm	micrometre or micron, 10^{-6} metre
USA	United States of America
UV light	ultraviolet light
X factor	haemin
ZN	Ziehl–Neelsen
°C	degrees Celsius

About the companion website

This book is accompanied by a companion website:

www.wiley.com/go/quinn/concise-veterinary-microbiology

The website includes:

- PowerPoint figures from the book for downloading

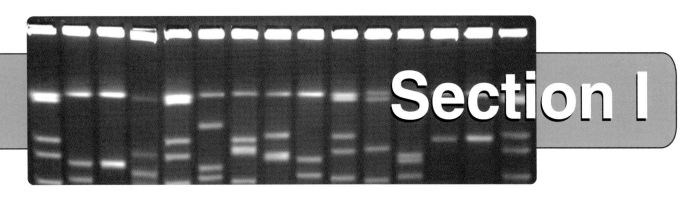

Section I

Introductory Bacteriology

1 Structure of bacterial cells

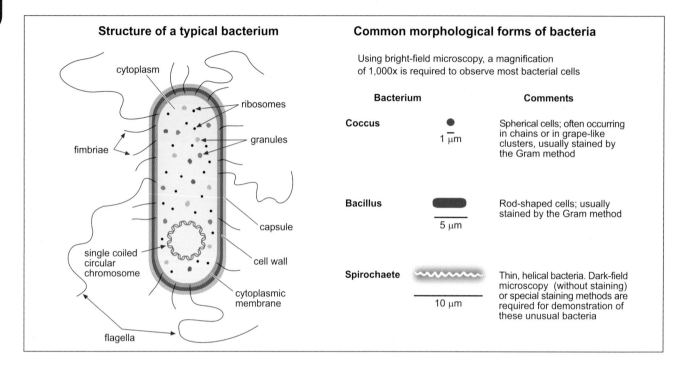

Structure of a typical bacterium

cytoplasm
ribosomes
granules
fimbriae
capsule
single coiled circular chromosome
cell wall
cytoplasmic membrane
flagella

Common morphological forms of bacteria

Using bright-field microscopy, a magnification of 1,000x is required to observe most bacterial cells

Bacterium		Comments
Coccus	1 μm	Spherical cells; often occurring in chains or in grape-like clusters, usually stained by the Gram method
Bacillus	5 μm	Rod-shaped cells; usually stained by the Gram method
Spirochaete	10 μm	Thin, helical bacteria. Dark-field microscopy (without staining) or special staining methods are required for demonstration of these unusual bacteria

Bacteria are unicellular organisms and usually occur in simple shapes such as rods, cocci, spiral forms and occasionally as branching filaments. They typically have rigid cell walls containing a peptidoglycan layer and multiply by binary fission. Bacteria are smaller and less complex than eukaryotic cells and do not contain membrane-bound organelles. Genetic information essential for organism survival, the core genome, is usually contained in a single circular chromosome; a nuclear membrane and a nucleolus are absent. Some bacteria have more than one chromosome and chromosomes in certain bacteria are linear. The accessory genome encodes non-essential cell functions and may include plasmids and bacteriophages (see Chapter 3). Despite their morphological diversity, most bacteria are between 0.5 and 5 μm in length. Motile bacteria possess flagella by which they can move through liquids *in vivo* and *in vitro*.

Most bacteria found in nature are not harmful to humans, animals or plants. Some bacteria make an important contribution to the utilization of nutrients in soil, in water and in the digestive tracts of animals. Bacteria which cause disease in animals or humans are referred to as pathogenic bacteria.

A typical bacterial cell is composed of a capsule, cell wall, cell membrane, cytoplasm (containing nuclear material) and

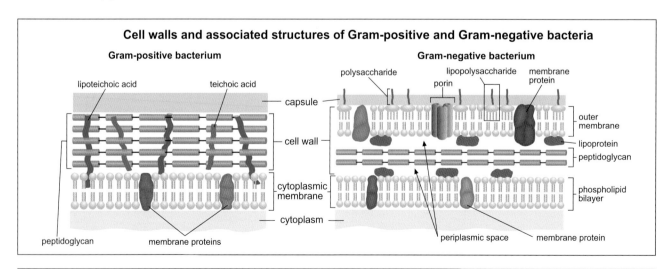

Cell walls and associated structures of Gram-positive and Gram-negative bacteria

Gram-positive bacterium

lipoteichoic acid
teichoic acid
capsule
cell wall
cytoplasmic membrane
cytoplasm
peptidoglycan
membrane proteins

Gram-negative bacterium

polysaccharide
lipopolysaccharide
membrane protein
porin
outer membrane
lipoprotein
peptidoglycan
phospholipid bilayer
periplasmic space
membrane protein

Concise Review of Veterinary Microbiology, Second Edition. P.J. Quinn, B.K. Markey, F.C. Leonard, E.S. FitzPatrick and S. Fanning.
© 2016 John Wiley & Sons, Ltd. Published 2016 by John Wiley & Sons, Ltd.
Companion website: www.wiley.com/go/quinn/concise-veterinary-microbiology

Table 1.1 Structural components of bacterial cells.

Structure	Chemical composition	Comments
Capsule	Usually polysaccharide; polypeptide in *Bacillus anthracis*	Often associated with virulence; interferes with phagocytosis; may prolong survival in the environment
Cell wall	Peptidoglycan and teichoic acid in Gram-positive bacteria. Lipopolysaccharide (LPS), protein, phospholipid and peptidoglycan in Gram-negative bacteria	Peptidoglycan is responsible for the shape of the organism. LPS is responsible for endotoxic effects. Porins – protein structures – regulate the passage of small molecules through the phospholipid layer
Cell membrane	Phospholipid bilayer	Selectively permeable membrane involved in active transport of nutrients, respiration, excretion and chemoreception
Flagellum (plural, flagella)	Protein called flagellin	Filamentous structure which confers motility
Pilus (plural, pili)	Protein called pilin	Also known as fimbria (plural, fimbriae). Thin, straight, thread-like structures present on many Gram-negative bacteria. Mediate attachment to host cells. Specialized pili are involved in conjugation
Chromosome	DNA	Single circular structure with no nuclear membrane
Ribosome	RNA and protein	Involved in protein synthesis
Storage granules or inclusions	Variable chemical composition	Present in some bacterial cells; may be composed of polyphosphate (volutin or metachromatic granules), poly-β-hydroxybutyrate (reserve energy source), glycogen

appendages such as flagella and pili. Some species of bacteria can produce dormant forms termed spores or endospores, structures which are resistant to environmental influences. The principal structural components of bacterial cells are presented in Table 1.1. Some bacteria can synthesize extracellular polymeric material, termed a capsule, which forms a well-defined structure, closely adherent to the cell wall. In the body, capsules of pathogenic bacteria interfere with phagocytosis. The tough, rigid cell walls of bacteria protect them from mechanical damage and osmotic lysis. Differences in the structure and chemical composition of the cell walls of bacterial species account for variation in their pathogenicity and influence other characteristics, including staining properties. Mycoplasmas, an important group of bacteria, lack rigid cell walls but have a flexible triple-layered outer membrane.

On the basis of colour when stained by the Gram method, bacteria can be divided into two major groups, Gram-positive and Gram-negative; this colour reaction is determined by the composition of the cell wall. Gram-positive bacteria, which stain blue, have a relatively thick uniform cell wall which is composed mainly of peptidoglycan and teichoic acids. In contrast, Gram-negative bacteria, which stain red, have cell walls with a more complex structure, consisting of an outer membrane and a periplasmic space containing a comparatively small amount of peptidoglycan.

The cell membranes of bacterial cells are flexible structures composed of phospholipids and proteins. Active transport of nutrients into the cell and elimination of waste metabolites are functions of the cell membrane and it is also the site of electron transport for bacterial respiration. The cytoplasm, which is enclosed by the cell membrane, is essentially an aqueous fluid containing the nuclear material, ribosomes, nutrients, enzymes and other molecules involved in synthesis, cell maintenance and metabolism.

In most bacteria, the bacterial genome is composed of a single haploid circular chromosome containing double-stranded DNA. Bacterial genomes differ in size depending on the species. Plas-

mids, small circular pieces of DNA which are separate from the core genome, are capable of autonomous replication. Plasmid DNA may encode characteristics such as antibiotic resistance and exotoxin production. All protein synthesis takes place on ribosomes, structures composed of ribonucleoproteins.

Motile bacteria possess flagella, attached to the cell wall, which are usually several times longer than the bacterial cell and are composed of a protein called flagellin. Fine, straight, hair-like structures called pili or fimbriae, composed of the protein pilin, are attached to the cell wall of many bacteria. In many pathogenic Gram-negative bacteria, adhesins present at the tips of pili function as attachment structures for mammalian cells.

Dormant, highly resistant structures, termed endospores, are formed by some bacteria to ensure survival during adverse environmental conditions. The only genera of pathogenic bacteria which contain endospore-forming species are *Bacillus* and *Clostridium*. The resistance of endospores is attributed to their layered structure, their dehydrated state, their negligible metabolic activity and their high content of dipicolinic acid. Because endospores are thermostable, moist heat at 121°C for 15 minutes is required for their inactivation.

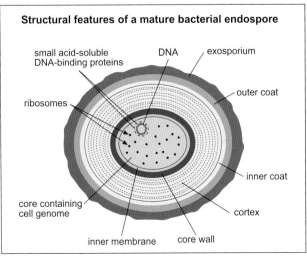

Structural features of a mature bacterial endospore

small acid-soluble DNA-binding proteins

DNA

exosporium

ribosomes

outer coat

core containing cell genome

inner coat

inner membrane

core wall

cortex

2 Cultivation, preservation and inactivation of bacteria

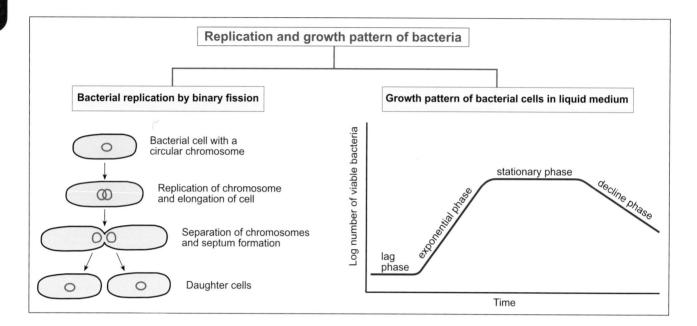

Appropriate conditions relating to moisture, pH, temperature, osmotic pressure, atmosphere and nutrients are required for bacterial growth. Bacteria replicate by binary fission. The generation time, the length of time required for a single bacterial cell to yield two daughter cells, ranges from 30 minutes to 20 hours. Long-term preservation of microorganisms usually involves freezing procedures. Heat treatment or chemicals can be used for inactivation of bacteria.

Following inoculation of bacterial cells into fresh broth medium, the growth curve of the culture exhibits lag, exponential and stationary phases and a final decline phase. During the lag phase, bacterial cells are metabolically active but not dividing; binary fission of cells results in an exponential increase in numbers. Procedures which can be used for total cell counting include direct microscopy, electronic methods and real-time quantitative polymerase chain reaction (PCR)-based methods. Viable bacterial numbers can be determined by colony counting and by membrane filtration. Accurate cell counts may be required for specific purposes such as vaccine preparation and for bacteriological testing of water.

Bacteria acquire nutrients from their immediate environment. Nutrient media for the isolation of pathogenic bacteria are formulated to supply particular growth factors for particular groups of organisms. Most bacteria require carbon and nitrogen in relatively large amounts. Trace elements and certain growth factors such as vitamins are also essential for bacterial growth.

In addition to nutritional factors, growth of bacteria is influenced by genetic factors and by chemical, physical and other environmental influences. Growth of bacteria in culture is

influenced by temperature, hydrogen ion concentration, availability of moisture, atmospheric composition and osmotic pressure. Most bacteria grow optimally at neutral pH. The majority of pathogenic bacteria can be grown aerobically on a nutrient agar medium at 37°C, close to the body temperature of humans and most domestic species. Bacteria with an optimal incubation temperature of 37°C are termed mesophiles and most pathogenic bacteria belong to this category. Based on their preference for particular levels of oxygen, bacteria can be assigned to four main groups, namely aerobes, anaerobes, facultative anaerobes and microaerophiles. A fifth group, capnophiles, are aerobic bacteria with a requirement for carbon dioxide. Anaerobic bacteria are unable to grow in an atmosphere containing oxygen. Strict anaerobes are cultured in tightly sealed jars in an atmosphere from which free oxygen has been removed.

Subculturing can be used for the short-term preservation of bacteria. Limitations of this procedure include death of some cells and a risk of contamination and mutation. Long-term methods of preservation include freeze-drying (lyophilization), freezing at –70°C and ultra-freezing in liquid nitrogen at –196°C. Freezing organisms in vials containing 20–30 porous polypropylene beads which can be removed and cultured singly is a convenient method of avoiding the need for repeated freezing and thawing of cultures. If properly used, these preservation methods can maintain organisms in a hypobiotic state for more than 30 years and ensure that the organisms remain unchanged and uncontaminated.

Sterilization is the method employed for the destruction of microorganisms on equipment used in microbiological and

Concise Review of Veterinary Microbiology, Second Edition. P.J. Quinn, B.K. Markey, F.C. Leonard, E.S. FitzPatrick and S. Fanning.
© 2016 John Wiley & Sons, Ltd. Published 2016 by John Wiley & Sons, Ltd.
Companion website: www.wiley.com/go/quinn/concise-veterinary-microbiology

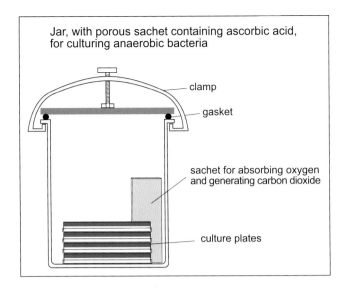

Jar, with porous sachet containing ascorbic acid, for culturing anaerobic bacteria

clamp

gasket

sachet for absorbing oxygen and generating carbon dioxide

culture plates

surgical procedures. Physical and chemical methods can be used for inactivation of microorganisms. Chemicals which inactivate bacteria include disinfectants and other compounds with bactericidal activity. Methods for preventing spoilage or limiting microbial growth in food are presented in Table 2.1. Physical methods for sterilizing equipment or fluids are presented in Table 2.2. Sterilization procedures are effective for the destruction of bacterial, fungal and viral agents. When dealing with bacterial endospores, such as those of *Clostridium* species, heating at a temperature of 121°C for 15 minutes in moist heat is required for their inactivation.

Table 2.2 Physical methods for sterilizing equipment or fluids; some can be used for disposing of contaminated material.

Method	Comments
Moist heat (autoclaving) employing steam under pressure to generate 121°C for 15 minutes or 115°C for 45 minutes	Used for sterilizing culture media, laboratory items and surgical equipment. Inappropriate for heat-sensitive plastics or fluids. Prions are not inactivated by this treatment
Dry heat in a hot-air oven at 160°C for 1–2 hours	Used for sterilizing metal, glass and other solid materials. Unsuitable for rubber and plastics
Incineration at 1,000°C	Used for destruction of infected carcasses and other contaminated material; environmental pollution a possible consequence
Flaming	Used for sterilizing inoculating loops in the naked flame of a Bunsen burner
Gamma irradiation	Ionizing rays used for sterilizing disposable plastic laboratory and surgical equipment. Unsuitable for glass and metal equipment
Ultraviolet (UV) light	Non-ionizing rays with poor penetration. Used in biosafety cabinets
Membrane filtration	Used for removing bacteria from heat-sensitive fluids such as serum and tissue culture media. Pore size of filter should be 0.22 μm or less

Table 2.1 Methods for preventing spoilage and limiting microbial growth in food.

Method	Application	Comments
Refrigeration at 4°C	Prevention of growth of spoilage organisms and pathogenic bacteria	Pathogens such as *Listeria monocytogenes*, *Yersinia* species and many fungal species can grow at 4°C
Freezing at –20°C	Long-term storage of food. Microbial multiplication prevented	Surviving microorganisms can multiply rapidly when thawed food is left at ambient temperatures
Boiling at 100°C	Inactivation of vegetative bacteria and fungi in food	Many endospores can withstand prolonged boiling
Pasteurization at 72°C for 15 seconds	Inactivation of most vegetative bacteria	Heat treatment should be followed by rapid cooling. If present in high numbers or located intracellularly, some bacteria may survive
Acidification	Adjustment of pH to a low level inhibits bacterial growth	Applicable to a limited range of foods such as vegetables
Increasing osmotic pressure	Inhibition of microbial multiplication; used for preservation of food	Addition of salts or sugars increases osmotic pressure; applicable to a limited range of foods
Vacuum packing	Packaging of meat and other perishable foods	Removal of oxygen prevents the growth of aerobes
Irradiation	Inactivation of spoilage organisms and pathogenic bacteria	Not permitted in some countries

3 Bacterial genetics and genetic variation

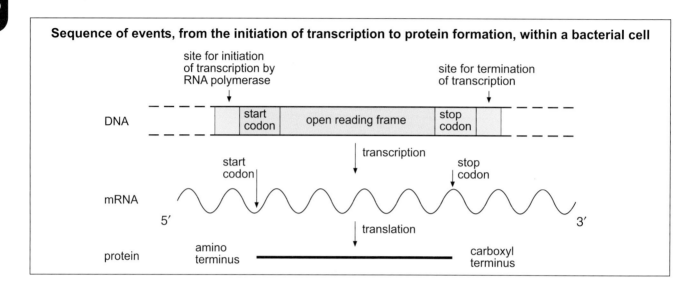

Sequence of events, from the initiation of transcription to protein formation, within a bacterial cell

Much of the genetic information in bacteria is contained on a single chromosome located in the cytoplasm of the cell. Bacterial genomes differ in size and express characteristic traits or phenotypes.

Properties of a bacterial cell, including those of veterinary interest such as antimicrobial resistance and virulence, are determined by the microbial genome. The genomic structure consists of three types of genetic information, the chromosome, plasmids and bacteriophages. A typical bacterium consists of a core genome, mainly composed of genes located on the chromosome consisting of double-stranded DNA, and an accessory genome comprising plasmid and bacteriophage DNA. In *Escherichia coli* K-12, the chromosome is a circular double-stranded DNA molecule of approximately 4.6×10^6 base pairs, containing 157 RNA-encoding genes including ribosomal and transfer RNA along with open reading frames (ORFs) coding for 4,126 bacterial proteins. Bacterial chromosomes typically contain sufficient DNA to encode between 1,000 and 4,000 different genes. Individual genes consist of a starting point, referred to as the start codon and composed of the nucleotides ATG, an ORF and a stop codon (TTA, TAG or TGA).

Although the bacterial chromosome exists free in the cytoplasm, it is compacted through supercoiling and looping of its structure. The central tenets of genetics consist of the expression of a gene from its locus on the chromosome or on a plasmid through transcription (production of messenger RNA or mRNA synthesis) and finally translation, decoding of the mRNA to produce a polypeptide. As the DNA is located in the bacterial cytoplasm, this facilitates the simultaneous transcription and translation of bacterial genes. The gene sequence and its subsequent expression through diverse biochemical pathways accounts for the phenotypic variation observed among bacteria. Recently, these specialized topics have given rise to defined areas of research, referred to as genomics, functional genomics or transcriptomics, and proteomics.

Bacteria replicate by binary fission and the daughter cells produced are usually indistinguishable genetically. Replication of the chromosome in bacteria begins at a specific location referred to as the origin of replication (or origin), at a locus referred to as *ori*. The two parental strands of the helical DNA unwind under the influence of the enzyme DNA helicase and two identical helical DNA molecules are formed through the action of the replicating enzyme, DNA polymerase. The ends of the newly synthesized strands are joined by DNA ligase, resulting in circular chromosomes.

Transcription and translation, the expression of genetic information

Transcription is an enzyme-mediated process that involves DNA being copied from the positive strand, forming an mRNA molecule. This process is mediated by the enzyme DNA-dependent RNA polymerase that binds to the promoter region of a gene, which is composed of two conserved DNA-binding sites referred to as the −35 and −10 promoter sequences. The two strands of DNA are partially unwound, and locally separate, following which mRNA is synthesized. The information encoded in the mRNA is translated into protein on a ribosome through the involvement of transfer RNA (tRNA), which delivers specific amino acids to the mRNA on the ribosome where the amino acids are enzymatically joined together, forming a peptide bond and extending the polypeptide chain.

Concise Review of Veterinary Microbiology, Second Edition. P.J. Quinn, B.K. Markey, F.C. Leonard, E.S. FitzPatrick and S. Fanning.
© 2016 John Wiley & Sons, Ltd. Published 2016 by John Wiley & Sons, Ltd.
Companion website: www.wiley.com/go/quinn/concise-veterinary-microbiology

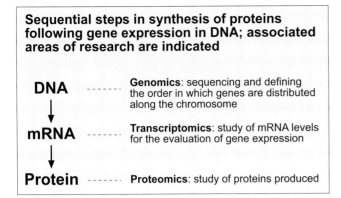

Sequential steps in synthesis of proteins following gene expression in DNA; associated areas of research are indicated

DNA -------- **Genomics**: sequencing and defining the order in which genes are distributed along the chromosome

↓

mRNA -------- **Transcriptomics**: study of mRNA levels for the evaluation of gene expression

↓

Protein ------- **Proteomics**: study of proteins produced

Genetic variation may occur following mutation in which a change occurs in the nucleotide sequence of a gene, or by recombination, whereby new groups of genes are introduced into the genome. A stable inheritable alteration in any genome is termed a mutation. A bacterium carrying a mutation is referred to as a mutant. When the original parent and mutant are compared, their genotypes differ and their phenotype may also differ depending on the nature of the mutation. Spontaneous mutations are the result of rare mistakes in DNA replication and occur at a frequency of about one in every 10^6 cell divisions. Because a gene with altered base pairs may code incorrectly for an amino acid in a protein, the mutation introduced may result in a phenotypic change that may be beneficial or harmful for the organism. Under defined environmental conditions, selected mutations may provide a growth advantage for the mutant over the parent or wild-type bacterium. Mutations can also be experimentally induced by physical, chemical or biological mutagens.

Many viruses that infect animals have RNA genomes which may also undergo mutation. The spontaneous mutation rate associated with these genomes is approximately 1,000-fold higher than that occurring in the host chromosome.

DNA may become damaged following contact with mutagenic chemicals, exposure to UV irradiation and by other means. Different mechanisms are available within the cell to organize the repair of damaged DNA and the choice of the appropriate method depends on the type of damage requiring correction.

Recombination occurs when sequences of DNA from two separate sources are integrated. In bacteria, recombination induces an unexpected inheritable change due to the introduction of new genetic material from a different cell. This new genetic material may be introduced by conjugation, transduction or transformation.

The transfer of genetic material in the form of plasmids of various sizes during conjugation is a complex process that has been extensively studied in the enteric bacterium *Escherichia coli*. During conjugation, F+ (male) bacteria synthesize a modified pilus, the F or sex pilus. This pilus allows direct contact to occur between the male (F+) and a suitable female (F−) bacterium during the process and provides a conduit through which a plasmid or an F-factor can be transferred. One strand of plasmid DNA is unwound and passed to the recipient female (F−) bacterium in which a complementary strand is later synthesized. Once a new plasmid is formed, the recipient cell is converted into an F+ bacterium. Individual bacteria may contain several different types of compatible plasmids.

Plasmid transfer by conjugation has important ecological significance, particularly when antibiotic resistance-encoding genes are involved. A plasmid containing an antibiotic resistance gene in a bacterial cell can, under appropriate conditions, convert the amenable bacterial population into similar plasmid-containing bacterial cells.

DNA acquired either from the original bacterial chromosome or plasmid in a previously infected bacterial cell can be incorporated into phage nucleic acid and transferred by progeny of the phage to susceptible recipient cells in a process called transduction.

Transformation is a process involving the transfer of free or 'naked' DNA containing genes on a segment of chromosomal or plasmid DNA from a lysed donor bacterium to a competent recipient. Natural transformation is uncommon and occurs only in a few bacterial genera.

Examples of mobile genetic elements

Plasmids

Although most bacteria carry all the genes necessary for survival on their chromosome, many bacteria contain small additional genetic elements, termed plasmids, which are also located in the cytoplasm and can replicate independently of the host chromosome. Many different plasmids are known in Gram-positive and Gram-negative bacteria. Most are closed, circular, double-stranded DNA molecules but some linear plasmids have been identified in bacteria. Depending on their genetic content, the size of a plasmid can vary from 1 kbp to more than 1 Mbp. Plasmids can carry genes that confer a wide variety of properties on the host bacterial cell. Most are not essential for normal survival of the bacterium, but they may offer a selective advantage under certain conditions, such as the ability to conjugate and transfer genetic information, encode resistance to antibiotics, produce bacteriocins and synthesize proteins inhibitory to other bacteria (Table 3.1). All plasmids carry the genes required for their stable maintenance. In some pathogenic bacteria, plasmids encode virulence factors and antibiotic resistance.

Plasmids that can coexist in the same host bacterium are referred to as compatible, whereas those that cannot are defined

Table 3.1 Virulence factors of pathogenic bacteria encoded by defined genetic elements.

Pathogen	Virulence factors / Genetic elements
Bacillus anthracis	Toxins, capsule / plasmids
Clostridium botulinum, types C, D and E	Neurotoxins / bacteriophages
Escherichia coli	Shiga-like toxin / bacteriophage Adherence factors, enterotoxins / plasmids Heat-stable toxin, siderophore production / transposons
Salmonella Dublin	Serum resistance factor / plasmid
Staphylococcus aureus	Enterotoxins (A, D, E), toxic shock syndrome factor-1 / bacteriophages Coagulase, exfoliating toxins, enterotoxins / plasmids
Yersinia pestis	Fibrinolysin, coagulase / plasmid

as incompatible. Incompatibility (Inc) group typing of plasmids has identified several different incompatibility groups in the *Enterobacteriaceae*.

The number of copies of a plasmid may vary, with some present in high numbers. Distribution of plasmids between daughter cells is random. Plasmids in the bacterial cytoplasm may be transferred not only during replication but also by conjugation and by transformation, as outlined in the previous section. The broad host range of some plasmids, together with their ability to be transferred, contributes to their wide dissemination, a fact that accounts for the spread of antibiotic resistance among bacterial strains. Emergence of bacteria resistant to one or more antibiotics is of particular significance in veterinary medicine. This correlates with the use of drugs for growth promotion in some instances and treatment of infectious diseases in animals. Importantly, in some circumstances, this may have an impact on human health where resistant zoonotic bacteria such as *Salmonella* and *Campylobacter* may be transferred to humans via the food chain.

Bacteriophages

Viruses that infect bacteria are termed bacteriophages or phages. Depending on their mode of replication, phages may be either virulent or temperate. Most phages attack a small number of strains of related bacteria and therefore can be described as having a narrow and specific host range. Virulent phages undergo a lytic cycle in bacteria, culminating in the production of phage progeny with lysis of host cells. Temperate phages, or prophages, are usually dormant and are integrated into the bacterial genome but they may also be present as circular DNA in the cytoplasm, like plasmids. Prophages can also express some of their genes, conferring additional properties on the host cell. The production of neurotoxins by certain types of *Clostridium botulinum* is associated with lysogenic conversion of host cells (Table 3.1).

Insertion sequences and transposons

Transposons are genetic elements that can move as a single unit from one replicon (chromosome, plasmid or bacteriophage) to another. This process is referred to as transposition. Transposons do not possess an origin of replication and consequently replicate as the bacterial host replicates. Transposons encode the necessary features to promote self-mobilization. An example of a simple transposon is an insertion sequence element, denoted as IS, that contains only a transposase-encoding gene required for insertion into new locations. Several IS elements are known and these differ in the numbers of nucleotides they contain. Many bacteria possess multiple IS copies inserted at different locations throughout their genomes.

Some transposons consist of a gene encoding resistance to an antibiotic such as kanamycin, flanked by two IS*50* elements, IS*50L* and IS*50R*, as in Tn*5*. Other transposons such as Tn*3* encode a β-lactamase gene along with other transposase genes (*tnpA* and *tnpR*) required to catalyse the molecular events involved in integration. The complex transposon Tn*1546* encodes genes conferring resistance to the glycopeptide antibiotics vancomycin, teicoplanin and the formerly used growth promoter avoparcin.

Integrons are derived from transposon Tn*21* and these elements can capture antibiotic resistance, encoding genes via an integron-encoded integrase (a member of the bacterial integrase superfamily) that catalyses a site-specific recombination. These integrons possess a conserved structure (CS) on the proximal end (known as the 5′-CS) containing an integrase gene (*int1*), a recombination site (*att1*) and a promoter (P_{ant}), along with a conserved distal region (3′-CS) containing a *qacEΔ1* [conferring resistance to quaternary ammonium compound(s), which are used as disinfectants] and a *sul1* determinant conferring resistance to sulphonamides. These CS regions flank a variable central locus into which gene cassettes are recombined. Gene cassettes are composed of one or more ORFs encoding antibiotic

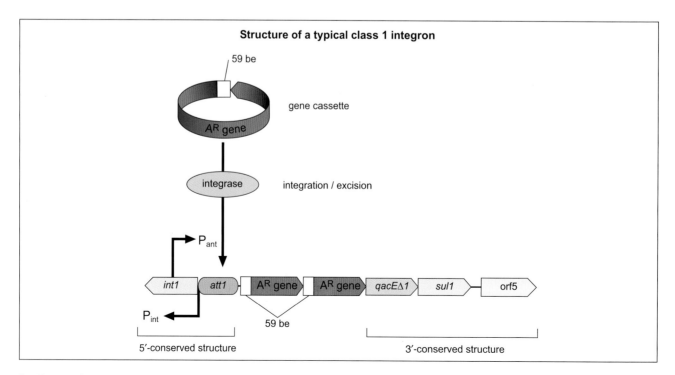

Structure of a typical class 1 integron

resistance gene(s) and a 59-base recognition sequence located at their 3'-end.

Integrons capture a variety of genes encoding resistance to antibiotics such as aminoglycosides and β-lactams, among others, and contribute to the mobilization of these integrons in response to environmental selective pressure. Some integrons possess multiple gene cassettes arranged in a classical 'head-to-tail' orientation.

Genetic engineering of bacteria in the laboratory

Useful genetic characteristics encoded by genes in the DNA of a naturally occurring organism can be cloned into a host bacterium in the laboratory, in a process referred to as genetic engineering. These genes can be inserted into cloning vectors, forming recombinant plasmids. They can then be introduced into bacterial cells (usually by transformation) and propagated. The DNA fragments carrying the genes that are selected are produced by either cleaving the donor DNA containing them, using suitable restriction endonuclease enzymes, or through direct amplification by the polymerase chain reaction (see Chapter 4).

Genetic engineering is currently used for the production of vaccines, hormones and other pharmaceutical products (see Chapter 78). Vaccines produced in this manner are potentially safer than conventional vaccines. The genes that code for the vaccine antigens can be cloned separately from genes associated with the parent organism. Genetically engineered vaccines may therefore stimulate an effective immune response without the risk of introducing a pathogen capable of replicating in animals which are being vaccinated.

Genetic databases and bioinformatics

In 1977, the entire DNA sequence of the phage ΦX174 was first published. Since that time there has been an exponential increase in DNA sequence information submitted to gene databases around the world. With increasing volumes of data entries, including high-throughput whole genome sequences for bacteria and other microorganisms, the first of which was *Haemophilus influenzae* (1.8 Mbp) completed in 1995, it has become impractical to analyse by manual methods these vast amounts of data. This has necessitated the development of specific computational tools to analyse DNA information and identify genes and their corresponding protein sequences, along with regulatory features, at a molecular level.

Bioinformatics is a new scientific discipline that relates to the development of computer algorithms and statistical techniques for analysing and managing genetic information. These tools facilitate the rapid annotation of genome sequences with identification of the position of ORFs within the genome, leading to the identification of genes encoding virulence factors associated with disease production.

Companies involved in the manufacture of pharmaceutical and diagnostic reagents often use bioinformatics to 'data mine' genomes, in an attempt to identify new therapeutic agents or useful diagnostic markers.

4 Molecular diagnostic methods

Summary of molecular methods for detection of diagnostic biomarkers

DNA

Molecular hybridization
 - Southern blotting
DNA sequencing
PCR
DNA fingerprinting
Microarrays
Whole genome sequencing

RNA

Molecular hybridization
 - northern blotting
 - *in situ* analysis (FISH)
RT-PCR
Microarrays

Protein

Molecular hybridization
 - western blotting
Protein sequencing
Mass spectrum analysis
Protein microarrays

Most of the characteristics of living bacteria are associated with the genes present on their bacterial chromosome. This structure consists of a double-stranded DNA helix, with all the properties required to control replication of the bacterium, store its genetic information and express some characteristics unique to the organism. All these properties are controlled by specific enzymes and the genetic message is, in some instances, subsequently decoded in a process involving other enzymes, leading to the synthesis of a bacterial protein (see Chapter 3).

The properties of DNA used for analytical purposes derive from its chemical structure. These have been used to develop many of the modern protocols for detection of bacterial pathogens in clinical specimens. A DNA molecule has three important analytical features that facilitate its utilization as a diagnostic target:

- Recognition properties: base-pairing rules in DNA underpin the analytical approach of molecular techniques including DNA probe hybridization, DNA sequencing, the polymerase chain reaction (PCR) and, more recently, microarrays.
- Stability and robust flexibility: the DNA molecule is inherently stable, which facilitates its recovery from degraded material.
- Sequence features: when the DNA sequence of any cell is closely examined, open reading frames (ORFs) encoding genes and other features can be determined.

Molecular hybridization

Any labelled DNA probe, under suitable experimental conditions, would be capable of binding or hybridizing to its complementary strand in solution (based on the DNA base-pairing rules). It is this binding event that is subsequently detected. Examples of molecular hybridization techniques include Southern and northern blotting.

DNA sequencing is the most powerful analytical/diagnostic approach that exists in the molecular armoury. Insight into the understanding of any DNA molecule derives from its nucleotide sequence. The nucleotide sequence can be used to deduce the primary protein structure of the corresponding protein which can

subsequently be compared with similar sequences from other organisms. DNA-binding sites and other regulatory features of genes can also be identified.

The DNA sequence of a gene, or the ORF, can be determined using either a chemical- or an enzyme-based approach. The technical principles of the latter method on which modern dideoxy DNA sequencing protocols are based involves the partial replication of a short DNA sequence using all four deoxyribonucleotides (dNTP) and a chemically modified dideoxyribonucleotide (ddNTP) lacking a hydroxyl group at the 2′-carbon on the ribose sugar ring. Like hybridization, this method is based on sequence recognition according to the base-pairing rules and accurate enzymatic synthesis, all of which are features of the naturally occurring replication event. To sequence a DNA molecule the following steps are usually required: primer hybridization, sequence reaction, detection and data analysis.

In a later development of this technology, fluorescent-based automated DNA sequencing was designed to reduce the manual manipulations involved whilst increasing sample throughput. More recent advances in DNA sequencing technology have produced instrumentation capable of sequencing a bacterial genome in a few hours (see Chapter 6).

The PCR assay was developed out of the strategies used for DNA sequencing. Typically a PCR protocol consists of three repeated steps, resulting in the amplification of a discrete segment of DNA (or RNA, after the addition of a reverse-transcription step, see following paragraphs). In the first of these, the template DNA, which has been recovered from a crude preparation of genomic DNA isolated from a microbial pathogen of veterinary interest or from blood or other tissue samples, is denatured, separating the two DNA strands. This is followed by an annealing step, wherein the reaction temperature is lowered, allowing two synthetic DNA primers or oligonucleotides to bind (hybridize) to the template. These primers are located on opposite DNA strands. Finally, the temperature is increased again (typically, 74°C) and a thermostable DNA polymerase enzyme begins a round of synthesis. These steps constitute one cycle and in a conventional PCR reaction up to 30 such cycles are carried

Concise Review of Veterinary Microbiology, Second Edition. P.J. Quinn, B.K. Markey, F.C. Leonard, E.S. FitzPatrick and S. Fanning.
© 2016 John Wiley & Sons, Ltd. Published 2016 by John Wiley & Sons, Ltd.
Companion website: www.wiley.com/go/quinn/concise-veterinary-microbiology

out. This repetitive cycling between temperatures facilitates the amplification of a specific DNA target by up to one million-fold.

A programmable thermal cycler controls the rate of temperature change, length of incubation at each temperature and the number of times each cycle is repeated. Multiple cycles produce an amplified PCR product, or amplicon, that can be detected by conventional agarose gel electrophoresis, stained with ethidium bromide and visualized using ultraviolet light.

Conventional PCR-based assays have been developed to detect a broad range of target genes in pathogenic bacteria associated with animals, including food-borne zoonotic pathogens. Commercial kits are also available for these and other pathogenic organisms.

A potential limitation of DNA-based diagnostic methods is that they detect both viable and non-viable bacterial cells. This limitation can be overcome either by using an enrichment step before nucleic acid extraction or by performing an RNA-based detection method using reverse transcriptase (RT)-mediated PCR, in a protocol known as RT-PCR. These assays can also be used to detect RNA deriving from viruses such as rotavirus, coronavirus and norovirus.

Detection and simultaneous quantification of amplicons in real time is an important enabling technology in molecular diagnostics. The method facilitates the determination of the absolute number of a specific DNA target, such as a virulence gene of veterinary importance, relative to a housekeeping gene, such as 16S rRNA, within a living cell. Quantitative real-time PCR (qPCR) can be used to quantify bacteria, other microorganisms and individual genes. Real-time PCR uses fluorescence to detect the presence or absence of a particular DNA or RNA target. It is this detection process that differentiates real-time from conventional PCR.

Expression of any gene in a microorganism or other cell can be determined by measuring the mRNA transcription, using RT-PCR. This technique is referred to as quantitative RT-PCR (qRT-PCR). Based on this protocol, commercial kits are now available to detect and quantify a range of pathogenic organisms relevant to veterinary medicine.

The development of DNA microarrays is based on the use of a solid support to which a series of genes or chemically synthesized segments of those genes can be attached. DNA microarrays can be used in several ways. The arrays can provide useful information for identifying those genes controlling growth of an organism under defined culturing conditions, including aerobic versus anaerobic environmental conditions. In environmental microbiology, DNA microarrays containing 16S rDNA sequences can be used to identify bacteria and other microorganisms present in a particular environment. This DNA microarray is termed a phylochip. Comparative genome analysis makes use of DNA microarrays to compare the gene index of different serovars of *Salmonella*. DNA chips have been developed to aid in the simultaneous identification of a number of important pathogens including bacteria and viruses that may share similar environmental niches.

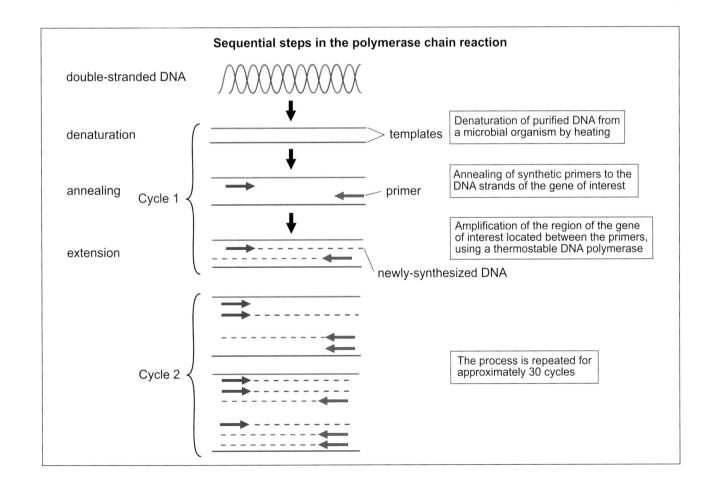

Sequential steps in the polymerase chain reaction

double-stranded DNA

denaturation — templates — Denaturation of purified DNA from a microbial organism by heating

annealing — Cycle 1 — primer — Annealing of synthetic primers to the DNA strands of the gene of interest

extension — Amplification of the region of the gene of interest located between the primers, using a thermostable DNA polymerase — newly-synthesized DNA

Cycle 2 — The process is repeated for approximately 30 cycles

5 Laboratory diagnosis of bacterial disease

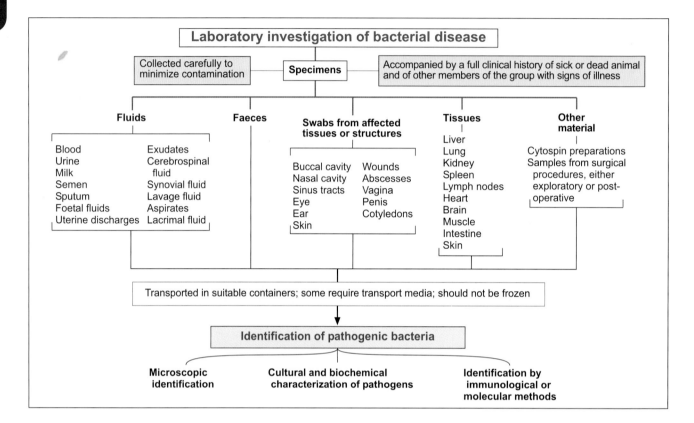

Laboratory investigation of bacterial disease is necessary for the identification of the aetiological agent and sometimes for determining the antimicrobial susceptibility of bacterial pathogens. A full clinical history, including the age and sex of the species affected together with the number of animals involved and any treatment administered, should accompany the specimens. A tentative clinical diagnosis should be included.

Care should be taken in the selection, collection and submission of specimens to the laboratory. Ideally, specimens should be obtained from live animals before administration of antimicrobial therapy. Samples from dead animals should be collected, if possible, before putrefactive changes occur. Procedures which minimize contamination should be used during specimen collection. Samples must be submitted in separate leak-proof containers, including secondary and tertiary packaging if submitted by post or courier. Each container should be labelled with the identity of the animal, the type of specimen and the date of collection.

If bacteria are present in large numbers, examination of stained smears prepared directly from clinical specimens may indicate the presence of pathogens; cultural and biochemical characteristics and immunological and molecular methods are used for specific identification. Staining methods routinely used

in diagnostic bacteriology are presented in Table 5.1. The Gram staining method is employed for the majority of pathogens. The Ziehl–Neelsen stain is used to detect acid-fast bacteria. *Coxiella burnetii*, *Brucella* species, *Nocardia* species and chlamydiae can be demonstrated in smears using the modified Ziehl–Neelsen stain. The fluorescent antibody staining method gives rapid specific identification of bacterial pathogens in smears and cryostat tissue sections.

The culture medium, atmospheric conditions and other requirements essential for bacterial isolation are determined by the characteristics of the suspected bacterium. Routine isolation of many pathogens involves inoculation of blood agar and MacConkey agar plates followed by incubation for 24–48 hours. Media used in diagnostic bacteriology are indicated in Table 5.2.

Plates should be inoculated using a streaking technique which facilitates growth of isolated colonies. This is an essential step for the identification of pathogens in clinical specimens which may contain microbial contaminants. In addition, clinical specimens from sites normally populated with commensal organisms, such as the upper respiratory or gastrointestinal tract, may yield a mixed flora on culture. Identification of the suspected pathogen may involve quantification to establish the dominant organism in the specimen and/or testing for virulence attributes

Concise Review of Veterinary Microbiology, Second Edition. P.J. Quinn, B.K. Markey, F.C. Leonard, E.S. FitzPatrick and S. Fanning.
© 2016 John Wiley & Sons, Ltd. Published 2016 by John Wiley & Sons, Ltd.
Companion website: www.wiley.com/go/quinn/concise-veterinary-microbiology

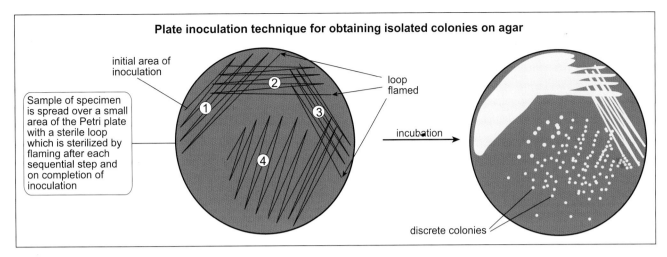

Plate inoculation technique for obtaining isolated colonies on agar

initial area of inoculation

Sample of specimen is spread over a small area of the Petri plate with a sterile loop which is sterilized by flaming after each sequential step and on completion of inoculation

loop flamed

incubation

discrete colonies

to prove pathogenicity. Definitive identification of a potential pathogen involves subculture of an isolated colony to obtain a pure growth which can then be subjected to biochemical or other tests. Morphological characteristics and biochemical tests allow presumptive identification of a bacterial pathogen. Biochemical tests relate to the catabolic activities of bacteria and an indicator system is usually employed to demonstrate utilization of a particular substrate.

Immunological techniques such as fluorescent antibody staining can be used for identifying bacterial pathogens. Serotyping is based on the immunological identification of surface antigens on pathogens such as *Escherichia coli* and *Pasteurella multocida*.

The fact that a particular bacteriophage (phage) is specific for a limited number of susceptible strains of bacteria allows differentiation by phage typing. This method is commonly used to differentiate isolates of *Staphylococcus aureus* and also serotypes of *Salmonella* Typhimurium.

Selected molecular techniques which can be used for the detection and typing of pathogenic bacteria are described in Chapters 4 and 6.

Table 5.2 Laboratory media commonly used for the isolation and presumptive identification of bacterial pathogens.

Medium	Comments
Nutrient agar	A basic medium on which non-fastidious bacteria can grow. Suitable for demonstrating colonial morphology and pigment production; also used for viable counting methods
Blood agar	An enriched medium which supports the growth of most pathogenic bacteria and is used for their primary isolation. Allows the recognition of haemolysin produced by bacteria
MacConkey agar	A selective medium containing bile which is especially useful for isolation of enterobacteria and some other Gram-negative bacteria. Allows differentiation of lactose fermenters and non-lactose fermenters. Colonies of lactose fermenters and the surrounding medium are pink
Selenite broth, Rappaport–Vassiliadis broth	Selective enrichment media used for the isolation of salmonellae from samples containing other Gram-negative enteric organisms
Edwards medium	A blood agar-based selective medium used for the isolation and recognition of streptococci
Chocolate agar	Heat-treated blood agar which supplies special growth requirements (X and V factors) for the isolation of *Haemophilus* species and for the culture of *Taylorella equigenitalis*
Brilliant green agar	An indicator medium for the presumptive identification of *Salmonella* species. *Salmonella* colonies and surrounding medium have a pink colour

Table 5.1 Routine staining methods for bacteria.

Method	Comments
Gram stain	Widely used for the routine staining of bacteria in smears. Gram-positive bacteria are stained blue by the crystal violet which is retained in their cell walls despite decolorization. In contrast, Gram-negative bacteria, which do not retain the crystal violet, are counterstained red
Giemsa	Useful for demonstrating *Dermatophilus congolensis*, rickettsiae and *Borrelia* species, which stain blue
Dilute carbol fuchsin	Especially useful for recognizing *Campylobacter* species, *Brachyspira* species and *Fusobacterium* species, which stain red
Polychrome methylene blue	Used for the identification of *Bacillus anthracis* in blood smears. The organisms stain blue with distinctive pink capsules
Ziehl–Neelsen stain	Hot concentrated carbol fuchsin which penetrates mycobacterial cell walls is retained after acid-alcohol decolorization. The red-staining bacteria are described as acid-fast or Ziehl–Neelsen positive
Modified Ziehl–Neelsen stain	Unlike the Ziehl–Neelsen stain, this method employs dilute carbol fuchsin with decolorization by acetic acid

6 Molecular subtyping of bacteria

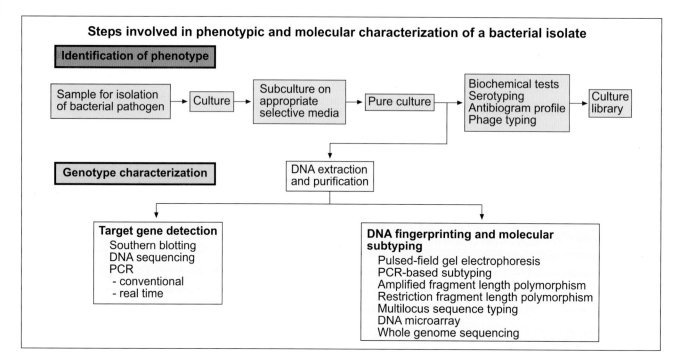

Steps involved in phenotypic and molecular characterization of a bacterial isolate

Identification of phenotype

Sample for isolation of bacterial pathogen → Culture → Subculture on appropriate selective media → Pure culture → Biochemical tests / Serotyping / Antibiogram profile / Phage typing → Culture library

Genotype characterization

DNA extraction and purification

Target gene detection
Southern blotting
DNA sequencing
PCR
 - conventional
 - real time

DNA fingerprinting and molecular subtyping
Pulsed-field gel electrophoresis
PCR-based subtyping
Amplified fragment length polymorphism
Restriction fragment length polymorphism
Multilocus sequence typing
DNA microarray
Whole genome sequencing

Infectious disease surveillance of pathogens of importance in veterinary medicine employs two strategies to detect cases and outbreaks, laboratory-based and syndrome-based surveillance. Of these, the former strategy is more accurate since definitive diagnosis of an infection requires laboratory confirmation. A range of methods is available in veterinary diagnostic laboratories, including conventional microbiological methods using traditional culture-based techniques, immunoassays to detect antigens associated with a pathogen of interest, and modern techniques that include analysis of bacterial nucleic acid. The emergence of novel bacteria challenges surveillance efforts and thus these protocols must constantly evolve to ensure the capability of identifying such pathogens. More than 60% of all emerging pathogens are zoonotic in origin.

Characterization of a veterinary pathogen is essential for the support of epidemiological investigations of a disease outbreak. Laboratory methods used must be capable of identifying those organisms linked to the outbreak while excluding isolates unrelated to the outbreak. Conventional laboratory approaches are summarized in the illustration.

Although some phenotype-based methods have been used successfully, many are not universally applicable and mutation or changes in gene complement can result in altered phenotypic expression, leading to incorrect bacterial identification. Accordingly, these former methods limit the reliability of phenotype-based identification for surveillance purposes.

The rapid development in molecular-based approaches has led to the design of new diagnostic protocols that are independent of the inherent limitations of traditional methods. Molecular subtyping methods target variation within the genomes of bacteria and also decrease the limitations encountered with more conventional phenotyping approaches.

Bacterial subtyping methods permit the identification of a bacterium below the species level and, in addition, provide methods for tracking an organism, describing its molecular epidemiology and defining its transmission routes. This modern analytical approach provides a more refined identification of a bacterium, based on its DNA fingerprint, than phenotype-based methods. Compared with traditional diagnostic methods, this facilitates the recognition of different *Escherichia coli* O157:H7 isolates and *Salmonella* Typhimurium subtypes among others. Transmission routes of methicillin-resistant *Staphylococcus aureus* (MRSA) between humans and animals have also been identified by subtyping isolates and comparing their DNA fingerprint patterns. In general, technical approaches to molecular subtyping include the use of restriction fragment length

Concise Review of Veterinary Microbiology, Second Edition. P.J. Quinn, B.K. Markey, F.C. Leonard, E.S. FitzPatrick and S. Fanning.
© 2016 John Wiley & Sons, Ltd. Published 2016 by John Wiley & Sons, Ltd.
Companion website: www.wiley.com/go/quinn/concise-veterinary-microbiology

Table 6.1 Molecular-based subtyping methods used for tracing bacterial pathogens associated with disease outbreaks in animal and human populations.

Sequential development of analytical methods	Molecular basis of subtyping methods
First-generation methods	Plasmid DNA profiling Restriction digestion of purified plasmids
Second-generation methods	Restriction endonuclease digestion of total DNA (including chromosomal and plasmid) Ribotyping
Third-generation methods	Pulsed-field gel electrophoresis (PFGE) PCR-based amplification Rapid amplification of polymorphic DNA (RAPD) PCR-RFLP analysis of conserved genes (*flaA*, *recN* and others) PCR ribotyping REP-PCR ERIC-PCR BOX-PCR AFLP
Fourth-generation methods	Multi-locus variable-number tandem repeat analysis (MLVA) Multi-locus sequence typing (MLST) Whole genome-based DNA sequencing

polymorphism (RFLP) analysis, PCR-based amplification of conserved repetitive sequences in bacterial genomes and whole bacterial genome DNA sequencing (Table 6.1).

Plasmid profiling, which can also be used to type organisms, involves the purification of plasmids from a bacterium of veterinary importance, followed by their separation on an agarose gel. Notwithstanding some limitations, plasmid profiling is important when characterizing genes encoding antibiotic resistance.

Comparative genomic hybridization

DNA microarrays (see Chapter 4) can also be used for subtyping purposes. Probes attached to the solid surface can detect complementary sequences in bacterial isolates of interest. DNA is purified from a bacterium and labelled either chemically or enzymatically, before being hybridized to the array. Unbound DNA is washed off and signals from hybridized probes are subsequently detected automatically by a scanner. These data are then analysed using suitable software. Together with other molecular methods, DNA microarrays are appropriate procedures for bacterial subtyping.

Commercial DNA microarrays are available and can be used for diagnostic testing and disease investigations. Similarly, the serotypes of *E. coli* and *Salmonella* species can now be identified using commercially available DNA microarrays.

Restriction fragment length polymorphism analysis

RFLP analysis requires the purification of the bacterial chromosome and associated plasmid(s), prior to enzymatic digestion with a restriction endonuclease. Electrophoresis produces a multi-band pattern or RFLP pattern in an agarose gel. The RFLP pattern produced is often too complex to serve as a fingerprint and is difficult to analyse, limiting the application of this subtyping method. Moreover, plasmids present initially in a strain may be lost later, altering the banding profile and complicating isolate comparison.

A high-resolution RFLP-based strategy known as optical mapping has been described. Following the gentle lysis of a bacterial cell, this technique facilitates the creation of a high resolution ordered genome map. Purified DNA is stretched out in a microfluidic chamber and digested with a restriction endonuclease enzyme. The resulting DNA fragments remain attached in the chamber in the same order as they appear in the genome. After staining with a DNA intercalating dye to allow visualization by fluorescent microscopy, the lengths of the DNA fragments are measured by fluorescent intensity. Using specialized software, the optical map is subsequently resolved.

Ribosomal-encoding DNA genes (rRNA) are naturally amplified in bacteria and have been used successfully as a target for identification. Large portions of these genes (the *rrs* genes code for 16S rRNA and the *rrl* genes code for 23S rRNA) have been conserved throughout evolution. In this procedure, chromosomal DNA is purified and digested with a suitable restriction enzyme, then Southern blotted, before hybridization with a species-specific rRNA probe. The pattern of fragments detected is referred to as the ribotype. Since these genes are highly conserved, pathogens can be identified using appropriately labelled 16S and 23S rRNA probes.

A major limitation with restriction enzyme-based methods is the complexity of the fragmentation patterns generated which renders their analysis difficult to interpret. Pulsed-field gel electrophoresis (PFGE) can overcome this limitation by taking advantage of the digestion of the bacterial chromosome and any associated plasmids using rare cutting restriction endonucleases, also known as macrorestriction analysis. These enzymes cut chromosomal DNA into a lower number of large DNA fragments which can be resolved using specialized electrophoresis equipment. PFGE is regarded as the gold standard in molecular subtyping.

PFGE is a highly discriminating subtyping protocol and is used to determine the genetic relationships between case-related and -unrelated isolates. As the method is relatively simple to perform, standardizing the technical elements facilitates the comparison of PFGE profiles between laboratories nationally and internationally. PulseNet (www.cdc.gov/pulsenet) is an example of a globally standardized and operated PFGE-based subtyping network used to track food-borne pathogens across countries and continents.

PCR-based subtyping methods

Several PCR-based subtyping methods have been developed. In general, these methods are simple to carry out and can be applied to any microbial genome. Some of these approaches are shown in Table 6.1. A brief outline of three methods is given below.

Rapid amplification of polymorphic DNA (RAPD) also known as arbitrarily primed-PCR (AP-PCR) was one of the first examples of PCR-based subtyping described. This method, which does not require any prior knowledge of the organism's DNA sequence, uses a randomly selected primer, along with a low-temperature annealing step during amplification to produce a DNA fingerprint pattern of a bacterium of particular interest.

PCR-RFLP can be applied to a gene target that exhibits a high degree of polymorphism and therefore can be used to discriminate between bacterial isolates. An example of this is *flaA* subtyping used to subtype *Campylobacter jejuni* isolates. In this example, the gene of interest, the flagellin A subunit encoding *flaA*, is amplified by PCR. The amplified PCR product is then subjected to digestion using a suitable restriction endonuclease, in this instance *Hinf*1, producing an RFLP profile. The RFLP profile is then used to compare different isolates of the same bacterium. Other targets used include 16S, 23S rRNA and the interspacial region 16–23S rRNA, *fliC* for *E. coli* O157 and the *coa*-encoding coagulase gene in *Staphylococcus aureus*.

Bacterial genomes contain several examples of repetitive sequences along their length. Examples of common repeats include the 38-bp repetitive extragenic palindromic sequence (REP), the 126-bp enterobacterial repetitive intergenic consensus (ERIC) and the 158-bp BOX repeat sequences (Table 6.1). REP-PCR utilizes the nucleotide sequences conserved within the repeat element to facilitate the design of primers located towards the extremities of these repeats and which amplify the DNA regions located between the repeats.

Amplification fragment length polymorphism (AFLP) does not require any prior knowledge of the target bacterial genome sequence. Bacterial genomic DNA is first digested with one or more restriction endonucleases to which synthetic short oligonucleotide adaptors of known sequence are attached using the cohesive ends generated by the restriction enzyme. This forms the sites to which adaptor-specific DNA primers are annealed and used to amplify the adaptor-ligated DNA fragment. A complex pattern of DNA fragments is produced following PCR, ranging in size from 50 to 100 bp with between 40 and 200 bands that are resolved by conventional agarose gel electrophoresis. DNA fragment profiles can be arranged as described earlier and compared with other bacterial isolates.

DNA sequence-based subtyping methods

DNA sequence-based subtyping has emerged as a new approach to distinguish isolates of the same bacterial species. Molecular subtyping methods based on a selected number of genes or the complete genome of a bacterium have been developed. Using purified DNA from their genomes, these methods are being utilized for identification of pathogenic bacteria in animals and humans (Table 6.1). Two of these methods are briefly described.

Multi-locus sequence typing (MLST) is an example of an approach whereby chromosomal DNA is purified and short segments of up to seven housekeeping genes are amplified prior to sequencing. The genes used for MLST analysis all encode protein products essential for bacterial viability and are there-

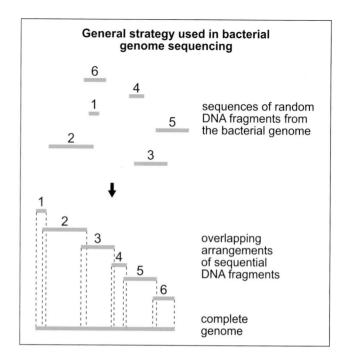

General strategy used in bacterial genome sequencing

sequences of random DNA fragments from the bacterial genome

overlapping arrangements of sequential DNA fragments

complete genome

fore subject to selective pressure. These DNA sequences are then compared. Based on the sequence differences or polymorphisms detected, each unique sequence is termed an allele and is identified by a unique sequence type (ST) number. ST numbers associated with these loci are then used to compare isolates and infer genetic relatedness. Bacterial isolates can be identified by a string of ST numbers and for two individual bacterial isolates where the same ST number strings occur, these isolates are confirmed as being indistinguishable by this method.

MLST protocols have been described for a variety of important veterinary pathogens. The method is easily standardized and detailed protocols have been described (www.mlst.net).

Recently, attempts have been made to develop MLST schemes that are based on virulence genes. Some multi-virulence locus sequence typing schemes are now available and can be applied to selected pathogens of veterinary importance.

Whole bacterial genome sequencing

Information obtained from genome sequencing projects can aid our understanding of infectious disease and microbial evolution. The first technical approach to determine the DNA sequence for a bacterium necessitated the construction of an extensive library of randomly generated DNA fragments. These short DNA fragments were then subjected to a high-throughput sequencing pipeline. Powerful bioinformatic computing tools were used to search this collection to identify overlapping sequences. These were then spliced together, until the complete genome of the bacterium was assembled.

Advances in sequencing technologies and computational analysis over the past few years have led to the development of faster analytical approaches, so-called next-generation sequencing technologies. These new methods significantly increase the volume of sequence data that can be evaluated. In addition, the methylation profile of a bacterial genome can be determined using single-molecule real-time DNA sequencing.

Surveillance strategies are now assessing metagenomics as a culture-independent method for identification of individual members of microbial populations, irrespective of source. This strategy aims to determine the sequence of all nucleic acids recovered from a sample of veterinary interest and it has the potential to revolutionize the detection of known pathogens and other microorganisms sharing the same ecological niche. Metagenomics offers the prospect of directly predicting antibiotic-resistant phenotypes along with the identification of virulence and other genes without the requirement for culturing bacteria.

7 Antibacterial agents

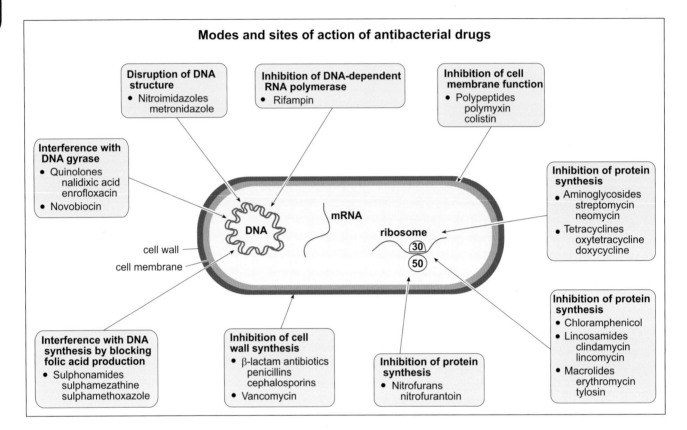

Modes and sites of action of antibacterial drugs

Disruption of DNA structure
- Nitroimidazoles
  metronidazole

Inhibition of DNA-dependent RNA polymerase
- Rifampin

Inhibition of cell membrane function
- Polypeptides
  polymyxin
  colistin

Interference with DNA gyrase
- Quinolones
  nalidixic acid
  enrofloxacin
- Novobiocin

Inhibition of protein synthesis
- Aminoglycosides
  streptomycin
  neomycin
- Tetracyclines
  oxytetracycline
  doxycycline

cell wall
cell membrane

DNA   mRNA   ribosome
30
50

Inhibition of protein synthesis
- Chloramphenicol
- Lincosamides
  clindamycin
  lincomycin
- Macrolides
  erythromycin
  tylosin

Interference with DNA synthesis by blocking folic acid production
- Sulphonamides
  sulphamezathine
  sulphamethoxazole

Inhibition of cell wall synthesis
- β-lactam antibiotics
  penicillins
  cephalosporins
- Vancomycin

Inhibition of protein synthesis
- Nitrofurans
  nitrofurantoin

Antibiotics are low-molecular-weight microbial metabolites which can kill or inhibit the growth of susceptible bacteria. The term 'antimicrobial agent' is sometimes used to include both antibiotics and synthetic compounds with antimicrobial activity. The therapeutic use of antibiotics depends on their selective toxicity: these drugs kill or inhibit bacterial pathogens without direct toxicity for animals receiving treatment. Individual antibacterial agents are not effective against all pathogenic bacteria. Some are active against a narrow range of bacterial species, while broad-spectrum antibiotics such as tetracyclines and chloramphenicol are active against many species.

The modes and sites of action of antibacterial drugs range from interference with DNA synthesis to inhibition of cell wall synthesis. The major classes of antimicrobial drugs and their modes of action are listed in Table 7.1. Because peptidoglycan is a unique component of bacterial cell walls, antibacterial agents which prevent cross-linking of peptidoglycan chains inhibit cell wall synthesis and are selectively toxic for bacteria. The penicillins and cephalosporins comprise the largest and most important class of antibacterial drugs which inhibit cell wall synthesis. A number of classes of antibacterial agents

inhibit protein synthesis. Aminoglycosides bind to 30S ribosomal subunits and affect a number of different steps in protein synthesis. Macrolide antibiotics inhibit protein synthesis by blocking 50S subunit activity. Many antibacterial agents including quinolones, novobiocin, rifampin, nitroimidazoles and sulphonamides inhibit nucleic acid synthesis. The activity of antibacterial drugs is influenced *in vivo* by the site and rate of absorption, the site of excretion and the tissue distribution and metabolism of a particular agent. In addition, antibacterial activity can be affected by interactions between pathogen and drug and between host and pathogen.

When antibacterial drugs are combined for treatment of disease, the outcome is influenced by the particular combinations employed. If a bacteriostatic drug is combined with a bactericidal drug, antagonism may occur. Bactericidal drugs, particularly the β-lactam antibiotics, are effective against actively dividing cells. If they are combined with a bacteriostatic drug which inhibits bacterial growth, their bactericidal activity may be abolished. Drugs which act synergistically include sulphonamides and trimethoprim, which act at two different sites in the folic acid pathway, and clavulanic acid and penicillin combinations,

Concise Review of Veterinary Microbiology, Second Edition. P.J. Quinn, B.K. Markey, F.C. Leonard, E.S. FitzPatrick and S. Fanning.
© 2016 John Wiley & Sons, Ltd. Published 2016 by John Wiley & Sons, Ltd.
Companion website: www.wiley.com/go/quinn/concise-veterinary-microbiology

Table 7.1 Major classes of antibacterial drugs and their modes of action.

Antibacterial drug	Mode of action	Effect	Comments
β-Lactam antibiotics Penicillins Cephalosporins	Inhibition of cell wall synthesis	Bactericidal	Low toxicity. Many are inactivated by β-lactamases
Glycopeptides Vancomycin	Inhibition of cell wall synthesis	Bactericidal	Used against methicillin-resistant *Staphylococcus aureus*
Polypeptides Polymyxin Colistin	Inhibition of cell membrane function	Bactericidal	Resistance slow to develop. Potentially nephrotoxic and neurotoxic
Nitrofurans Nitrofurantoin	Inhibition of protein synthesis	Bacteriostatic	Synthetic agents with broad-spectrum activity. Relatively toxic
Aminoglycosides Streptomycin Neomycin	Inhibition of protein synthesis Block 30S ribosomal activity	Bactericidal	Active mainly against Gram-negative bacteria. Ototoxic and nephrotoxic
Tetracyclines Oxytetracycline Doxycycline	Inhibition of protein synthesis Block 30S ribosomal activity	Bacteriostatic	Formerly used in feed for prophylactic medication. Development of resistance common
Chloramphenicol **Florfenicol**	Inhibition of protein synthesis Block 50S ribosomal activity	Bacteriostatic	Use prohibited in food-producing animals in some countries. Potentially toxic
Lincosamides Clindamycin Lincomycin	Inhibition of protein synthesis Block 50S ribosomal activity	Bactericidal or bacteriostatic	May be toxic in many species. Contraindicated in horses and neonatal animals. Oral administration is hazardous in ruminants
Macrolides Erythromycin Tylosin	Inhibition of protein synthesis Block 50S ribosomal activity	Bacteriostatic	Active against Gram-positive bacteria. Some macrolides active against mycoplasmal pathogens
Quinolones Nalidixic acid Enrofloxacin	Inhibition of nucleic acid synthesis by blocking DNA gyrase	Bactericidal	Synthetic agents used for treating enteric infections and for intracellular pathogens
Novobiocin	Inhibition of nucleic acid synthesis by blocking DNA gyrase	Bactericidal or bacteriostatic	Often used along with other compatible drugs for treatment of mastitis
Rifampin	Inhibition of nucleic acid synthesis by blocking DNA-dependent RNA polymerase	Bacteriostatic	Antimycobacterial activity; used with erythromycin for treating *Rhodococcus equi* infections
Sulphonamides Sulphamezathine Sulphamethoxazole	Inhibition of nucleic acid synthesis by competitive blocking of *para*-aminobenzoic acid (PABA) incorporation into folic acid	Bacteriostatic	Synthetic structural analogues of PABA active against rapidly growing bacteria
Trimethoprim	Inhibition of nucleic acid synthesis by combining with the enzyme dihydrofolate reductase	Bacteriostatic	Usually administered with sulphamethoxazole. This combination, referred to as a potentiated sulphonamide, is bactericidal
Nitroimidazoles Metronidazole	Disruption of DNA structure and inhibition of DNA repair	Bactericidal	Particularly active against anaerobic bacteria; also active against some protozoa

in which clavulanic acid inhibits β-lactamase activity, preventing inactivation of penicillin.

Antimicrobial drugs can alter the host's immune response and may change the normal flora, particularly on the skin and in the intestinal tract. Disturbance of the normal intestinal flora following therapy for enteric pathogens, such as *Salmonella* species, may allow the development of an extended carrier state and prolonged therapy may predispose the recipient to fungal infections.

8 Antimicrobial susceptibility testing

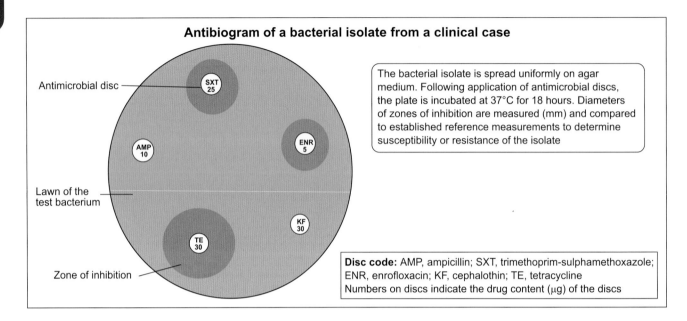

Antibiogram of a bacterial isolate from a clinical case

Antimicrobial disc — SXT 25

AMP 10

ENR 5

Lawn of the test bacterium

KF 30

TE 30

Zone of inhibition

The bacterial isolate is spread uniformly on agar medium. Following application of antimicrobial discs, the plate is incubated at 37°C for 18 hours. Diameters of zones of inhibition are measured (mm) and compared to established reference measurements to determine susceptibility or resistance of the isolate

Disc code: AMP, ampicillin; SXT, trimethoprim-sulphamethoxazole; ENR, enrofloxacin; KF, cephalothin; TE, tetracycline
Numbers on discs indicate the drug content (μg) of the discs

Tests to determine the most suitable antibiotic for effective treatment of a given bacterial infection can be conducted on bacterial isolates cultured from clinical cases. These tests, which are carried out *in vitro*, assist the clinician in selecting a therapeutic agent which may be effective *in vivo*. However, the tests cannot allow for the various factors which may affect antibacterial activity in an infected animal and the results obtained following treatment may not reflect the susceptibility pattern of an isolate as determined in the laboratory. The antibacterial susceptibility tests available include broth dilution, disc diffusion, agar gradient and some automated methods. The Kirby–Bauer disc diffusion method is a flexible and relatively inexpensive technique

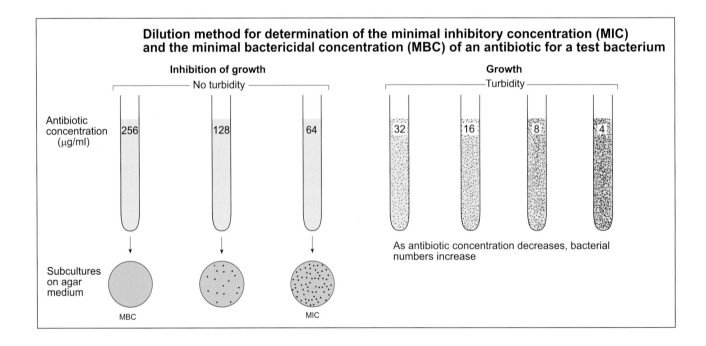

Dilution method for determination of the minimal inhibitory concentration (MIC) and the minimal bactericidal concentration (MBC) of an antibiotic for a test bacterium

Inhibition of growth — No turbidity

Growth — Turbidity

Antibiotic concentration (μg/ml): 256, 128, 64 | 32, 16, 8, 4

As antibiotic concentration decreases, bacterial numbers increase

Subcultures on agar medium

MBC   MIC

Concise Review of Veterinary Microbiology, Second Edition. P.J. Quinn, B.K. Markey, F.C. Leonard, E.S. FitzPatrick and S. Fanning.
© 2016 John Wiley & Sons, Ltd. Published 2016 by John Wiley & Sons, Ltd.
Companion website: www.wiley.com/go/quinn/concise-veterinary-microbiology

which is commonly used in diagnostic laboratories. Standardized methods for conducting these techniques and interpretive standards for reading the tests have been developed by organizations such as the Clinical and Laboratory Standards Institute (CLSI) and the European Committee on Antimicrobial Susceptibility Testing (EUCAST). Using this disc diffusion method, susceptibility to an antibacterial drug indicates that the infection caused by the bacterium may respond to treatment if the drug reaches therapeutic levels in the affected tissues. Increasingly, laboratories are employing methods which allow determination of the minimal inhibitory concentration (MIC) of an antibiotic for a test bacterium. Methods such as the broth microdilution technique provide such data and are available commercially in 96-well plate formats and in formats which can be used in automated systems. Commercially available E test strips provide an alternative system for determining MICs and are suitable for use in small laboratories. MIC data, in combination with knowledge of the pharmacodynamics and pharmacokinetics of a particular antimicrobial agent, can be used to more accurately select the most effective drug and its dosage. In addition, MIC data are more valuable than qualitative data for monitoring trends in antimicrobial resistance.

Although phenotypic methods are commonly used in diagnostic laboratories for the detection of antimicrobial resistance, procedures for identification of resistance genes have been developed. These methods are usually based on conventional or real-time PCR and can be used to detect the presence of resistance genes in an organism isolated from a clinical specimen or even in the clinical specimen itself. The principal advantage of molecular methods is the speed with which results become available especially for organisms which are difficult to culture. Molecular methods allow the rapid selection of antibiotics

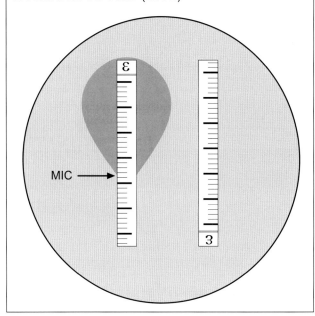

Inert plastic strips incorporating predetermined antibiotic gradients are placed on a bacterial culture and incubated. Following incubation, the MIC value is read from the scale (arrow)

which are likely to be effective. The disadvantage of these methods is that the presence of a gene does not necessarily confirm its phenotypic expression and thus inaccurate clinical information could be generated using such methods. In addition, if molecular detection of resistance is determined directly from the clinical specimens, isolates of the suspected bacterial pathogens will not be available for MIC testing.

9 Bacterial resistance to antimicrobial drugs

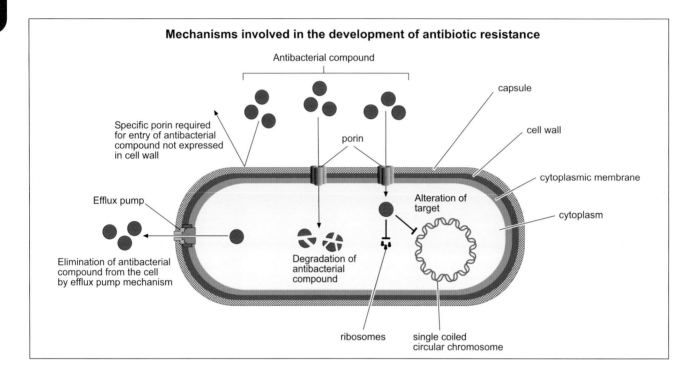

Mechanisms involved in the development of antibiotic resistance

Antibacterial compound

Specific porin required for entry of antibacterial compound not expressed in cell wall

porin

capsule

cell wall

cytoplasmic membrane

Alteration of target

cytoplasm

Efflux pump

Elimination of antibacterial compound from the cell by efflux pump mechanism

Degradation of antibacterial compound

ribosomes

single coiled circular chromosome

Resistance to antibacterial drugs is an important problem in both animals and humans. The widespread and sometimes indiscriminate use of these drugs results in the selection of bacteria which are inherently resistant. Not only may these resistant bacteria become the predominant species in a population, but they may also transfer genetic material to other bacterial species which confers resistance on recipients. In broad terms, resistance of an organism can be defined as either innate (intrinsic) or acquired (extrinsic). Innate resistance is chromosomally encoded and relates to the general physiology of an organism arising from its existing properties such as cell wall complexity, efflux mechanisms or enzymatic inactivation of an antibiotic. In contrast, acquired resistance can arise from a mutation in a resident gene or the transfer of genetic material encoding resistance genes via plasmids, bacteriophages carrying resistance genes or transposons containing integron sequences (Table 9.1 and Chapter 3). Resistance to an antibacterial agent often results in cross-resistance to other agents in the same class. Carriage of several resistance genes by plasmids and transposable elements often enable bacteria to become resistant to a number of drugs of different classes. This type of resistance can be transferred rapidly between different bacterial genera and species, creating multi-drug resistant isolates such as *Salmonella* Typhimurium DT104. This strain is characterized by a penta-resistant phenotype ACSSuT (conferring resistance to ampicillin, chloramphenicol, streptomycin, sulphonamide and tetracycline).

The resistance genes corresponding to the ACSSuT phenotype are encoded on the Salmonella Genomic Island 1 which is located on the chromosome but can be transferred between organisms within this bacterial genus. A monophasic variant of *Salmonella* Typhimurium, *Salmonella* 4,[5],12:i:-, is increasing in prevalence worldwide and exhibits an ASSuT resistance phenotype; the genes encoding resistance in these isolates are located on a chromosomal genomic island also. Multiple drug resistance is of particular concern in zoonotic pathogens and in nosocomial pathogens. The latter cause disease in hospitalized humans and animals where the selection pressure is high. These nosocomial pathogens are sometimes referred to as 'superbugs' and generally fall into one of two categories: widely recognized pathogens such as methicillin-resistant *Staphylococcus aureus* which have acquired resistance to multiple antimicrobial agents, and environmental organisms such as *Pseudomonas aeruginosa* which are intrinsically resistant to many agents and cause opportunistic infections.

In general terms, resistance to antibiotics occurs as a result of drug inactivation, drug-target modification and decreased intracellular accumulation associated with reduced membrane permeability or increased drug efflux. Mechanisms producing resistance to antibacterial drugs include production of enzymes by bacteria which destroy or inactivate the drug. Production of β-lactamases renders bacteria resistant to β-lactam antibiotics. The mode of action of these antibiotics involves interacting

Concise Review of Veterinary Microbiology, Second Edition. P.J. Quinn, B.K. Markey, F.C. Leonard, E.S. FitzPatrick and S. Fanning.
© 2016 John Wiley & Sons, Ltd. Published 2016 by John Wiley & Sons, Ltd.
Companion website: www.wiley.com/go/quinn/concise-veterinary-microbiology

Table 9.1 Antibacterial drug resistance.

Drug	Target	Examples of resistant bacteria / Genetic basis	Comments
Fluoroquinolones	DNA gyrase Topoisomerase	Gram-positive, Gram-negative / Chromosomally-based	Mutation results in structurally altered enzyme
	Cell membrane	*Enterobacteriaceae* / Chromosomally-based	Decreased permeability
Rifampin	DNA-dependent RNA polymerase	*Enterobacteriaceae* / Chromosomally-based	Mutation results in structurally altered enzyme
Erythromycin	Ribosomal protein	*Staphylococcus aureus* / Chromosomally-based	Due to structural change, ribosomes unaffected by drug action
Streptomycin	Ribosomal protein	*Enterobacteriaceae* / Chromosomally-based	Mutation results in altered ribosome
Tetracycline	Ribosomal protein	*Enterobacteriaceae* / Plasmid-mediated	Ribosome protection proteins produced
	Transport mechanisms	*Enterobacteriaceae* / Plasmid-mediated	Decreased absorption or development of energy-dependent efflux mechanism
Chloramphenicol	Peptidyltransferase	*Staphylococcus* species, streptococci / Plasmid- or chromosomally-based	Inactivation of drug by a specific acetyltransferase
Sulphonamides	Dihydropteroate synthetase	*Enterobacteriaceae* / Plasmid- or chromosomally-based	New folic acid synthetic pathway employing sulphonamide-resistant enzyme
β-Lactam antibiotics	Penicillin-binding proteins (PBP)	*Staphylococcus aureus* / Chromosomally-based	Decreased affinity of PBP for drug
	Penicillin-binding proteins	*Enterobacteriaceae* / Chromosomally-based	Outer membrane of most Gram-negative bacteria inherently impermeable to drug
	Penicillin-binding proteins	*Staphylococcus aureus*, *Enterobacteriaceae* / Plasmid- or chromosomally-based	Enzymatic degradation of drug by β-lactamases

with penicillin-binding proteins which interfere with transpeptidation. β-Lactamases cleave the β-lactam ring, rendering the antibiotic ineffective. These enzymes may be plasmid-mediated, as in staphylococci, or they may be chromosomally encoded, as in Gram-negative bacteria. Sulphonamides interfere with the formation of folic acid, an essential precursor for nucleic acid synthesis. Their action relates to their structural similarity to *para*-aminobenzoic acid. When present at sufficient concentrations, sulphonamides are utilized by the enzyme dihydropteroate synthetase instead of *para*-aminobenzoic acid, forming non-functional analogues of folic acid.

Bacteria may also develop alternative metabolic pathways to those inhibited by the drug. An antibiotic may be eliminated from the cell through the action of a range of membrane-bound efflux pumps or the target site of the drug may be structurally altered (Table 9.1).

Antibacterial resistance is widespread in many regions of the world and control measures in a particular country may not be effective if resistant bacteria in food or in the normal flora of animals or humans are imported from countries with less stringent controls. Effective surveillance systems for collecting data on resistant organisms should be established at local, national and international levels. The supply and use of antibacterial drugs should be closely monitored to facilitate evaluation of the risks and benefits of therapy and there should be strict adherence to the recommended therapeutic dose for the prescribed period of time. Adherence to drug withdrawal periods following treatment of food-producing animals should be strictly enforced. Antimicrobial agents should not be used for growth promotion and greater reliance should be placed on improved hygiene measures, disinfection and vaccination for the prevention and control of infectious diseases in animals.

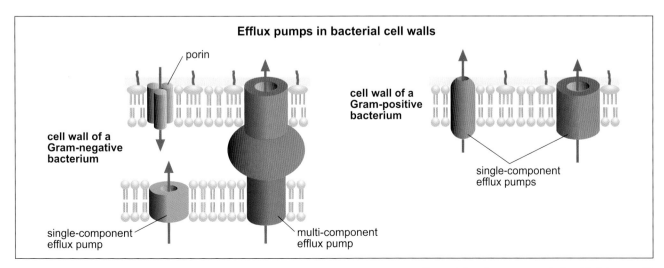

10 Bacterial infections

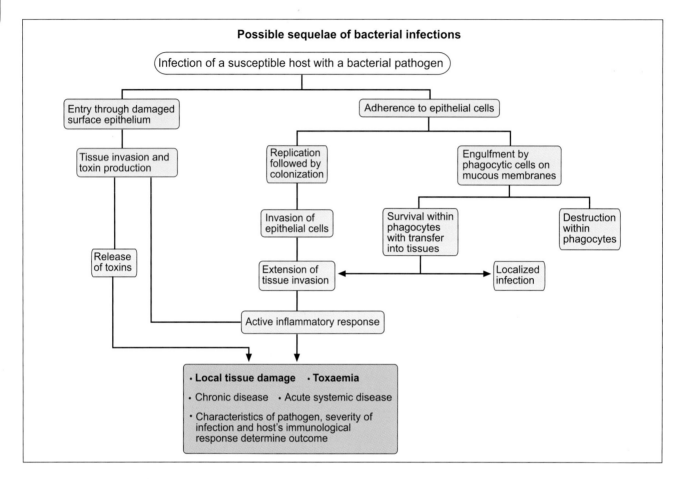

Possible sequelae of bacterial infections

Infection of a susceptible host with a bacterial pathogen

Entry through damaged surface epithelium

Adherence to epithelial cells

Tissue invasion and toxin production

Replication followed by colonization

Engulfment by phagocytic cells on mucous membranes

Invasion of epithelial cells

Survival within phagocytes with transfer into tissues

Destruction within phagocytes

Release of toxins

Extension of tissue invasion

Localized infection

Active inflammatory response

- **Local tissue damage** • **Toxaemia**
- Chronic disease • Acute systemic disease
- Characteristics of pathogen, severity of infection and host's immunological response determine outcome

Although most bacteria are saprophytes which grow on organic matter in the environment, a small number, referred to as bacterial pathogens, produce infection and disease in animals and humans. The development and severity of infections with many pathogenic bacteria are influenced by host-related determinants such as physiological status and immune competence.

Animals may be exposed to infection from exogenous or endogenous sources. Exogenous infections occur after direct or indirect transmission from an infected animal or from the environment. Endogenous infections can be caused by commensal bacteria when an animal is subjected to stressful environmental factors. Infections can be acquired by a number of routes. In exogenous infections, pathogens may enter the host through the skin, the conjunctiva or the mucous membranes of the respiratory, gastrointestinal or urogenital tracts or be vector-borne. Other possible routes of entry include the teat canal and the umbilicus.

The virulence of a bacterium relates to its ability to invade and produce disease in a normal animal. Highly virulent organisms produce serious disease or death in many affected animals

whereas bacteria of low virulence rarely produce serious illness. Factors which influence the outcome of interactions between host and pathogen are illustrated.

Avoidance of defence mechanisms is essential for successful invasion of the host by pathogens. Some of the mechanisms which assist bacterial survival in animals are presented in Table 10.1. Certain bacteria remain at the site of primary infection with local extension only. This localized invasion may be facilitated through breakdown of host tissues by collagenases, lipases, hyaluronidases and fibrinolysin produced by bacterial pathogens. Bacteria can be carried throughout the body in the bloodstream. In bacteraemia, bacteria are present transiently in the bloodstream without replication, whereas in septicaemia pathogenic organisms multiply and persist in the bloodstream, producing systemic disease.

Bacteria can damage host tissues directly through the effect of exotoxins and endotoxins. Bacterial exotoxins and endotoxins differ in their structures and modes of action (Table 10.2). Exotoxins are produced by Gram-positive and Gram-negative bacteria. The effects of exotoxins, which include cell

Concise Review of Veterinary Microbiology, Second Edition. P.J. Quinn, B.K. Markey, F.C. Leonard, E.S. FitzPatrick and S. Fanning.
© 2016 John Wiley & Sons, Ltd. Published 2016 by John Wiley & Sons, Ltd.
Companion website: www.wiley.com/go/quinn/concise-veterinary-microbiology

Table 10.1 Mechanisms which assist bacterial survival in the host.

Mechanism	Comments
O antigen polysaccharide chain	Length of polysaccharide chain hinders binding of the membrane attack complex of complement to the outer membrane of many Gram-negative bacteria
Capsule production	Antiphagocytic role in many bacteria
M protein production	Antiphagocytic activity in *Streptococcus equi*
Production of Fc-binding proteins	Staphylococci and streptococci produce proteins which bind to the Fc region of IgG and prevent interaction with the Fc receptor on membranes of phagocytes
Production of leukotoxins	Cytolysis of phagocytes by toxins produced by *Mannheimia haemolytica*, *Actinobacillus* species and other pathogenic bacteria
Interference with phagosome–lysosome fusion	Allows the survival of pathogenic mycobacteria within phagocytes
Escape from phagosomes	Survival mechanism used by *Listeria monocytogenes* and rickettsiae
Resistance to oxidative damage	Allows survival of salmonellae and brucellae within phagocytes
Antigenic mimicry of host antigens	Adaptation of surface antigens by *Mycoplasma* species to avoid recognition by the immune system
Antigenic variation of surface antigens	*Mycoplasma* species and borrelliae can partially evade detection by the host's immune response
Coagulase production	Conversion of fibrinogen to fibrin by *Staphylococcus aureus* can isolate site of infection from effective immune responses

Table 10.2 Comparison of exotoxins and endotoxins.

Exotoxins	Endotoxins
Produced by live bacteria, both Gram-positive and Gram-negative	Component of the cell wall of Gram-negative bacteria released following cell death
Proteins, usually of high molecular weight	Lipopolysaccharide complex containing lipid A, the toxic component
Heat labile	Heat stable
Potent toxins, usually with specific activity; not pyrogenic. Highly antigenic; readily converted into toxoids which induce neutralizing antibodies	Toxins with moderate, non-specific generalized activity; potent pyrogens, weakly antigenic; not amenable to toxoid production. Neutralizing antibodies not associated with natural exposure
Synthesis determined extrachromosomally	Encoded in chromosome

membrane damage or interference with protein synthesis, are summarized in Box 10.1. Endotoxins of Gram-negative bacteria contain a hydrophobic glycolipid (lipid A) and a hydrophilic polysaccharide composed of a core oligosaccharide and an O-polysaccharide (O antigen). The toxicity of this complex lipopolysaccharide molecule resides in the lipid A portion. The effects of endotoxins are summarized in Box 10.2.

Some individual pathogens tend to produce a predictable clinical picture following infection of a susceptible animal. Anthrax in ruminants is invariably peracute and fatal. In contrast, infections with bacteria such as *Salmonella* Dublin in cattle may produce many different forms of disease. Bacterial infections can be conveniently categorized as acute, subacute, chronic or persistent. Acute infections usually have a short clinical course and the invading bacteria are often cleared from the body by the host's immune response. Chronic infections tend to occur when the host fails to eliminate the pathogen. Persistent infections may occur in certain sites such as the uriniferous tubules and the central nervous system in which cell-mediated and humoral immunity are unable to exert their full effect.

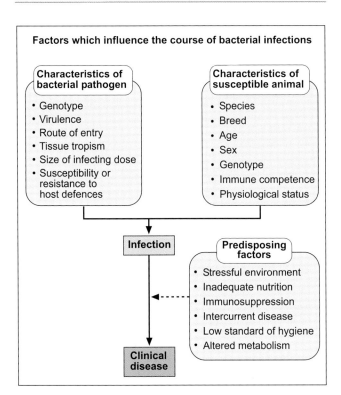

Factors which influence the course of bacterial infections

Characteristics of bacterial pathogen
- Genotype
- Virulence
- Route of entry
- Tissue tropism
- Size of infecting dose
- Susceptibility or resistance to host defences

Characteristics of susceptible animal
- Species
- Breed
- Age
- Sex
- Genotype
- Immune competence
- Physiological status

Infection

Predisposing factors
- Stressful environment
- Inadequate nutrition
- Immunosuppression
- Intercurrent disease
- Low standard of hygiene
- Altered metabolism

Clinical disease

Box 10.1 Effects of exotoxins

- Cell membrane damage
  - Enzymatic digestion
  - Formation of pores
- Interference with protein synthesis
- Elevation of cAMP levels
- Disruption of functions relating to nervous tissue
- Digestion of components of interstitial tissue: collagen, elastin, hyaluronic acid

Box 10.2 Effects of endotoxins

- Activation of polymorphonuclear and mononuclear phago-cytes, platelets and B lymphocytes
- Release of interleukin-1, leading to fever
- Activation of complement, promoting inflammatory changes
- Elevated concentrations produce a dramatic drop in blood pressure (endotoxic shock)

11 Structure and components of the immune system

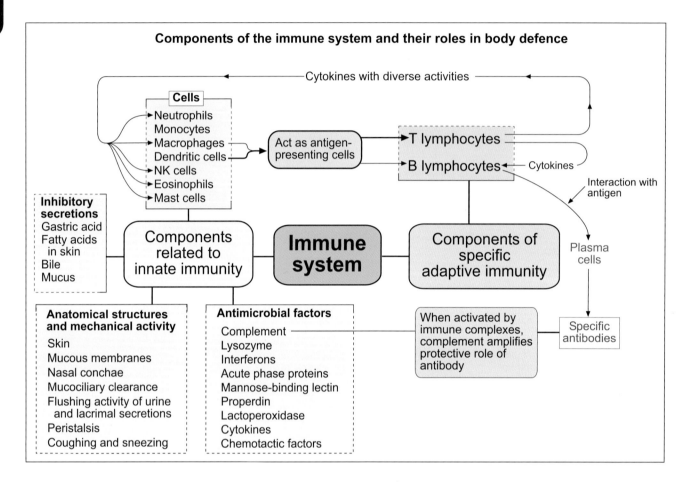

Components of the immune system and their roles in body defence

Cytokines with diverse activities

Cells
- Neutrophils
- Monocytes
- Macrophages
- Dendritic cells
- NK cells
- Eosinophils
- Mast cells

Act as antigen-presenting cells

T lymphocytes

B lymphocytes — Cytokines

Interaction with antigen

Plasma cells

Inhibitory secretions
Gastric acid
Fatty acids in skin
Bile
Mucus

Components related to innate immunity

Immune system

Components of specific adaptive immunity

Specific antibodies

Anatomical structures and mechanical activity
Skin
Mucous membranes
Nasal conchae
Mucociliary clearance
Flushing activity of urine and lacrimal secretions
Peristalsis
Coughing and sneezing

Antimicrobial factors
Complement
Lysozyme
Interferons
Acute phase proteins
Mannose-binding lectin
Properdin
Lactoperoxidase
Cytokines
Chemotactic factors

When activated by immune complexes, complement amplifies protective role of antibody

In biology, the term 'immunity' is used to describe resistance to infectious disease. The cells, tissues, structures and secretions which mediate this resistance to infectious agents are collectively referred to as the immune system. Like other body systems, the immune system is composed of an array of structures, cells and secretions, but unlike other systems it provides defence not only against opportunistic infections but also against pathogenic microorganisms which can cause life-threatening infections in susceptible animals. Vertebrates and invertebrates possess intrinsic mechanisms for defending themselves against microbial infections. Because these defence mechanisms are always present, they constitute what is referred to as innate immunity. Adaptive immunity is activated initially by the response of the innate immune system following invasion of host tissues by pathogenic microorganisms. Although responses occur more slowly with adaptive immunity, this branch of the immune system provides a specific effective defence against invading pathogens.

Cells of the immune system derive from multipotent stem cells which develop in the bone marrow during haematopoiesis.

Apart from erythrocytes and platelets which are also produced at this phase of foetal development, each of the other cell types has a distinctive role in innate and adaptive immune responses. The origin, lineage, characteristics and distribution of cells of the immune system are summarized in Table 11.1.

Innate immunity

The first line of defence against invading microorganisms, which is present at birth and persists for life, derives from components of innate immunity. Unlike adaptive immunity, innate immunity has limited specificity and exhibits limited immunological memory for infectious agents previously encountered. Innate immunity has four components: (1) epithelial barriers and mechanical activity of particular structures; (2) secretions with inhibitory activity against microorganisms; (3) antimicrobial factors present in blood, body fluids and secretions; and (4) cells with phagocytic and other properties which confront invading pathogens. In addition to providing protection against infection at an early stage if host tissues are invaded, innate

Concise Review of Veterinary Microbiology, Second Edition. P.J. Quinn, B.K. Markey, F.C. Leonard, E.S. FitzPatrick and S. Fanning.
© 2016 John Wiley & Sons, Ltd. Published 2016 by John Wiley & Sons, Ltd.
Companion website: www.wiley.com/go/quinn/concise-veterinary-microbiology

Table 11.1 Origin, lineage, distribution and other characteristics of cells of the immune system.

Cells	Origin	Lineage	Morphology	Distribution	Comments
Basophils	Bone marrow	Myeloid	Lobed nuclei, metachromatic cytoplasmic granules	Blood	Non-phagocytic circulating granulocytes, structurally and functionally similar to mast cells
B lymphocytes	Bone marrow	Lymphoid	Round or slightly indented condensed nuclei	Blood and tissues	In mammals, these cells mature in the bone marrow; in birds, in the cloacal bursa. B lymphocytes express membrane-bound antibody; following interaction with antigen, they differentiate into plasma cells
Dendritic cells	Bone marrow	Some arise from myeloid stem cells, others from lymphoid stem cells	Large mononuclear cells with thin processes	Found in skin, most organs, lymphoid tissue, blood and lymph	Specialized group of antigen-presenting cells which present antigen to T helper cells; a distinct group of these cells, follicular dendritic cells, present antigen to B lymphocytes
Eosinophils	Bone marrow	Myeloid	Bilobed nuclei, large cytoplasmic granules with affinity for acidic dyes	Blood and tissues	Motile granulocytes with some phagocytic activity; participate in immediate-type hypersensitivity reactions
Macrophages	Bone marrow	Myeloid	Mononuclear cells with nuclei which have irregular outlines	Present in tissues throughout body	Tissue-based mononuclear phagocytes which derive from blood monocytes; named according to location; have a central role in innate and adaptive immune responses
Mast cells	Bone marrow	Myeloid	Mononuclear cells, metachromatic cytoplasmic granules	Connective tissue near blood vessels and nerves	Contain numerous mediator-filled granules rich in histamine and heparin; express high-affinity receptors for IgE
Monocytes	Bone marrow	Myeloid	Large mononuclear cells with kidney-shaped nuclei	Blood	Motile mononuclear phagocytic cells which circulate briefly in the bloodstream before differentiating into tissue macrophages
Natural killer cells	Bone marrow	Lymphoid	Large granular mononuclear cells	Blood and peripheral tissues	Cytotoxic lymphocytes, distinct from T lymphocytes and B lymphocytes; can destroy virus-infected cells; activate macrophages by secreting interferon γ
Neutrophils	Bone marrow	Myeloid	Multilobed nuclei, pale staining cytoplasmic granules	Blood, migrate into tissues in response to chemotactic stimuli	Short-lived circulating motile phagocytic cells which engulf and destroy bacterial pathogens
Plasma cells	Bone marrow	Lymphoid	Basophilic cells, prominent endoplasmic reticulum, eccentric cartwheel-shaped nuclei	Connective tissue, secondary lymphoid organs and bone marrow	Antibody-secreting cells derived from B lymphocytes
Platelets	Bone marrow, from megakaryocytes	Myeloid	Cytoplasmic fragments	Blood	Platelets are small cytoplasmic fragments produced by megakaryocytes under the influence of thrombopoietin. Adhesion of platelets to subendothelium of damaged blood vessels initiates blood clotting
T lymphocytes	Arise from lymphoid stem cells in bone marrow, mature in the thymus	Lymphoid	Round or slightly indented condensed nuclei	Blood and tissues	Participate in cell-mediated immune responses; functional subsets express CD4 or CD8 membrane glycoprotein molecules and possess receptors for antigen recognized in association with major histocompatibility complex molecules

immunity, through the participation of the antigen-presenting cells, macrophages and dendritic cells, alerts lymphocytes to the threat of invading pathogens, thereby initiating specific adaptive immune responses against the invading infectious agents.

The three major routes of entry of pathogens into the body are the skin, the gastrointestinal tract and the respiratory tract. Because these three routes are composed of or lined by continuous epithelia which interfere with the entry of microbial pathogens, loss of skin integrity or damage to the epithelial lining of the respiratory or gastrointestinal tracts predisposes host tissues to microbial invasion. In addition to the mechanical protection offered by the skin against bacterial and fungal invasion, skin secretions, which include sebum and fatty acids, inhibit bacterial and fungal growth. Trauma involving the skin and non-infectious diseases of the skin allow tissue invasion by opportunistic pathogens. Because they are covered by a layer of mucus which traps microorganisms, mucous membranes provide protection against entry of opportunistic pathogens. Mucus also contains antibacterial substances such as lysozyme. The pulmonary airways are coated with mucus and trapped particles are propelled towards the pharynx by ciliated epithelial cells. Mechanical activity such as the flushing of urine and lacrimal secretions dislodges bacteria from tissue surfaces. Inhibitory secretions such as gastric acid, fatty acids in the skin and bile inhibit growth of many potential pathogens. Some pathogenic bacteria, especially members of the *Enterobacteriaceae*, can survive gastric acidity and tolerate bile salts in the intestinal tract.

Antimicrobial factors present in blood, body fluids and secretions include complement, lysozyme, interferons and lactoferrin. The complement system consists of approximately 30 serum and membrane proteins which can contribute to a variety of immune reactions, including promotion of inflammatory responses, chemotaxis, opsonization and destruction of cell membranes. The majority of complement components circulate as functionally inactive forms, proenzymes, until proteolytic cleavage removes an inhibitory fragment and exposes the active site of the molecule. The complement system can be activated by microorganisms in the absence of antibody and also by antibodies attached to foreign antigenic material derived from infectious agents. Complement components are designated by the letter C and numerals from 1 to 9. The number assigned to each component refers to the order in which individual proteins were discovered. The biochemical reaction sequence is C1–C4–C2–C3–C5–C6–C7–C8–C9. Upper case letters identify factors that interact with complement components. Lower case letters after a complement component, such as C3b, are used to identify peptide fragments formed by activation of that component. There are three pathways of complement activation: two, called the alternative and lectin pathways, are initiated by microorganisms without the requirement of antibody; a third pathway, called the classical pathway, is initiated by immune complexes. The three pathways converge on a common terminal pathway that leads to the formation of a membrane attack complex which produces transmembrane pores in the membranes of target cells resulting in osmotic lysis of these cells.

Lysozyme, a highly cationic low-molecular-weight antimicrobial factor present in body fluids and secretions, acts directly on the cell wall of Gram-positive bacteria and enzymatically cleaves the bonds between *N*-acetylglucosamine and *N*-

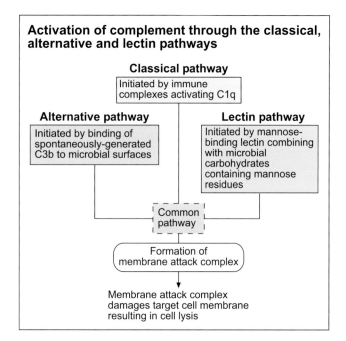

Activation of complement through the classical, alternative and lectin pathways

Classical pathway
Initiated by immune complexes activating C1q

Alternative pathway
Initiated by binding of spontaneously-generated C3b to microbial surfaces

Lectin pathway
Initiated by mannose-binding lectin combining with microbial carbohydrates containing mannose residues

Common pathway

Formation of membrane attack complex

Membrane attack complex damages target cell membrane resulting in cell lysis

acetylmuramic acid which stabilize the peptidoglycan layer. This antimicrobial factor is present in the granules of neutrophils and is a secretory product of macrophages. It is present in most body fluids including saliva and tears.

Interferons α and β, referred to as type I interferons, are produced by cells of the innate immune system following viral invasion of tissues and also by epithelial cells and other cells invaded by viruses. Interferon γ, which has immunomodulatory activity, is produced by T lymphocytes and natural killer cells in response to antigenic or mitogenic stimulation. Interferons bind to the interferon receptor on adjacent host cells and induce production of antiviral protein, enabling them to resist infection. Interferons do not directly block viral replication but activate genes which can confer direct antiviral capability on the cells.

Cells involved in innate immune responses

The ability to ingest and kill pathogens is an essential component of host defence and cells that participate in the recognition, removal and destruction of bacterial or fungal invaders are referred to as phagocytes. Neutrophils, monocytes, macrophages and dendritic cells are the principal cell types involved in phagocytosis, a process in which relatively large particles such as bacteria or yeasts are engulfed by these phagocytic cells. Phagocytosis is a receptor-mediated process in which specific recognition of a particle by receptors on a phagocytic cell leads to the engulfment of the particle and fusion of the vesicle containing the engulfed particle with specialized intracellular organelles, lysosomes. The stages involved in phagocytosis of pathogens include activation, chemotaxis and attachment of the organisms, followed by their ingestion and destruction.

Neutrophils are short-lived motile phagocytic cells that can engulf and destroy bacterial and fungal pathogens. In many mammals, neutrophils constitute the majority of circulating leukocytes. After differentiation in the bone marrow, neutrophils released into the peripheral blood circulate for up to ten hours before migrating into the tissues where they have a life span of a few days. In response to many types of infections, particularly those caused by pyogenic bacteria, the number of neutrophils increases significantly. The resultant transient increase in neutrophil numbers, termed leucocytosis, is usually indicative of a pyogenic infection. At the site of a bacterial infection, neutrophils phagocytose and destroy invading bacteria. Neutrophil granules contain a wide range of antimicrobial proteins and degradative enzymes including acid hydrolases, elastase and lysozyme.

Up to 10% of white blood cells are monocytes, a heterogeneous group of cells which differentiate into phagocytic cells including macrophages and dendritic cells. When monocytes migrate into tissues in response to infection, they can differentiate into tissue macrophages. Unlike neutrophils, macrophages are long-lived cells, well equipped to engulf and destroy microorganisms. Some macrophages become established residents in particular organs or tissues where they may contribute to tissue repair and regeneration. Macrophages, which participate in innate immune responses, undergo a number of structural and functional changes when they encounter microbial pathogens in tissues. Microglial cells in the central nervous system and alveolar macrophages in the lung are examples of such cell types. Activated macrophages exhibit greater phagocytic activity and an enhanced ability to kill engulfed pathogens than resting macrophages. In addition, these activated cells have increased secretion of inflammatory and cytotoxic mediators and function more effectively as antigen-presenting cells for helper T cells.

Dendritic cells are a specialized group of phagocytic cells with long membranous extensions which resemble the dendrites on nerve cells, hence their name. These cells are present in the skin, lymph nodes, in close association with mucosal surfaces and many subsets are described. Through their ability to bind, process and ultimately present antigens to T lymphocytes and in some instances to B lymphocytes, dendritic cells act as important antigen-presenting cells with a central role in the initiation of adaptive immune responses.

Natural killer (NK) cells are lymphoid cells which are closely related to B lymphocytes and T lymphocytes. Formerly referred to as large granular lymphocytes, because of their microscopic appearance, these cells do not express antigen-specific receptors and are considered part of the innate immune system. Up to 10% of lymphocytes in the peripheral circulation are NK cells. These cells exhibit cytotoxicity for tumour cells and virus-infected cells. Receptors for immunoglobulins on the surface of NK cells allow these cells to recognize and bind to target cells bearing bound antibodies on their surfaces. When the NK cells make contact with the target cells, they release granules which induce death of the target cells. In some species of animals, NK cells are reported to have limited immunological memory.

Cells and secretions of the innate immune system constitute a major component of the inflammatory response to infectious agents and lead to the activation of adaptive immune responses.

12 Adaptive immunity

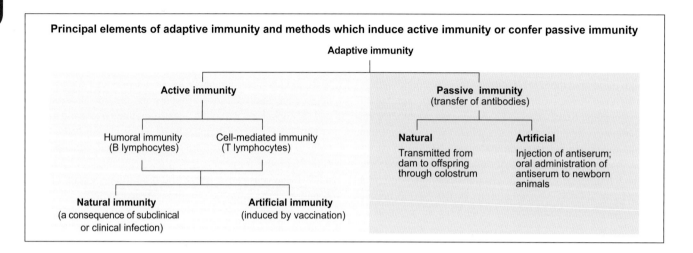

Principal elements of adaptive immunity and methods which induce active immunity or confer passive immunity

Adaptive immunity

Active immunity

Humoral immunity
(B lymphocytes)

Cell-mediated immunity
(T lymphocytes)

Natural immunity
(a consequence of subclinical
or clinical infection)

Artificial immunity
(induced by vaccination)

Passive immunity
(transfer of antibodies)

Natural

Transmitted from
dam to offspring
through colostrum

Artificial

Injection of antiserum;
oral administration of
antiserum to newborn
animals

The organs of the lymphoid system are traditionally divided into primary and secondary organs. The primary lymphoid organs in mammals are the bone marrow and thymus. In these locations, lymphocytes are produced and differentiate into mature naïve lymphocytes. Secondary lymphoid tissues in mammals consist of lymph nodes located in strategic sites around the body, the spleen and Peyer's patches. Although secondary lymphoid organs such as the spleen and lymph nodes are not essential for the generation of lymphocytes, they have a central role in the maturation of these cells and the development of immunity. In particular anatomical sites, lymph nodes have specialized roles. Those associated with the upper and lower respiratory tract are referred to as mucosa-associated lymphoid tissue (MALT) and those in close proximity to the intestine are termed gut-associated lymphoid tissue (GALT). Secondary lymphoid organs have important functions in the development of adaptive immunity. They are reservoirs of T and B lymphocytes and they are sites at which antigenic material is recognized and presented to T and B cells. Immune responses to invading pathogens or foreign material recognized by antigen-presenting cells usually occur in lymphoid organs.

The names assigned to lymphocytes reflects the tissue or organ in which they mature after leaving the bone marrow, or in the case of natural killer (NK) cells, to their immunological activity. Thus, the designation of T cell relates to lymphocytes that mature in the thymus and the name B cell relates to lymphocytes that mature in the avian cloacal bursa or in its equivalent in mammals, the bone marrow. Additional sites in mammals where B-lymphocyte maturation may take place include Peyer's patches or other GALT. Although lymphocytes are morphologically heterogeneous, B cells and T cells can be differentiated by their antigen receptors and by the characteristics of their surface markers. The primary role of B lymphocytes

is antibody production. Each B cell is genetically programmed to express surface receptors for a particular antigen. When stimulated by an antigen for which they have receptors, B cells differentiate into plasma cells which produce large amounts of specific antibody. Mature T lymphocytes, which comprise functionally distinct populations, are involved in the activation of many cell types including B lymphocytes, macrophages and other cell types involved in inflammatory responses. Subsets of T cells express different markers and, through the release of cytokines, T lymphocytes are responsible for the activation and control of many specific immune responses. Lymphocytes which are distinct from T and B lymphocytes, referred to as NK cells, have some characteristics in common with T cells but do not exhibit antigenic specificity. These large granular lymphocytes are part of the innate immune system and do not express clonally distributed antigen receptors.

The only cells in the body capable of recognizing antigenic determinants in a highly specific manner are T and B lymphocytes. In addition, these lymphocytes produce memory cells following an encounter with antigenic material. Accordingly, specificity and memory are two fundamental features of adaptive immune responses. As a consequence of immunological memory, a more rapid and effective immune response occurs with a second or subsequent encounter with an infectious agent than on primary exposure. This contrasts with innate immune responses which do not alter following repeated exposure to the same infectious agent (Table 12.1). Adaptive immune responses occur in two phases: recognition of the infectious agent's surface antigens and development of specific immune responses aimed at clearing the microbial pathogen from the tissues. In the first phase, selection of lymphocytes involves the recognition of antigen with subsequent clonal expansion of T and B lymphocytes with surface receptors for the antigen.

Concise Review of Veterinary Microbiology, Second Edition. P.J. Quinn, B.K. Markey, F.C. Leonard, E.S. FitzPatrick and S. Fanning.
© 2016 John Wiley & Sons, Ltd. Published 2016 by John Wiley & Sons, Ltd.
Companion website: www.wiley.com/go/quinn/concise-veterinary-microbiology

Table 12.1 Comparative features of innate and adaptive immunity.

Feature	Innate immunity	Adaptive immunity
Occurrence	Ancient form of protection present in all members of the animal kingdom	Evolved in vertebrates much later than the innate immune system
Induction	Present at birth and functions without any previous interaction with infectious agents	Develops in response to antigenic challenge postnatally
Rate of response	Rapid response to infection; ranges from minutes to hours	Relatively slow; protective immune response may take up to 7 days to develop
Physical barriers	Skin, mucous membranes, mucociliary clearance, nasal conchae	Not applicable
Mechanical action	Flushing activity of tears and urine, peristalsis, coughing and sneezing	Not applicable
Physiological influences	Low pH values on skin, gastric acidity, bile, mucus	Not applicable
Specificity	Relatively non-specific	Highly specific
Recognition of infectious agents	Infectious agents are recognized by pattern recognition receptors on many different cell types	Antigen recognition occurs through membrane-bound immunoglobulins on B lymphocytes and through T-cell receptors on T lymphocytes
Nature of recognition molecules	Pattern recognition receptors recognize conserved microbial structures and there are probably a few hundred receptors for pathogens	Immunoglobulins recognize determinants on the surface of infectious agents or in a soluble form; T-cell receptors recognize peptides bound to MHC molecules on host cells
Immunological memory	Absent	Immunological memory is present, and on repeated exposure the response becomes faster and stronger
Contribution to body defences	First line of defence against opportunistic pathogens; offers limited protection against virulent microorganisms	Produces a long-lasting protective response to a wide range of virulent microorganisms
Participating cells	Polymorphonuclear leukocytes, monocytes, macrophages, NK cells, dendritic cells, mast cells and epithelial cells	B lymphocytes; T lymphocytes in association with antigen-presenting cells
Principal soluble factors	Complement, lysozyme, interferons, acute phase proteins, cytokines and antimicrobial peptides	Cytokines produced by T lymphocytes and also cytotoxic mediators; antibodies secreted by plasma cells

In the second phase, differentiation of the lymphocytes into effector cells and memory cells results in the development of humoral and cell-mediated immune responses.

Subsets of T lymphocytes with helper or cytotoxic activity can be distinguished by the presence or absence of CD4 or CD8 membrane glycoproteins. Most CD4$^+$ T cells are helper T cells; lymphocytes which are CD8$^+$ generally function as cytotoxic T cells. Lymphocytes with regulatory activity are identified by the presence of both CD4 and CD25 markers on their membranes. These T_{REG} cells tend to suppress immune responses and act as cellular regulators of the immune system. All T cells express antigen-binding T-cell receptors which functionally resemble membrane-bound antibodies on B lymphocytes but differ from them structurally. Before antigenic material can be recognized by the T-cell receptor, it must be bound to the major histocompatibility complex molecules on the surface of antigen-presenting cells. The major histocompatibility complex (MHC) is a collection of genes arranged within a continuous segment of DNA encoding three classes of molecules. MHC class I genes encode glycoproteins expressed on the surface of most nucleated cells. The major function of class I gene products is the presentation of antigenic fragments to cytotoxic T lymphocytes, CD8$^+$ cells. MHC class II genes encode glycoproteins expressed on antigen-presenting cells such as macrophages, dendritic cells and B cells.

These antigen-presenting cells present processed antigenic peptides to T helper cells, CD4$^+$ T cells. MHC class I molecules bind peptides derived from cytosolic proteins, referred to as endogenous proteins, while MHC class II molecules bind peptides taken into the cell by phagocytosis or endocytosis. MHC class III genes encode secreted molecules with immune functions such as cytokines.

Cell-mediated immunity is a term reserved for a form of adaptive immunity which is mediated by T lymphocytes and serves as a defence strategy against microorganisms which survive within phagocytes or which infect other host cells. Antibodies are ineffective against microbial or parasitic pathogens which replicate in phagocytes or in non-phagocytic host cells. Cell-mediated immune responses include CD4$^+$ T cell-mediated activation of macrophages which have engulfed pathogens and CD8$^+$ cytotoxic T lymphocyte killing of cells infected with intracellular pathogens, usually viruses.

With its capacity to recognize a vast array of antigenic determinants on infectious agents, the immune system can respond to tissue invasion with effective humoral and cell-mediated responses. Cooperation between components of innate and adaptive immunity is a requirement for effective protection against pathogenic microorganisms.

13 Protective immune responses against infectious agents

Resistance to infectious agents is a requirement for survival in all species of animals. Characteristics of infectious agents, including virulence, route of entry, tissue tropism and ability to resist host defences, often influence the course of an infection. However, the species, breed, age and immunological competence of the host may also influence the progress of infection and, ultimately, its outcome. Although innate immune responses usually lack specificity and do not exhibit immunological memory, they constitute the first line of defence against invading microorganisms. The rate of response to infection by components of the innate immune system is relatively fast and offers protection against opportunistic pathogens. Cooperation between innate immunity and adaptive immunity is a requirement for protection against highly virulent pathogens which can resist phagocytosis and intracellular killing by macrophages and for microbial pathogens which elaborate potent toxins. Antibodies produced by B lymphocytes can neutralize viruses and bacterial toxins and, through the activity of IgA on mucosal surfaces, can protect the respiratory and alimentary tracts against microbial attack. The protective role of antibodies, however, is limited to extracellular pathogens as humoral immunity is ineffective against microbial and parasitic pathogens which replicate within host cells. Protection against intracellular pathogens including viruses, bacteria such as *Mycobacterium bovis* and *Listeria monocytogenes* and fungal pathogens such as *Histoplasma capsulatum* is dependent on effective cell-mediated immune responses which involve T helper cells and cytotoxic T lymphocytes. If, following intracellular infection by a microbial pathogen, the infected cells are unable to kill the invading agent, the only means of eradication of the infection is by destruction of the infected host cells. Accordingly, cell-mediated immunity is an essential part of adaptive immune responses to infectious agents.

Adaptive immunity can be divided into two branches, active immunity and passive immunity. Active immunity results from exposure to foreign antigenic material which activates B lymphocytes and T lymphocytes and induces an active immune response to the material encountered by the animal. Passive immunity refers to the transfer of antibodies from an actively immune animal to a susceptible animal. Antiserum specific for a particular pathogen or toxin can be administered by injection to give immediate short-term protection against infectious agents. Natural passive immunity is transmitted from dam to offspring through the ingestion of colostrum. Antibodies produced by the dam and secreted in colostrum passively protect newborn animals against a wide range of respiratory and enteric pathogens. These antibodies have the ability to neutralize bacterial toxins and viruses and can opsonize microbial pathogens for phagocytosis by macrophages and neutrophils. By activating the classical complement pathway, antibodies can opsonize pathogenic agents through fixation of C3b, leading to lysis of microbial pathogens.

Immunity to bacteria

Innate defences against bacterial invasion include epithelial barriers, mucociliary clearance of bacteria and inhibitory secretions such as gastric acid and bile. Although not considered part of innate defences, normal flora can compete with and sometimes prevent colonization by pathogenic microorganisms. Antimicrobial factors present in body fluids include complement, acute phase proteins, lysozyme and transferrin. Macrophages and neutrophils are two phagocytic cell types which are especially important in innate immunity (Box 13.1). The type of adaptive immune responses required for protection against a bacterial infection is determined by the virulence of the organism, tissue tropism and the pathogen's resistance to host defences. Cell-mediated immunity is essential for the control of intracellular bacteria such as *Mycobacterium bovis* and *Listeria monocytogenes*. Humoral immunity has a major protective role against extracellular bacteria. Secretory IgA can bind to bacterial adhesins and block bacterial attachment to mucosal surfaces. The presence of a capsule may render bacteria resistant to phagocytosis but when opsonized by specific antibody and C3b, such encapsulated bacteria can be ingested and destroyed by phagocytes. Specific antibody can agglutinate and immobilize motile bacteria, activate complement and neutralize bacterial toxins and enzymes which promote bacterial spreading in tissues (Box 13.2).

Box 13.1 Innate defences against bacteria causing systemic infections

- Surface barriers: skin, mucous membranes
- Mucociliary clearance
- Flushing activity of urine and lacrimal secretions
- Inhibitory secretions: gastric acid, bile, mucus, fatty acids in skin
- Antimicrobial factors in body fluids: complement, lysozyme, acute phase proteins, cytokines, IFN-γ, chemotactic factors, mannose-binding lectin, transferrin, lipopolysaccharide-binding protein
- NK cells
- Phagocytic cells: neutrophils, monocytes, macrophages, dendritic cells

---

Concise Review of Veterinary Microbiology, Second Edition. P.J. Quinn, B.K. Markey, F.C. Leonard, E.S. FitzPatrick and S. Fanning.
© 2016 John Wiley & Sons, Ltd. Published 2016 by John Wiley & Sons, Ltd.
Companion website: www.wiley.com/go/quinn/concise-veterinary-microbiology

Box 13.2 Adaptive immune responses to bacteria causing systemic infections

Antibodies
- Specific antibodies (IgM, IgG and IgA) opsonize bacteria, prevent binding of bacteria to mucosal surfaces, agglutinate and immobilize motile bacteria. These antibodies also neutralize toxins and enzymes which promote spreading of the pathogens. IgM and IgG activate complement, leading to bacteriolysis

Cells
- Priming of CD4$^+$ T cells by dendritic cells promotes helper T-cell development with release of cytokines which promote B-cell differentiation into plasma cells. These T cells also release IFN-γ which activates macrophages, leading to enhanced intracellular killing of engulfed bacteria. Presentation of intracellular bacterial antigens to CD8$^+$ cytotoxic T cells activates these cells which release proinflammatory and macrophage-enhancing cytokines; they also release cytotoxic mediators which kill infected host cells

Immunity to fungi

A relatively small number of fungal species cause disease in humans and animals. Tissue invasion by fungi is usually indicative of immunological incompetence, immunosuppression or, in the case of yeast infections, a consequence of prolonged antibacterial therapy. Innate defences offer the first and often the most important protection against many opportunistic fungal invaders. Intact skin, with its low pH and secreted fatty acids, and mucosal surfaces with their antimicrobial secretions are major barriers to fungal invasion. Competition from normal commensal microflora on the skin and on mucosal surfaces is important for its inhibitory effect on yeast proliferation on mucosal surfaces. Antimicrobial factors in body fluids, phagocytic cells and pathogen-recognition receptors on host cells provide both protection against fungal invasion and detection of their presence on mucosal surfaces (Box 13.3).

Box 13.3 Innate defences against fungi causing systemic infections

- Surface barriers: skin, mucous membranes
- Mucociliary clearance
- Inhibitory secretions: fatty acids in skin, gastric acid, bile, mucus
- Antimicrobial factors in body fluids:
  - C-reactive proteins
  - Complement
  - Dectin-1
  - Mannose-binding lectin
  - Receptor for β-glucans
  - Toll-like receptors
- Phagocytic cells:
  - Neutrophils
  - Macrophages
  - Dendritic cells
- NK cells

Adaptive immune responses to fungi involve cell-mediated immune responses and humoral responses. Although specific antibodies may opsonize fungal structures in host tissues and

contribute to their clearance by neutrophils, protective immunity does not usually rely on humoral immune responses. Resistance to most fungal pathogens is dependent on T cell-mediated immunity, particularly CD4$^+$ T$_H$1 cells secreting interferon γ with the participation of macrophages, dendritic cells and natural killer (NK) cells (Box 13.4).

Box 13.4 Adaptive immune response to fungi causing systemic infections

Antibodies
- Although specific antibodies may act as opsonins and facilitate clearance of invading yeast cells, fungal spores and hyphal elements, antibody production does not confer protection

Cells
- In response to fungal invasion, macrophages release interleukin (IL)-13, which acts on T lymphocytes and NK cells. These cells in turn release IFN-γ which acts on macrophages promoting destruction of engulfed fungal structures. For most fungal pathogens, T cell-mediated immunity is required for elimination of infection and development of protective immunity

Immunity to viruses

Induction of innate immune responses to viral infections result in the production of type I interferons and activation of NK cells. Type I interferons, a family of related polypeptides, include interferon (IFN)-α, IFN-β, IFN-κ and a number of other cytokines with similar biological activities. The stimulus for type I interferon synthesis is viral infection. Within hours of viral infection, IFN-α and IFN-β are produced by infected cells or by sentinel cells of the innate immune system. IFN-α is produced by leukocytes, especially macrophages, following viral infection. Fibroblast and epithelial cells produce IFN-β. Interferons bind to the interferon receptor on adjacent host cells and induce production of antiviral protein, enabling them to resist infection.

Within days of a viral infection, activated NK cells are present in the tissues. By killing host cells expressing viral antigen on their surfaces, NK cells contribute to the elimination of cellular reservoirs of infection. The ability of NK cells to protect host cells against infection is enhanced by cytokines secreted by macrophages and dendritic cells. Macrophages contribute to antiviral immunity through phagocytosis of viruses and virus-infected cells, sometimes with the involvement of specific antibody and complement (Box 13.5).

Box 13.5 Innate defences against viruses causing systemic infections

- Surface barriers: skin, mucous membranes
- Phagocytic cells: macrophages, dendritic cells, neutrophils
- NK cells
- Antiviral cytokines:
  - IFN-α
  - IFN-β
  - IFN-γ
- Antimicrobial factors:
  - Complement
  - Chemotactic factors
  - Cytidine deaminases
  - Endonuclease

Antibodies
- Specific antibodies neutralize virus particles in tissues and body fluids
- Secretory IgA can prevent attachment of viruses to host cell receptors on mucosal surfaces
- When activated by IgM or IgG antibodies, complement can lyse enveloped virions
- Antibodies and complement can opsonize virus particles facilitating clearance by phagocytosis
- Virus-infected cells coated with IgG antibodies can be destroyed through antibody-dependent cell-mediated cytotoxicity by NK cells

Cells
- Presentation of viral antigen to naïve T cells by dendritic cells results in $CD4^+$ T helper cells releasing antiviral cytokines, followed by activation of $CD8^+$ T cells and B-cell development
- Cytotoxic $CD8^+$ T cells destroy virus-infected cells directly, release IFN-γ and tumour necrosis factor α which recruit macrophages, NK cells and T cells to the site of viral invasion

Innate immune responses to viral invasion are succeeded by adaptive immune responses. Antibodies, which block virus binding and entry into host cells, and cytotoxic T lymphocytes, which can eliminate infection by killing virus-infected cells, are the principal components involved in adaptive antiviral responses (Box 13.6). Antiviral antibodies function mainly as neutralizing antibodies which prevent virus attachment and entry into host cells. These antibodies bind to the viral envelope, capsid antigens and other surface antigenic components. Secreted antibodies of the IgA isotype prevent attachment of viruses to host cells on mucosal surfaces. Antibodies can promote clearance of virus particles from the circulation by clumping viruses and facilitating their removal by phagocytic cells. Lysis of some enveloped viruses by the membrane attack complex can occur when IgG or IgM antibodies bind to viral surface antigens and activate the complement system. In the course of a viral infection, $CD8^+$ T cells undergo rapid proliferation. Expansion of the T-cell population is accompanied by differentiation into effector cytotoxic $CD8^+$ T cells which release cytokines, particularly IFN-γ and tumour necrosis factor and kill infected cells directly through the release of perforin and granzymes.

Although the immune system has the ability to protect the host against a wide range of pathogenic microorganisms, the characteristics of individual infectious agents such as RNA viruses and retroviruses, with their high mutation rates, can limit the effectiveness of immune responses and long-lasting protection against some of these pathogens is difficult to achieve. The immune system itself is not exempt from defects, either developmental or acquired. Defects in one or more component of the immune system can result in increased susceptibility to opportunistic infections. A deficit affecting components of the immune system essential for the development of protective immunity invariably leads to overwhelming infection. A gradual decline in immunological competence of individual animals occurs as they approach the end of their normal lifespan.

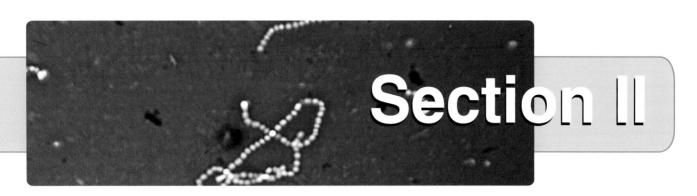

Section II

Pathogenic Bacteria

14 *Staphylococcus* species

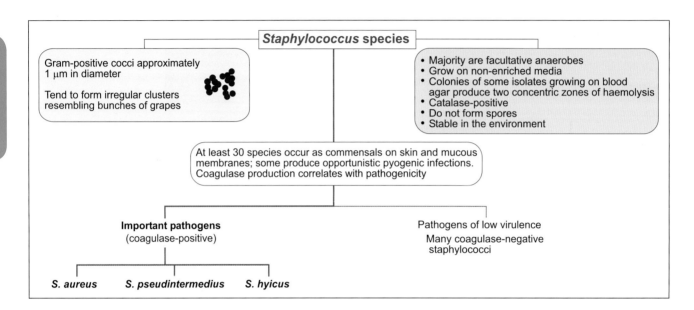

Staphylococci are Gram-positive cocci, approximately 1 μm in diameter, which form irregular clusters resembling bunches of grapes. They occur as commensals on skin and mucous membranes; some act as opportunistic pathogens causing pyogenic infections. They are comparatively stable in the environment. The coagulase-positive *S. aureus* subsp. *aureus* (referred to as *S. aureus*) and *S. pseudintermedius* and the coagulase-variable *S. hyicus* are important pathogens of domestic animals. Coagulase, which converts fibrinogen in plasma to fibrin, is a virulence factor of these organisms which correlates with pathogenicity. Coagulase-negative staphylococci are usually of low virulence. In clinical specimens, *Staphylococcus* species must be differentiated from *Streptococcus* species and from *Micrococcus* species. Staphylococci are generally catalase-positive and streptococci catalase-negative. *Staphylococcus* species are usually identified by the appearance of their colonies, haemolytic pattern and biochemical profiles. Molecular typing methods are increasingly being used to assign *S. aureus* and *S. pseudintermedius* to clonal complexes. Such methods include multi-locus sequence typing, analysis of patterns following enzymatic digestion and pulsed-field gel electophoresis and staphylococcal protein A typing.

Because staphylococci are pyogenic bacteria, they often cause suppurative lesions. Minor trauma or immunosuppression may predispose to the development of infection. Virulence factors of *S. aureus* and their pathogenic effects are indicated in Table 14.1. Although some virulence factors are plasmid-mediated, many are encoded in the staphylococcal core genome. Staphylococcal diseases of importance in domestic animals include mastitis, tick pyaemia, exudative epidermitis, botryomycosis and pyoderma (Table 14.2).

Staphylococcal mastitis, usually caused by specific clones of *S. aureus* adapted to the bovine mammary gland, is a common form of bovine mastitis worldwide. Infection occurs mainly by contact at milking through contaminated milker's hands, teat cup liners and udder cloths. The disease may be subclinical, acute or chronic. Most infections are subclinical. Peracute and gangrenous forms are associated with severe systemic reactions and can be life-threatening. In chronic or subclinical staphylococcal mastitis, episodes of bacterial shedding from affected quarters occur along with elevated somatic cell counts. Bacterial multiplication occurs principally in the collecting ducts and to a limited extent in the alveoli. Influx of phagocytic cells may lead to abscess formation and fibrosis, which further limits effective clearance of the organisms and also interferes with antibiotic penetration during treatment. The majority of *S. aureus* intramammary infections become chronic, low-grade or subclinical, resulting in substantial production losses.

Tick pyaemia, an infection of lambs with *S. aureus*, is confined to hill-grazing regions of Britain and Ireland where there are suitable habitats for the tick *Ixodes ricinus*. Lambs can carry *S. aureus* on their skin and nasal mucosa and infection occurs through minor skin trauma, including tick bites. Tick pyaemia is characterized either by septicaemia and rapid death or by localized abscess formation in many organs. Clinical manifestations include arthritis, posterior paresis and ill-thrift. Microscopic demonstration of the bacteria in pus, followed by isolation and identification of *S. aureus* from lesions, is confirmatory.

Concise Review of Veterinary Microbiology, Second Edition. P.J. Quinn, B.K. Markey, F.C. Leonard, E.S. FitzPatrick and S. Fanning.
© 2016 John Wiley & Sons, Ltd. Published 2016 by John Wiley & Sons, Ltd.
Companion website: www.wiley.com/go/quinn/concise-veterinary-microbiology

Table 14.1 Virulence factors, including toxins, of *Staphylococcus aureus* and their pathogenic effects.

Virulence factor	Pathogenic effects
Coagulase	Conversion of fibrinogen to fibrin. Fibrin deposition may shield staphylococci from phagocytic cells
Lipase, esterases, elastase, staphylokinase, deoxyribonuclease, hyaluronidase, phospholipase	These factors facilitate dissemination and enhance toxicity of the organisms
Protein A	Surface component which binds the Fc portion of IgG and inhibits opsonization
Leukocidin	Cytolytic destruction of phagocytes of some animal species
Alpha-toxin (α-haemolysin)	The major toxin in gangrenous mastitis. It causes spasm of smooth muscle and is necrotizing and potentially lethal
Beta-toxin (β-haemolysin)	A sphingomyelinase which damages cell membranes
Toxic shock syndrome toxin (TSST)-1	Superantigen activity
Exfoliative toxins	Responsible for desquamation in staphylococcal 'scalded skin syndrome' in humans
Enterotoxins	Heat-stable toxins associated with staphylococcal food poisoning in humans

Table 14.2 Coagulase-positive staphylococci and their clinical importance.

Species	Hosts	Clinical conditions
Staphylococcus aureus	Cattle	Mastitis, udder impetigo
	Sheep	Mastitis Tick pyaemia (lambs) Benign folliculitis (lambs) Dermatitis
	Goats	Mastitis Dermatitis
	Pigs	Botryomycosis of mammary glands Impetigo on mammary glands
	Horses	Scirrhous cord (botryomycosis of the spermatic cord), mastitis
	Dogs, cats	Suppurative conditions similar to those caused by *S. pseudintermedius*
	Poultry	Arthritis and septicaemia in turkeys Bumblefoot Omphalitis in chicks
S. pseudintermedius	Dogs	Pyoderma, endometritis, cystitis, otitis externa, and other suppurative conditions
	Cats	Various pyogenic conditions
S. schleiferi subsp. *coagulans*	Dogs	Otitis externa
S. hyicus	Pigs	Exudative epidermitis (greasy pig disease) Arthritis

Treatment is of limited value in severely affected lambs. Efforts should be directed at control within the flock and tick-control measures such as dipping should be introduced.

Exudative epidermitis, caused by *S. hyicus*, occurs worldwide in piglets and weaned pigs up to three months of age. This highly contagious disease is characterized by widespread excessive sebaceous secretion, exfoliation and exudation on the skin surface. Affected pigs, which are anorexic, depressed and febrile, have an extensive non-pruritic dermatitis with a greasy exudate. Morbidity rates range from 20 to 100% and mortality rates can reach 90% in severely affected litters. Predisposing stress factors include agalactia in the sow, intercurrent infections and weaning. *Staphylococcus hyicus* can be isolated from the vaginal mucosa and skin of healthy sows and transmission to piglets occurs at or shortly after birth. The organism probably

causes infection following entry through minor abrasions such as bite wounds. Isolation and identification of *S. hyicus* from dermal lesions is confirmatory.

Botryomycosis, a chronic suppurative granulomatous condition often caused by *S. aureus*, can occur in horses after castration, due to infection of the stump of the spermatic cord. The lesion is composed of a mass of fibrous tissue containing foci of pus and sinus tracts.

Staphylococcus pseudintermedius is commonly isolated from pyoderma, otitis externa and other suppurative conditions including mastitis, endometritis, cystitis, osteomyelitis and wound infections in dogs and cats. Occasionally, similar suppurative conditions are caused by *S. aureus*.

Antimicrobial resistance is a major problem with some staphylococcal isolates, particularly *S. aureus* and *S. pseudintermedius*. Both of these organisms can acquire the *mecA* gene encoding penicillin-binding protein 2a, which renders them methicillin-resistant. Frequently, methicillin-resistant strains are resistant to many other classes of antimicrobial agent, in addition to all β-lactam drugs. Methicillin-resistant *S. aureus* (MRSA) isolated from dogs are often similar to MRSA isolated from hospitalized humans. Isolates of MRSA from horses appear to be species adapted to horses and those working with horses, although it is likely these strains originated in humans. Livestock-associated MRSA isolates are found principally in pigs but also in poultry, veal calves and dairy cows.

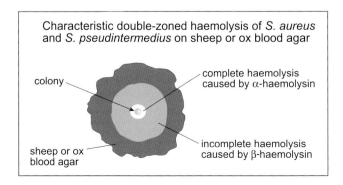

Characteristic double-zoned haemolysis of *S. aureus* and *S. pseudintermedius* on sheep or ox blood agar

colony

complete haemolysis caused by α-haemolysin

sheep or ox blood agar

incomplete haemolysis caused by β-haemolysin

15 Streptococci

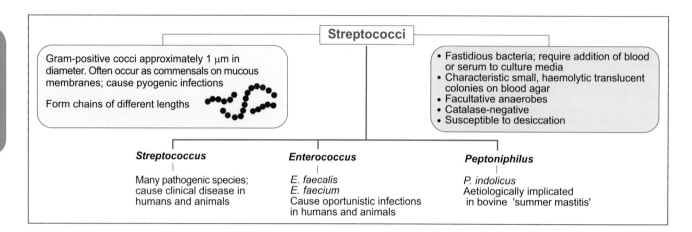

Streptococci are a group of bacteria which can cause pyogenic infections in many animal species. These Gram-positive cocci, which form chains of different lengths, are fastidious and require the addition of blood or serum to culture media for growth *in vitro*. *Streptococcus* species are non-motile, facultative anaerobes which are catalase-negative. *Enterococcus* species are enteric streptococci found in the intestine of humans and animals.

Three laboratory procedures are used for differentiating streptococci: type of haemolysis, Lancefield grouping and biochemical testing. On sheep or ox blood agar, β-haemolysis refers to complete haemolysis indicated by clear zones around colonies; α-haemolysis is partial haemolysis indicated by greenish or hazy zones around colonies. Lancefield grouping is a serological method of classification based on group-specific C-substance (polysaccharide) in the cell wall; latex agglutination test kits for Lancefield grouping are commercially available. Pyogenic streptococci are associated with abscess formation, other suppurative conditions and septicaemia. Streptococci producing β-haemolysis are usually more pathogenic than those producing α-haemolysis. Virulence factors include enzymes and exotoxins such as streptolysins (haemolysins), hyaluronidase, DNase, streptokinase and proteases. The polysaccharide capsule of some strains of *S. equi* is antiphagocytic and M proteins which project from the surface of the organism interfere with the activation of complement. Identification criteria for streptococcal isolates include the presence of small translucent colonies, some of which may be mucoid. Chains of Gram-positive cocci which are catalase-negative and the type of haemolysis produced on blood agar may be indicative of streptococcal organisms. Definitive identification requires a biochemical test profile of the isolate and Lancefield typing. A number of molecular methods have been used for typing of streptococci, including multi-locus sequence typing and analysis of patterns following enzymatic digestion and pulsed-field gel electophoresis. Isolates of *S. equi*. subsp. *equi* may be typed by sequencing the variable region of the *SeM* gene which encodes the M protein.

Streptococci are often commensals on mucous membranes and, consequently, many streptococcal infections are opportunistic. Infections may be primary, as in strangles, or secondary as in streptococcal pneumonia following viral infection. Lymph nodes, genital tract or mammary glands may become infected. Strangles, porcine streptococcal meningitis and bovine streptococcal mastitis are important specific infections. Vaccines for the control of streptococcal infections are usually ineffective. Pathogenic streptococci and their clinical consequences are listed in Table 15.1.

Strangles is a highly contagious disease of horses caused by *S. equi* subsp. *equi*. It is a febrile disease involving the upper respiratory tract with abscessation of regional lymph nodes. Outbreaks of disease most commonly occur in young horses. Assembling horses at sales, shows and racecourses increases the risk of acquiring infection. As *S. equi* subsp. *equi* is not a commensal organism, subclinically or clinically affected animals constitute the main source of infection. Transmission is via purulent exudates from the upper respiratory tract or from discharging abscesses. Infected animals may shed *S. equi* for at least four weeks after development of clinical signs. A chronic carrier state develops in some animals in which the organism is present in the guttural pouch for many months. The incubation period is up to six days and the course of uncomplicated disease is about 10 days. There is a high fever, depression and anorexia followed by oculonasal discharge that becomes purulent. Characteristically, the submandibular nodes are affected and they may eventually rupture, discharging purulent, highly infectious material. Guttural pouch empyema is a common finding. The morbidity may be up to 100% and mortality is usually less than 5%. Following outbreaks of the disease, buildings and

Concise Review of Veterinary Microbiology, Second Edition. P.J. Quinn, B.K. Markey, F.C. Leonard, E.S. FitzPatrick and S. Fanning.
© 2016 John Wiley & Sons, Ltd. Published 2016 by John Wiley & Sons, Ltd.
Companion website: www.wiley.com/go/quinn/concise-veterinary-microbiology

Table 15.1 Pathogenic streptococci of animals, their habitats, hosts and consequences of infection.

Species	Lancefield group	Haemolysis on blood agar	Hosts	Consequences of infection	Usual habitat
S. agalactiae	B	β (α, γ)	Cattle, sheep, goats	Chronic mastitis	Milk ducts
			Humans, dogs	Neonatal septicaemia	Vagina
S. dysgalactiae	C	α (β, γ)	Cattle	Acute mastitis	Buccal cavity, vagina, environment
			Lambs	Polyarthritis	
S. equi (*S. equi* subsp. *equi*)	C	β	Horses	Strangles, suppurative conditions, purpura haemorrhagica	Upper respiratory tract, guttural pouch
S. zooepidemicus (*S. equi* subsp. *zooepidemicus*)	C	β	Horses	Mastitis, pneumonia, navel infections	Mucous membranes
			Cattle, lambs, pigs, poultry	Suppurative conditions, septicaemia	Skin, mucous membranes
S. suis	D	α (β)	Pigs	Septicaemia, meningitis, arthritis, bronchopneumonia	Tonsils, nasal cavity
			Humans	Septicaemia, meningitis	
S. canis	G	β	Carnivores	Neonatal septicaemia, suppurative conditions, toxic shock syndrome	Vagina, anal mucosa
S. uberis	Not assigned	α (γ)	Cattle	Mastitis	Skin, vagina, tonsils

equipment should be cleaned and disinfected. Live attenuated vaccines, which reduce the severity of clinical signs but do not prevent infection, are available.

Streptococcus suis is recognized worldwide as a cause of significant losses in the pig industry. It is associated with meningitis, arthritis, septicaemia and bronchopneumonia in pigs of all ages and with sporadic cases of endocarditis, neonatal deaths and abortion. At least 35 serotypes of varying virulence have been recognized. About 70% of *S. suis* isolates belong to serotypes 1–9. Of these, serotype 2 is the most prevalent serotype, with carrier rates up to 90%. This serotype is associated with meningitis in both pigs and humans. Asymptomatic pigs harbour *S. suis* in tonsillar tissue. Disease outbreaks are most common in intensively reared pigs when they are subjected to overcrowding, poor ventilation and other stress factors. Sows carrying the organisms can infect their litters. Meningitis, which is often fatal, is characterized by fever, tremors, incoordination, opisthotonos and convulsions. As these bacteria tend to become endemic in a herd, eradication is not feasible. Improved husbandry methods may decrease the prevalence of clinical disease.

Streptococcus agalactiae, *S. dysgalactiae* and *S. uberis* are the principal pathogens involved in streptococcal mastitis. *Streptococcus agalactiae* is an obligate pathogen of the mammary gland in which it multiplies and invades the lactiferous ducts. An influx of neutrophils into the mammary gland follows and the inflammatory reaction results in blockage of teat ducts and atrophy of secretory tissue. These inflammatory cycles occur periodically with progressive loss of secretory tissue. *Streptococcus dysgalactiae*, which is found in the buccal cavity and genitalia and on the skin of the mammary gland, causes acute mastitis. *Streptococcus uberis*, a normal inhabitant of the skin, tonsils and vaginal mucosa, is an important cause of clinical mastitis, usually in housed cows. Contamination of teat ends due to poor environmental hygiene is a major predisposing factor in the development of mastitis caused by *S. dysgalactiae* and *S. uberis*. Differentiation of the mastitis-producing streptococci is based on the type of haemolysis produced on blood agar, aesculin hydrolysis in Edwards medium, identification of the Lancefield group to which they belong and biochemical testing. Both *S. dysgalactiae* and *S. uberis* produce α-haemolysis while *S. agalactiae* produces β-haemolysis. Aesculin is hydrolysed by *S. uberis*.

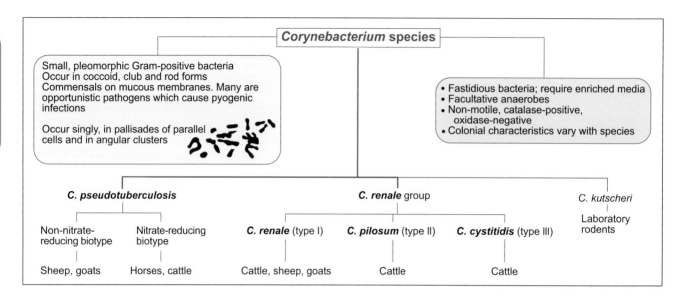

Corynebacterium species

Corynebacterium species are small, pleomorphic, Gram-positive bacteria which occur in coccoid, club and rod forms. In stained smears they may occur in angular clusters resembling Chinese letters. Most corynebacteria are catalase-positive, oxidase-negative, non-spore-forming facultative anaerobes which require enriched media for growth. Colonies are small with variable haemolysis, depending on species. Many *Corynebacterium* species are commensals on mucous membranes. Most pathogenic corynebacteria are relatively host-specific and produce identifiable clinical syndromes. The host species and the nature of the disease may suggest the causal agent. Identification critieria include bacterial cell morphology, colonial appearance and biochemical reactions. Molecular detection and typing methods have been developed for some corynebacterial species, particularly for *C. pseudotuberculosis*. Two biotypes of *C. pseudotuberculosis* are recognized. The ovine/caprine strains lack nitrate-reducing capacity, while the equine/bovine strains usually reduce nitrate. The biotypes differ in their geographical distribution.

Table 16.1 The pathogenic corynebacteria, their hosts, usual habitats and the disease conditions which they produce.

Pathogen	Host	Disease condition	Usual habitat
Corynebacterium bovis	Cattle	Subclinical mastitis	Teat cistern
C. kutscheri	Laboratory rodents	Superficial abscesses, caseopurulent foci in liver, lungs and lymph nodes	Mucous membranes, environment
C. pseudotuberculosis			
Non-nitrate-reducing biotype	Sheep, goats	Caseous lymphadenitis	Skin, mucous membranes, environment
Nitrate-reducing biotype	Horses, cattle	Ulcerative lymphangitis, abscesses	Environment
C. renale group			
C. renale (type I)	Cattle	Cystitis, pyelonephritis	Lower urogenital tracts of cows and bulls
	Sheep and goats	Ulcerative (enzootic) balanoposthitis	Prepuce
C. pilosum (type II)	Cattle	Cystitis, pyelonephritis	Bovine urogenital tract
C. cystitidis (type III)	Cattle	Severe cystitis, rarely pyelonephritis	Bovine urogenital tract
C. ulcerans	Cattle	Mastitis	Human pharyngeal mucosa
	Cats	Rare cases of upper respiratory tract infections	

Concise Review of Veterinary Microbiology, Second Edition. P.J. Quinn, B.K. Markey, F.C. Leonard, E.S. FitzPatrick and S. Fanning.
© 2016 John Wiley & Sons, Ltd. Published 2016 by John Wiley & Sons, Ltd.
Companion website: www.wiley.com/go/quinn/concise-veterinary-microbiology

SECTION II

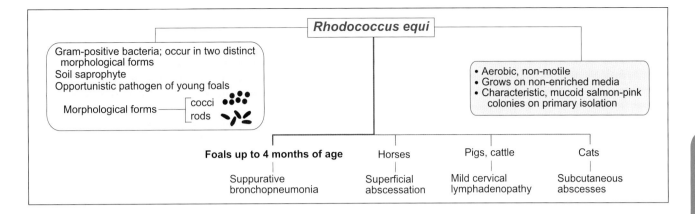

Rhodococcus equi

Gram-positive bacteria; occur in two distinct
  morphological forms
Soil saprophyte
Opportunistic pathogen of young foals

Morphological forms ─── cocci
                         rods

• Aerobic, non-motile
• Grows on non-enriched media
• Characteristic, mucoid salmon-pink
  colonies on primary isolation

Foals up to 4 months of age | Horses | Pigs, cattle | Cats

Suppurative bronchopneumonia | Superficial abscessation | Mild cervical lymphadenopathy | Subcutaneous abscesses

Many corynebacteria are opportunistic pathogens. With the exception of *C. bovis*, these organisms are pyogenic and cause a variety of suppurative conditions in domestic animals. Urease is produced by all pathogenic corynebacteria except *C. bovis* and fimbriae are important virulence attributes of the uropathogenic corynebacteria. The main diseases caused by infections with *Corynebacterium* species are summarized in Table 16.1.

Caseous lymphadenitis is a chronic suppurative condition of sheep and goats caused by *C. pseudotuberculosis*; cattle are rarely affected. Sheep become infected through contamination of shearing wounds, by arthropod bites or from contaminated dips or shearing equipment. Infection results in abscessation and enlargement of superficial or internal lymph nodes. The incubation period is about three months. The organism is a facultative intracellular pathogen, which can survive and replicate in phagocytes. Its major virulence factors include its cell wall lipid and an exotoxin, phospholipase D. The disease, which is prevalent in Australia, New Zealand, the Middle East, Asia, Africa and parts of North and South America, is being reported with greater frequency in Britain and other European countries. Ill-thrift may be evident in affected animals and the disease invariably results in condemnation of carcasses and devaluation of hides. Infection is spread by pus from ruptured abscesses and from nasal and oral secretions. The organism can survive in the environment for several months. Affected lymph nodes are enlarged and exhibit characteristic encapsulated abscesses containing greenish pus. They often have an 'onion ring' appearance on their cut surfaces. The visceral form of the disease may not be detectable antemortem. Goats usually develop the superficial form of the disease. The disease may be suspected on clinical grounds or at postmortem examination. Smears from lesions may reveal Gram-positive coryneform bacteria. Isolation and identification of *C. pseudotuberculosis* from abscess material is confirmatory. Because of the chronic nature of lesions and the ability of the organisms to survive intracellularly, therapy is usually ineffective. Appropriate control measures for individual countries are determined by the prevalence of the disease. Owing to the difficulties of detecting infection in the live animal, a number of different ELISA methods have been developed. Serologically positive animals may be culled. Vaccines are available in some countries.

The nitrate-reducing biotype of *C. pseudotuberculosis* causes sporadic cases of ulcerative lymphangitis in horses and cattle.

This disease occurs in Africa, the Americas, the Middle East and India. Infection occurs through skin wounds, arthropod bites or by contact with contaminated harness. The condition presents as either lymphangitis of the lower limbs or abscessation in the pectoral region. Organisms belonging to the *C. renale* group can be isolated from the vulva, vagina and prepuce of apparently normal cattle. The stress of parturition and the shortness of the urethra in the cow predispose to infection of the urinary tract. Ascending infection from the bladder through the ureters can result in pyelonephritis. Clinical signs of pyelonephritis include fever, anorexia, restlessness due to pain and decreased milk production. Dysuria, an arched back and blood-tinged urine are invariably present. Culture of *C. renale* from urinary deposits, in association with the presence of characteristic clinical signs, is confirmatory.

Rhodococcus equi

Rhodococcus equi is a Gram-positive, aerobic soil saprophyte which occurs worldwide. It is an opportunisitic pathogen of foals under six months of age. *Rhodococcus equi* grows on non-enriched media and produces characteristic mucoid salmon-pink colonies. Some strains of *R. equi* appear as cocci, and others as rods up to 5 μm in length.

Suppurative bronchopneumonia of foals is the major disease caused by this pyogenic organism. Infection is generally acquired by inhalation of dust contaminated with *R. equi*, either from dusty pastures in warmer climates or indoors from dust in poorly ventilated, dusty stables in temperate regions. The organism is often present in large numbers in the faeces of healthy foals and also in the faeces of older horses. A build-up of *R. equi* can occur on pastures heavily stocked with horses. Only virulent *R. equi*, which possess a large plasmid containing the *vapA* gene, are associated with disease. Virulent organisms can survive and multiply within macrophages. Acute disease often occurs in one-month-old foals, with sudden onset of fever, anorexia and signs of bronchopneumonia. In older foals, the disease tends to be insidious and lesions can be well advanced before animals exhibit coughing, dyspnoea, weight loss and characteristic loud, moist rales on auscultation of the lungs. A history of the disease on the farm, the age of the affected foal and clinical signs may suggest infection with *R. equi*. Culture or PCR-based detection of *R. equi* from tracheal aspirates and pus from lesions, in association with clinical signs, is confirmatory.

17 *Actinobacteria*

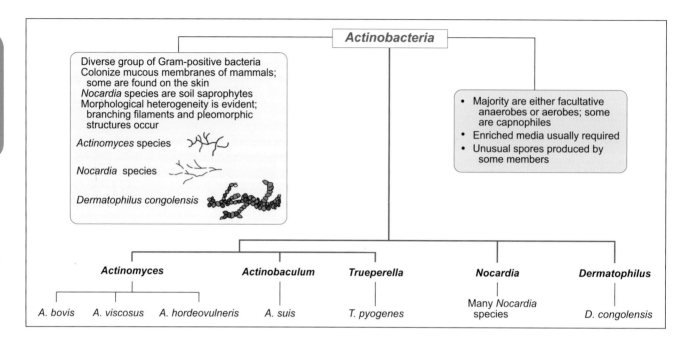

The actinobacteria are a phylogenetically diverse group of Gram-positive bacteria which tend to grow slowly and produce branching filaments. The bacteria in this group which cause disease in domestic animals belong to the genera *Actinomyces*, *Trueperella*, *Actinobaculum*, *Nocardia* and *Dermatophilus*. The genera are classified within three different bacterial families. Morphological and cultural characteristics of actinobacteria are presented in Boxes 17.1 and 17.2. Comparative features of actinobacteria of veterinary importance are presented in Table 17.1.

Box 17.1 Morphology of actinobacteria

- Diverse group of bacteria including Gram-positive, partially acid-fast and acid-fast organisms
- Morphologically heterogeneous:
  - Branching filaments
  - Pleomorphic forms
  - Typical rod-shaped bacteria

Box 17.2 Cultural characteristics of actinobacteria

- Atmospheric requirements vary widely; some are strict aerobes, others are facultative anaerobes or capnophiles
- Enriched media or specialized media incorporating specific supplements required for particular species
- Atypical spores produced by some members

Actinomyces, *Trueperella* and *Actinobaculum* species

Species in these genera are non-motile, non-spore-forming, Gram-positive bacteria which require enriched media for growth. *Trueperella pyogenes* was formerly called *Arcanobacterium pyogenes* and *Actinobaculum suis* was formerly known by other names. The species of veterinary importance in the group are *Trueperella pyogenes*, *Actinobaculum suis*, *Actinomyces bovis*, *Actinomyces viscosus* and *Actinomyces hordeovulneris*. Apart from *A. hordeovulneris*, pathogenic members of these genera colonize mucous membranes of mammals. Differentiating features of the genera are presented in Table 17.2. Disease conditions produced by *Actinomyces*, *Trueperella* and *Actinobaculum* species in domestic animals are summarized in Table 17.3.

Trueperella pyogenes is a common cause of suppurative lesions in many domestic species worldwide, especially cattle, pigs and sheep. The principal virulence factor produced by *T. pyogenes* is pyolysin which is cytolytic for several cell types including neutrophils and macrophages. This organism also produces proteases and a number of adhesins. Lymphadenitis, osteomyelitis, peritonitis and neural abscessation are commonly associated with tissue invasion by this pathogen. This organism is also implicated in pyometra, metritis and acute mastitis in dairy cows. In the acute bovine mastitis referred to as 'summer mastitis' in Britain and Ireland, the anaerobic bacterium *Peptoniphilus indolicus* is usually associated

---

Concise Review of Veterinary Microbiology, Second Edition. P.J. Quinn, B.K. Markey, F.C. Leonard, E.S. FitzPatrick and S. Fanning.
© 2016 John Wiley & Sons, Ltd. Published 2016 by John Wiley & Sons, Ltd.
Companion website: www.wiley.com/go/quinn/concise-veterinary-microbiology

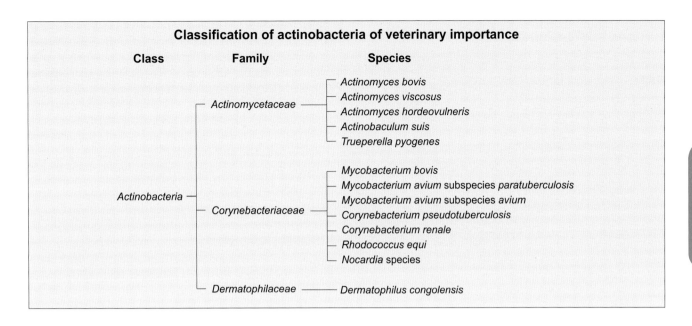

Classification of actinobacteria of veterinary importance

Class	Family	Species
Actinobacteria	Actinomycetaceae	*Actinomyces bovis* *Actinomyces viscosus* *Actinomyces hordeovulneris* *Actinobaculum suis* *Trueperella pyogenes*
	Corynebacteriaceae	*Mycobacterium bovis* *Mycobacterium avium* subspecies *paratuberculosis* *Mycobacterium avium* subspecies *avium* *Corynebacterium pseudotuberculosis* *Corynebacterium renale* *Rhodococcus equi* *Nocardia* species
	Dermatophilaceae	*Dermatophilus congolensis*

Table 17.1 Comparative features of actinobacteria of veterinary importance.

Feature	*Actinomyces* species	*Trueperella pyogenes*	*Actinobaculum suis*	*Nocardia* species	*Dermatophilus congolensis*
Atmospheric growth requirements	Anaerobic or facultatively anaerobic and capnophilic	Facultatively anaerobic and capnophilic	Anaerobic	Aerobic	Aerobic and capnophilic
Aerial filament production	–	–	–	+	–
Modified Ziehl–Neelsen staining	–	–	–	+	–
Growth on Sabouraud dextrose agar	–	–	–	+	–
Usual habitat	Nasopharyngeal and oral mucosae	Nasopharyngeal mucosa of cattle, sheep and pigs	Prepuce and preputial diverticulum of boars	Soil	Skin of carrier animals, scabs from lesions
Site of lesions	Many tissues including bone	Soft tissues	Urinary tract of sows	Thoracic cavity, skin and other tissues	Skin

Table 17.2 Differentiation of *Actinomyces*, *Trueperella* and *Actinobaculum* species of veterinary importance.

Characteristic	*Actinomyces bovis*	*Actinomyces viscosus*	*Actinomyces hordeovulneris*	*Trueperella pyogenes*	*Actinobaculum suis*
Morphology	Filamentous, branching, some short forms	Filamentous, branching, short forms	Filamentous, branching, short forms	Coryneform	Coryneform
Atmospheric requirements	Anaerobic + CO_2	10% CO_2	10% CO_2	Aerobic	Anaerobic
Haemolysis on sheep blood agar	±	–	±	+	±
Catalase production	–	+	+	–	–
Pitting of Loeffler's serum slope	–	–	–	+	–
Granules in pus	'Sulphur granules'	White granules	No granules	No granules	No granules

Species	Hosts	Disease conditions
Trueperella pyogenes	Cattle, sheep, pigs	Abscessation, mastitis, suppurative pneumonia, endometritis, pyometra, arthritis, umbilical infections
Actinomyces hordeovulneris	Dogs	Cutaneous and visceral abscessation, pleuritis, peritonitis, arthritis
Actinomyces bovis	Cattle	Bovine actinomycosis ('lumpy jaw')
Actinomyces viscosus	Dogs	Canine actinomycosis: • cutaneous pyogranulomas • pyothorax and proliferative pyogranulomatous pleural lesions • disseminated lesions (rare)
	Horses	Cutaneous pustules
	Cattle	Abortion
Actinomyces species (unclassified)	Pigs	Pyogranulomatous mastitis
	Horses	Poll evil and fistulous withers
Actinobaculum suis	Pigs	Cystitis, pyelonephritis

with *T. pyogenes*. In foot lesions in ruminants and in other mixed infections, *T. pyogenes* also occurs in association with anaerobes. Diagnosis is based on the typical pleomorphic cell morphology in Gram-stained smears from specimens, colonial characteristics and the ability of *T. pyogenes* to pit a Loeffler's serum slope.

Invasion of the mandible and, less commonly, the maxilla of cattle by *A. bovis* causes a chronic rarefying osteomyelitis referred to as 'lumpy jaw'. The organsim is presumed to invade the tissues following trauma to the mucosa from rough feed or through dental alveoli during tooth eruption. A painless swelling of the affected bone enlarges over a period of several weeks. The swelling becomes painful and fistulous tracts, discharging exudate containing 'sulphur granules' with characteristic club colonies, develop. Spread to contiguous soft tissues may occur, but there is minimal involvement of regional lymph nodes. Surgery is the treatment of choice when lesions are small and circumscribed. In advanced cases, surgical treatment may be ineffective.

Porcine cystitis and pyelonephritis caused by *Actinobaculum suis* affects the urinary tract of pregnant sows. The pathogen, which is transmitted by carrier boars at coitus, causes a potentially fatal infection. Anorexia, arching of the back, dysuria and haematuria are prominent signs. If both kidneys are extensively damaged, death may result.

Actinomyces viscosus affects dogs and usually presents in one of two forms. It may cause subcutaneous pyogranulomatous lesions or extensive fibrovascular proliferation on the peritoneal or pleural surfaces with sanguinopurulent exudate in the affected cavity. The thoracic lesions closely resemble those of canine nocardiosis.

Nocardia species

Members of *Nocardia* species are Gram-positive, aerobic, saprophytic actinobacteria. In smears of exudate from infected tissue, they appear as long, slender, branching filaments with a tendency to fragment into rods and cocci. When cultured, these organisms produce aerial filaments which may form spores. Components of the cell wall render *Nocardia* species partially acid-fast (modified Ziehl–Neelsen positive). *Nocardia asteroides* is the pathogen of greatest significance in this genus, although a number of other pathogenic species have been identified following reclassification of nocardial organisms using molecular methods.

Table 17.4 Disease conditions produced by *Nocardia* species in domestic animals.

Species	Hosts	Disease conditions
Nocardia species	Dogs	Canine nocardiosis: • cutaneous pyogranulomas • pyogranulomatous pleural lesions and pyothorax • disseminated lesions
	Cattle	Chronic mastitis, abortion
	Pigs	Abortion
	Sheep, goats, horses	Wound infections, mastitis, pneumonia, other pyogranulomatous conditions
Nocardia farcinica	Cattle	Bovine farcy

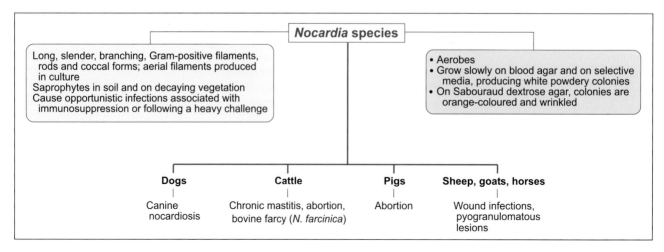

Nocardia species are saprophytes found in soil and decaying vegetation. Infection, which is opportunistic, is usually associated with immunosuppression or, alternatively, may follow a heavy challenge. The usual mode of infection is by inhalation but it may also occur through skin wounds or via the teat canal. Virulent strains of *N. asteroides* survive intracellularly. Cell-mediated immunity is essential for protection against infection by this facultative intracellular bacterium.

Nocardial infections in domestic animals are presented in Table 17.4. The most commonly encountered conditions are cutaneous and systemic infections in dogs and mastitis in dairy cattle. Outbreaks of nocardial mastitis are often associated with contaminated intramammary tubes. Canine nocardiosis, due to *N. asteroides*, is acquired by inhalation, through skin wounds or by ingestion. Thoracic, cutaneous and disseminated forms of the disease are recognized. The thoracic form is characterized by fever, anorexia and respiratory distress. Sanguinopurulent fluid accumulates in the thoracic cavity. The cutaneous form presents either as an indolent ulcer or as a granulomatous swelling with discharging fistulous tracts. *Nocardia asteroides* strains show marked variation in their susceptibility to antibiotics. A presumptive diagnosis of infection with *N. asteroides* is based on clinical findings and laboratory procedures. Smears of exudate should be stained by the Gram and modified Ziehl–Neelsen methods. *Nocardia asteroides* is modified Ziehl–Neelsen positive. When cultured aerobically on blood agar, colonies are usually visible after five days. They are white, powdery and firmly adherent to the agar.

Nocardia farcinica is implicated in bovine farcy and occurs only in tropical climates. Because a number of organisms, including *N. farcinica*, have been isolated from the lesions, the aetiology of the disease is uncertain. Chronic infection of superficial lymphatic vessels and lymph nodes occurs. Early lesions consist of small cutaneous nodules, often on the medial aspects of the legs and on the neck. These nodules enlarge slowly and coalesce, forming large swellings which rarely ulcerate. Lymphatic vessels become thickened and cord-like. Internal organs may be affected occasionally with lesions resembling tuberculosis.

Dermatophilus congolensis

This member of the actinobacteria is a Gram-positive, filamentous, branching organism. It is unusual because it produces motile zoospores about 1.5 μm in diameter. Mature zoospores produce germ tubes which develop into filaments. Within these filaments, transverse and longitudinal divisions form segments which ultimately develop into zoospores. Mature filaments may be more than 5 μm in width and contain columns of zoospores which impart a 'tram-track' appearance to the filaments. Skin infections caused by *D. congolensis* occur worldwide but are most prevalent in tropical and subtropical regions. The organism seems to persist in foci in the skin of many clinically normal animals, particularly in endemic areas. Although zoospore survival in the environment is usually limited, there may be extended survival in dry scabs.

Trauma and persistent wetting predispose to skin invasion. When activated, zoospores produce germ tubes and these develop into filaments, which invade the epidermis. Pathogenic factors include an alkaline ceramidase and a number of proteases which facilitate invasion of the epidermis. Invasion leads to an acute inflammatory response, characterized by large numbers of neutrophils which ultimately form microabscesses in the epidermis. Factors which depress specific immune responses, including intercurrent diseases and pregnancy, may increase host susceptibility to dermatophilosis. Infections with *D. congolensis* are usually confined to the epidermis. When skin of the lower limbs of sheep is involved, the condition is termed 'strawberry footrot'.

Although the disease affects animals of all ages, it is more prevalent and often more severe in young animals. Zoospores are most often transmitted by direct contact with infected animals. A number of blood-sucking insects may be important in disease transmission in the tropics. Economic loss derives from damage to hides and fleece.

Lesion distribution usually correlates with those areas of skin predisposed to infection. Heavy prolonged rainfall in association with warm environmental temperatures can result in lesions predominantly affecting the dorsum of farm animals. Trauma to the face and limbs of animals grazing in thorny scrub can predispose to lesions in these sites. Early lesions present as papules and are often detectable only by palpation. As lesions progress, serous exudate causes matting of hairs, resulting in a tufted appearance. Lesions may coalesce, forming irregular elevated crusty scabs. Tufts of hair can be readily plucked from the lesions along with adherent scab material and underlying exudate. Scab formation tends to be more pronounced in cattle and sheep than in horses. In severe infections, lesions may be extensive and deaths may occur occasionally in calves and lambs. Diagnosis is based on clinical appearance of lesions and demonstration of *D. congolensis* in scabs. Isolation of the organisms is confirmatory.

The outcome of treatment is influenced by the severity and extent of lesions. Parenterally administered antibiotics such as long-acting oxytetracycline are usually effective. Control measures are based on minimizing the effects of predisposing factors and early treatment of clinical cases. Where feasible, grazing areas should be cleared of thorny scrub and tick infestation should be reduced by dipping or spraying with acaricides. Control of intercurrent disease reduces the severity of dermatophilosis.

18 Listeria species

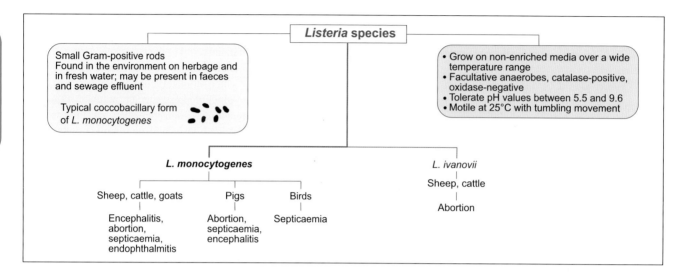

Listeria species

Small Gram-positive rods
Found in the environment on herbage and in fresh water; may be present in faeces and sewage effluent

Typical coccobacillary form of *L. monocytogenes*

- Grow on non-enriched media over a wide temperature range
- Facultative anaerobes, catalase-positive, oxidase-negative
- Tolerate pH values between 5.5 and 9.6
- Motile at 25°C with tumbling movement

L. monocytogenes

Sheep, cattle, goats | Pigs | Birds

Encephalitis, abortion, septicaemia, endophthalmitis | Abortion, septicaemia, encephalitis | Septicaemia

L. ivanovii

Sheep, cattle

Abortion

Most *Listeria* species are small, Gram-positive, coccobacillary rods up to 2 μm in length. The genus is composed of 10 species, two of which are pathogenic. *Listeria monocytogenes*, the more important of these two pathogens, has been implicated worldwide in diseases of many animal species and humans. *Listeria ivanovii* occasionally causes abortions in cattle and sheep. The organism can grow over a wide temperature range, from 4 to 45°C, and can tolerate pH values between 5.5 and 9.5 and up to 10% sodium chloride. *Listeria* species can replicate in the environment and are widely distributed in herbage, faeces of healthy animals, sewage effluent and bodies of fresh water. Based on cell wall and flagellar antigens, 16 serotypes are recognized with serotypes 4b and 1/2 responsible for most cases of disease in animals and humans.

Infection with *L. monocytogenes* usually follows ingestion of contaminated feed and may result in septicaemia, encephalitis or abortion. Organisms probably penetrate the M cells in Peyer's patches in the intestine. Spread occurs via lymph and blood to various tissues. In pregnant animals, infection results in transplacental transmission. There is evidence that the organism can invade through breaks in the oral or nasal mucosa. From this site, migration in cranial nerves is thought to be the main route of infection in neural listeriosis. Lesions in the brainstem are composed of microabscesses and perivascular lymphatic cuffs. *Listeria monocytogenes* has the ability to invade both phagocytic and non-phagocytic cells with the aid of specific proteins known as internalins. Listeriolysin O and phospholipases mediate escape from the phagosome and cell-to-cell spread following intracellular replication of the organism.

Listeriosis in ruminants may present as encephalitis, abortion, septicaemia or endophthalmitis. Usually only one form of disease occurs in a group of affected animals. Outbreaks of lis-

teriosis tend to be seasonal in European countries and to affect silage-fed animals in late pregnancy. *Listeria monocytogenes* can replicate in poor-quality silage with pH values above 5.5. The incubation period for neural listeriosis ranges from 14 to 40 days. Dullness, circling and tilting of the head are common clinical signs. Unilateral facial paralysis results in drooling of saliva and drooping of the eyelid and ear. Abortion with evidence of systemic illness may occur up to 12 days after infection. Septicaemic listeriosis, with a short incubation period, is most commonly encountered in lambs. *Listeria monocytogenes* is an important food-borne pathogen of pregnant women and immunocompromised humans.

Characteristic neurological signs or abortion in association with silage feeding may suggest listeriosis. Appropriate specimens for laboratory examination include cerebrospinal fluid and tissue from the medulla and pons of animals with neurological signs and cotyledons, foetal abomasal contents and uterine discharges from cases of abortion. Suitable samples from septicaemic cases include fresh liver, spleen or blood. *Listeria* species cultured on blood agar have small, haemolytic, translucent colonies which can be definitively identified using biochemical tests. However, many PCR-based methods have been described for detection of *Listeria* species in clinical specimens and foods. In addition to serotyping, molecular techniques such as multi-locus sequence typing, pulsed-field gel electrophoresis-based methods and amplified fragment length polymorphism are used for characterization of isolates.

Response to antibiotic therapy may be poor in neural listeriosis and prolonged treatment may be required. In the early stages of septicaemic listeriosis, response to therapy is usually satisfactory. Poor-quality silage should not be fed to pregnant ruminants.

Concise Review of Veterinary Microbiology, Second Edition. P.J. Quinn, B.K. Markey, F.C. Leonard, E.S. FitzPatrick and S. Fanning.
© 2016 John Wiley & Sons, Ltd. Published 2016 by John Wiley & Sons, Ltd.
Companion website: www.wiley.com/go/quinn/concise-veterinary-microbiology

19 *Erysipelothrix rhusiopathiae*

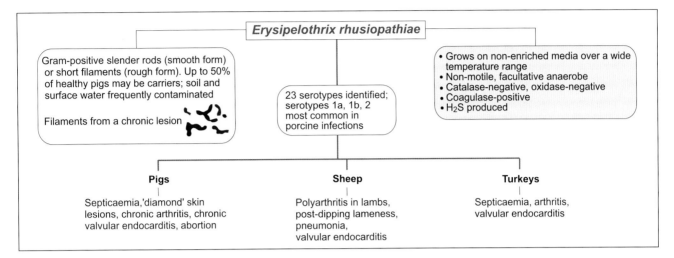

Erysipelothrix rhusiopathiae

Gram-positive slender rods (smooth form) or short filaments (rough form). Up to 50% of healthy pigs may be carriers; soil and surface water frequently contaminated

Filaments from a chronic lesion

23 serotypes identified; serotypes 1a, 1b, 2 most common in porcine infections

- Grows on non-enriched media over a wide temperature range
- Non-motile, facultative anaerobe
- Catalase-negative, oxidase-negative
- Coagulase-positive
- H_2S produced

Pigs

Septicaemia, 'diamond' skin lesions, chronic arthritis, chronic valvular endocarditis, abortion

Sheep

Polyarthritis in lambs, post-dipping lameness, pneumonia, valvular endocarditis

Turkeys

Septicaemia, arthritis, valvular endocarditis

Erysipelothrix rhusiopathiae is a non-motile, Gram-positive, facultative anaerobe. It is catalase-negative, oxidase-negative, resistant to high salt concentrations and grows in the temperature range of 5–42°C and in the pH range of 6.7–9.2. It can survive for several weeks in the environment but does not replicate outside the animal host. Isolates from animals with acute infections form smooth colonies, while isolates from chronically infected animals form rough colonies. Smears from smooth colonies yield slender rods whereas rough colonies are usually composed of short filaments which decolorize readily. The bacterium grows on nutrient agar but growth is improved in media containing blood or serum.

Erysipelothrix rhusiopathiae causes erysipelas in pigs and turkeys worldwide. Sheep and other domestic animals are occasionally infected. Up to 50% of healthy pigs may harbour *E. rhusiopathiae* in their tonsils. Carrier pigs may excrete the organism in faeces and in oronasal secretions.

Infection is usually acquired by ingestion of material contaminated with pig faeces. Entry may occur through the tonsils, skin or mucous membranes. Virulence factors include a capsule which protects the organism against phagocytosis and several exoenzymes. The enzyme neuraminidase assists in adherence to, and penetration of, endothelial cells and hyaluronidase facilitates dissemination into host tissues. Swine erysipelas can occur in four forms. The septicaemic and cutaneous ('diamond') forms are acute, while arthritis and vegetative endocarditis are chronic forms of the disease. Chronic arthritis has the most significant negative impact on productivity. Septicaemia occurs after an incubation period of about three days. Some pigs may be found dead; others are febrile and depressed. Mortality may be high in some outbreaks and pregnant sows may abort. In the diamond-skin form, systemic signs are less severe. Pigs are febrile and cutaneous lesions progress from small, light pink or purple,

raised areas to more extensive diamond-shaped erythematous plaques. Arthritis, which is commonly encountered in older pigs, can present as stiffness, lameness or reluctance to bear weight on affected limbs. Joint lesions can progress to erosion of articular cartilage with eventual fibrosis and ankylosis. In vegetative endocarditis, the least common form, wart-like thrombotic masses are present usually on the mitral valves. Many affected animals are asymptomatic but some may develop congestive heart failure or die suddenly if stressed by physical exertion or by pregnancy. Clinical presentation and the type and location of lesions may suggest swine erysipelas. Diamond-shaped lesions are pathognomonic. *Erysipelothrix rhusiopathiae* can be isolated on blood agar and identified using biochemical tests. However, PCR-based procedures, including a combination of enrichment broth cultivation and PCR, have been described for detection of the pathogen and for identification. Typing procedures include serotyping and, more recently, molecular techniques such as pulsed-field gel electrophoresis and nucleotide sequencing of the *spaA* gene. The latter encodes the spaA surface protein, a major protective antigen. Live and attenuated vaccines are available for the prevention of erysipelas in pigs, although some workers suggest that the use of live vaccines may be associated with chronic arthritic forms of the disease.

Turkey erysipelas affects birds of all ages. Toms may excrete the organisms in their semen and turkey hens may die suddenly within five days of artificial insemination.

Non-suppurative polyarthritis of lambs may result from entry of *E. rhusiopathiae* through the navel or, more commonly, through docking or castration wounds. Post-dipping lameness, which affects older lambs and adult sheep, is due to cellulitis and laminitis associated with contamination of the dipping fluid by the pathogen.

Concise Review of Veterinary Microbiology, Second Edition. P.J. Quinn, B.K. Markey, F.C. Leonard, E.S. FitzPatrick and S. Fanning.
© 2016 John Wiley & Sons, Ltd. Published 2016 by John Wiley & Sons, Ltd.
Companion website: www.wiley.com/go/quinn/concise-veterinary-microbiology

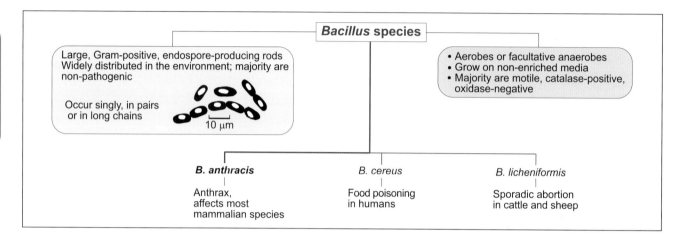

Most *Bacillus* species are large, Gram-positive, endospore-producing rods up to 10 μm in length. In smears from tissues or cultures, cells occur singly, in pairs or in long chains. The genus comprises more than 200 species with diverse characteristics. *Bacillus* species are catalase-positive, aerobic or facultatively anaerobic and, with the exception of *Bacillus anthracis* and *B. mycoides*, motile. Most species are saprophytes with no pathogenic potential. *Bacillus anthracis* is the most important pathogen in the group.

Because they produce highly resistant endospores, *Bacillus* species are widely distributed in the environment. In soil, endospores of *B. anthracis* can survive for more than 50 years. The ability to grow aerobically and to produce catalase distinguishes *Bacillus* species from clostridia, which are also Gram-positive, endospore-forming rods. Differentiation of *Bacillus* species is largely based on colonial characteristics and biochemical tests or on molecular methods.

The major disease conditions caused by bacteria in this group are listed in Table 20.1. Anthrax is the most important of these diseases. *Bacillus licheniformis* can be a significant cause of abortion in sheep and cattle and is associated with the feeding of poorly preserved silage or hay. Because they have some similar phenotypic characteristics, *B. anthracis* and *B. cereus* require careful differentiation (Table 20.2).

Anthrax

Anthrax is a severe disease which affects virtually all mammalian species including humans and is an important agent of bioterrorism. The disease, which occurs worldwide, is endemic in some countries. Ruminants are highly susceptible, often developing a rapidly fatal septicaemic form of the disease. Pigs and horses are moderately susceptible to infection, while carnivores are comparatively resistant. Birds are almost totally resistant to infection.

Endospore formation is the most important factor in the persistence and spread of anthrax. Outbreaks of disease in herbivores can occur when pastures are contaminated by spores originating from buried carcasses. Spores may be brought to the surface by flooding, excavation, subsidence, or by the activity of earthworms. Concentration of spores may also occur in some geographical regions with alkaline soils and following repeated cycles of flooding and evaporation in low-lying areas. Sporadic outbreaks of disease in non-endemic areas have been associated with the importation of contaminated meat-and-bone meal, fertilizers of animal origin and hides. Infection in animals is

Table 20.1 Clinical manifestations of diseases caused by *Bacillus anthracis* and other *Bacillus* species.

Bacillus species	Susceptible species	Clinical manifestations
B. anthracis	Cattle, sheep	Fatal peracute or acute septicaemic anthrax
	Pigs	Subacute anthrax with oedematous swelling in pharyngeal region; an intestinal form with higher mortality is less common
	Horses	Subacute anthrax with localized oedema; septicaemia with colic and enteritis sometimes occurs
	Humans	Skin, pulmonary and intestinal forms of anthrax are recorded in humans periodically
B. cereus	Cattle	Mastitis (rare)
	Humans	Food poisoning, eye infections
B. licheniformis	Cattle, sheep	Sporadic abortion

Concise Review of Veterinary Microbiology, Second Edition. P.J. Quinn, B.K. Markey, F.C. Leonard, E.S. FitzPatrick and S. Fanning.
© 2016 John Wiley & Sons, Ltd. Published 2016 by John Wiley & Sons, Ltd.
Companion website: www.wiley.com/go/quinn/concise-veterinary-microbiology

Table 20.2 Differentiating features of *Bacillus anthracis* and *B. cereus*.

Feature	*B. anthracis*	*B. cereus*
Motility	Non-motile	Motile
Appearance on sheep blood agar	Non-haemolytic	Haemolytic
Susceptibility to penicillin (10 unit disc)	Susceptible	Resistant
Lecithinase activity on egg yolk agar	Weak and slow	Strong and rapid
Effect of gamma phage	Lysis	Lysis rare
Pathogenicity for animals (application to scarified area at tail base of mouse)	Death in 24–48 hours	No effect

Chains of *Bacillus anthracis* as they appear in a thin blood smear stained with polychrome methylene blue

The blue-staining, square-ended organisms are surrounded by pink capsules

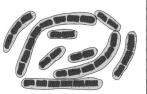

usually acquired by ingestion of spores and, less commonly, by inhalation or through skin abrasions.

The virulence of *B. anthracis* derives from the presence of a capsule and the ability to produce a complex toxin. Both virulence factors are encoded by plasmids and are required for disease production. The capsule, composed of poly-D-glutamic acid, inhibits phagocytosis. The complex toxin consists of three antigenic components: protective antigen, oedema factor and lethal factor. Protective antigen functions as the host cell-binding moiety for both oedema factor and lethal factor. Oedema factor is an adenylate cyclase enzyme which increases cAMP levels in the cell with resultant disturbance of water homeostasis. Lethal factor is a zinc metalloprotease which targets macrophages, dendritic cells, neutrophils and some epithelial and endothelial cells. In naturally occurring disease, local effects of the complex toxin include swelling and darkening of tissues due to oedema and necrosis. When septicaemia occurs, increased vascular permeability and extensive haemorrhage lead to shock and death.

The incubation period of anthrax ranges from hours to days. In cattle and sheep, the disease is usually septicaemic and rapidly fatal. Although most animals are found dead without premonitory signs, pyrexia, with temperatures up to 42°C, depression, congested mucosae and petechiae may be observed antemortem. In cattle, postmortem findings include rapid bloating, incomplete rigor mortis, widespread ecchymotic haemorrhages and oedema, dark unclotted blood and blood-stained fluid in body cavities. An extremely large soft spleen is characteristic of the disease in cattle. Splenomegaly and oedema are less prominent postmortem features in affected sheep. In pigs, infection generally results in oedematous swelling of the throat and head along with regional lymphadenitis. Some affected pigs may survive.

Carcasses of animals which have died from anthrax are bloated, putrefy rapidly and do not exhibit rigor mortis. Dark unclotted blood may issue from the mouth, nostrils and anus. The carcasses of such animals should not be opened because this will facilitate sporulation with the risk of long-term environmental contamination. Peripheral blood from the tail vein of ruminants or peritoneal fluid from pigs should be collected into a sterile syringe. Thin smears of blood or fluid, stained with polychrome methylene blue, reveal chains of square-ended, blue-staining rods surrounded by a pink capsule (M'Fadyean reaction). Blood and MacConkey agars are inoculated with the suspect specimens and incubated aerobically at 37°C for 24–48 hours. Identification criteria for isolates include colonial morphology, microscopic appearance in Gram-stained smears, absence of growth on MacConkey agar and other test procedures (Table 20.2). New molecular diagnostic methods based on PCR to amplify specific virulence-related plasmid markers have been developed and include real-time PCR procedures which are highly sensitive. *Bacillus anthracis* isolates are highly clonal but can be differentiated into different phylogenetic groups based on techniques such as multi-locus variable number tandem repeat analysis, with lineage A being the most widely distributed worldwide. Further subdivision of groups using techniques based on single nucleotide polymorphisms is possible and is useful in epidemiological investigations.

If administered early in the course of the disease, high doses of penicillin G or oxytetracycline may prove effective. Suspect cases of anthrax must be reported immediately to appropriate regulatory authorities. In endemic regions, annual vaccination of sheep and cattle with the Sterne strain spore vaccine is advisable. In non-endemic regions, movement of animals, feed and bedding is prohibited following a disease outbreak. Personnel implementing control measures should wear protective clothing and footwear. Carcasses should be incinerated or buried deeply away from watercourses. Contaminated equipment should be disinfected with 10% formalin. In-contact animals should be isolated and kept under close observation for at least two weeks. Contaminated buildings should be sealed and fumigated with formaldehyde before removal of bedding. Following removal of fittings and bedding, the building should be sprayed with 5% formalin which should be left to act for 10 hours before final washing.

Three main forms of anthrax occur in humans. Cutaneous anthrax (malignant pustule) is the result of endospores entering abraded skin. If not treated promptly, this localized lesion can progress to septicaemia. Pulmonary anthrax (wool-sorters' disease) follows inhalation of spores, while intestinal anthrax results from the ingestion of infective material. In the absence of early treatment, the disease may prove fatal.

21 *Clostridium* species

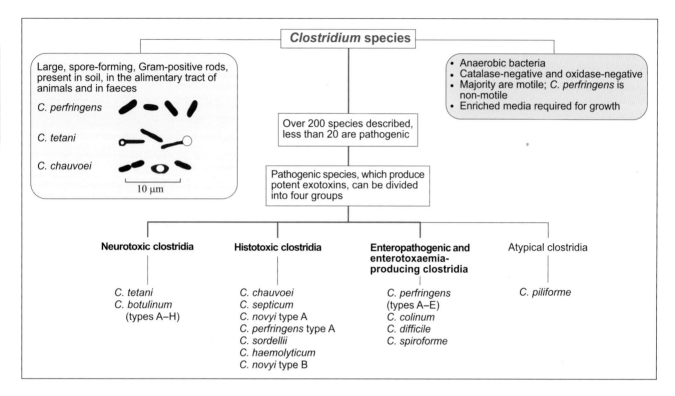

Clostridium species

- Large, spore-forming, Gram-positive rods, present in soil, in the alimentary tract of animals and in faeces

  C. perfringens

  C. tetani

  C. chauvoei

  10 μm

- Anaerobic bacteria
- Catalase-negative and oxidase-negative
- Majority are motile; *C. perfringens* is non-motile
- Enriched media required for growth

Over 200 species described, less than 20 are pathogenic

Pathogenic species, which produce potent exotoxins, can be divided into four groups

Neurotoxic clostridia

C. tetani
C. botulinum
    (types A–H)

Histotoxic clostridia

C. chauvoei
C. septicum
C. novyi type A
C. perfringens type A
C. sordellii
C. haemolyticum
C. novyi type B

Enteropathogenic and enterotoxaemia-producing clostridia

C. perfringens
    (types A–E)
C. colinum
C. difficile
C. spiroforme

Atypical clostridia

C. piliforme

Clostridia are saprophytes which are found in soil, fresh water and marine sediments. They constitute part of the normal intestinal flora of humans and animals and some may be sequestered as endospores in muscle or liver. Enriched blood agar is suitable for the culture of clostridia. Anaerobic jars containing hydrogen supplemented with 5–10% carbon dioxide provide a suitable atmosphere for growth.

Differentiation of clostridia

Clostridia can be differentiated by their colonial morphology, biochemical tests, by toxin neutralization methods and by molecular methods. Specific toxins in body fluids or intestinal contents can be identified by toxin neutralization or protection tests in laboratory animals, usually mice. Immunoassay methods such as ELISA can also be used for toxin detection and these tests have replaced many mouse bioassay tests. However, ELISA procedures may not be sufficiently sensitive for toxin detection in some circumstances. The presence of histotoxic clostridia in lesions can be demonstrated rapidly by fluorescent antibody techniques.

Neurotoxic clostridia

The neurotoxic clostridia, *C. tetani* and *C. botulinum*, elaborate potent neurotoxins. The neurotoxin of *C. tetani* is produced by organisms replicating locally in damaged tissues. When

absorbed, toxin exerts its effect on synaptic junctions remote from the site of toxin production. The neurotoxin of *C. botulinum* is usually produced by bacteria replicating in organic matter or in the anaerobic conditions in contaminated cans of meat or vegetables. When absorbed from the gastrointestinal tract into the bloodstream, the toxin affects the functioning of neuromuscular junctions. The toxins of both *C. tetani* and *C. botulinum* are similar in structure and function and the differing clinical signs caused by the toxins are due to differences in their sites of action.

Tetanus

This acute and potentially fatal intoxication is caused by the toxin of *C. tetani* which affects many species including humans. Species susceptibility to toxin varies: horses and humans are highly susceptible, ruminants and pigs are moderately susceptible while poultry are resistant.

Infection occurs when endospores of *C. tetani* from soil or faeces are introduced into damaged tissue. The presence of necrotic tissue or contaminating facultative anaerobes may create the anaerobic conditions in a wound in which *C. tetani* spores can germinate. Vegetative bacteria multiplying in necrotic tissue produce the potent neurotoxin tetanospasmin, which is responsible for the clinical signs of tetanus. Although 10 serological types of *C. tetani* can be distinguished by their flagellar antigens,

Concise Review of Veterinary Microbiology, Second Edition. P.J. Quinn, B.K. Markey, F.C. Leonard, E.S. FitzPatrick and S. Fanning.
© 2016 John Wiley & Sons, Ltd. Published 2016 by John Wiley & Sons, Ltd.
Companion website: www.wiley.com/go/quinn/concise-veterinary-microbiology

the neurotoxin produced is antigenically uniform and antibodies induced by one neurotoxin neutralize the neurotoxins produced by others. The neurotoxin binds irreversibly to ganglioside receptors. Toxin is transferred trans-synaptically to its site of action in the terminals of inhibitory neurons where it blocks presynaptic transmission of inhibitory signals through hydrolysis of synaptobrevin, a vesicle-associated membrane protein. Because release of inhibitory neurotransmitters is prevented, spastic paralysis results. Bound toxin is not neutralized by antitoxin.

The incubation period of tetanus may be up to 10 days but can extend to three weeks. Clinical effects of the neurotoxin, which are similar in all domestic animals, include stiffness, localized spasms, altered heart and respiratory rates, dysphagia and altered facial expression. Mild tactile or auditory stimuli may precipitate tonic contraction of muscles. Spasm of masticatory muscles may lead to 'lockjaw'. In horses, generalized muscle stiffness can result in a 'saw-horse' stance. Animals which recover from tetanus are not necessarily immune, as the low dose of toxin capable of producing disease may not induce neutralizing antibodies. Diagnosis is based on clinical signs, a history of recent trauma, Gram-stained smears from lesions and anaerobic culture of *C. tetani* from wound tissue. The presence of neurotoxin in serum from affected animals can be demonstrated by inoculating mice with the serum and observing the development of spastic paralysis.

Treatment procedures include prompt antitoxin administration, large doses of penicillin to inhibit growth of *C. tetani* in lesions and surgical debridement of wounds. Prevention of tetanus in farm animals is based on routine vaccination with tetanus toxoid, followed by booster doses at specified intervals.

Botulism

This potentially fatal intoxication is usually acquired by ingestion of preformed toxin. The endospores of *C. botulinum* are distributed in soils and aquatic environments worldwide. Nine types of *C. botulinum* are recognized on the basis of toxins which they produce (A, B, C_α, C_β, D, E, F, G, H). *Clostridium botulinum* type G has been renamed *C. argentinense*. The usual sources of toxins of *C. botulinum* types A–H for susceptible species are summarized in Table 21.1. *Clostridium botulinum* types C and D cause most outbreaks of botulism in domestic animals. Outbreaks of disease occur most commonly in waterfowl, cattle, horses, sheep, mink, poultry and farmed fish. Botulism in cattle has been associated with ingestion of poultry carcasses present in ensiled poultry litter used as bedding or spread on pasture. Waterfowl and other birds can acquire toxin from dead invertebrates, decaying vegetation or from the consumption of maggots containing toxin.

The neurotoxins of *C. botulinum* are the most potent biological toxins known. When absorbed from the gastrointestinal tract, preformed toxin acts at the neuromuscular junctions of cholinergic nerves and at peripheral autonomic synapses. Hydrolysis of synaptobrevins causes irreversible interference with the release of the transmitter, acetylcholine, resulting in flaccid paralysis. Death results from paralysis of respiratory muscles.

The clinical signs of botulism, which develop within days after toxin ingestion, are similar in all species and reflect the prevention of acetylcholine release at the sites of action. Dilated pupils, dry mucous membranes, decreased salivation, tongue

Table 21.1 Toxins produced by *Clostridium botulinum*.

Toxin	Source	Susceptible species
Type A	Meat, canned products Toxico-infection Meat, carcasses	Humans Infants Mink, dogs, pigs
Type B	Meat, canned products Toxico-infection Toxico-infection	Humans Infants Foals (up to 2 months of age)
Type C	Dead invertebrates, maggots, rotting vegetation and carcasses of poultry	Waterfowl, poultry
	Ensiled poultry litter, baled silage (poor quality), hay or silage contaminated with rodent carcasses	Cattle, sheep, horses
	Meat, especially chicken carcasses	Dogs, mink, lions, monkeys
Type D	Carcasses, bones Feed contaminated with carcasses	Cattle, sheep Horses
Type E	Dead invertebrates, sludge in earth-bottomed ponds Fish	Farmed fish Fish-eating birds, humans
Type F	Meat, fish	Humans
Type G	Soil-contaminated food	Humans (in Argentina)
Type H	Toxico-infection	Infants

flaccidity and dysphagia are features of the disease in farm animals. Incoordination and knuckling of the fetlocks is followed by flaccid paralysis and recumbency. Death may follow within days. In birds, there is progressive flaccid paralysis which initially affects legs and wings. Paralysis of neck muscles ('limberneck') is evident only in long-necked species.

Clinical signs and the history may suggest botulism. Confirmation requires the demonstration of toxin in the serum of affected animals by mouse inoculation. ELISA methods are not usually sufficiently sensitive for detection of toxin in serum but may be used for toxin demonstration in intestinal contents which have been frozen immediately post collection to prevent postmortem multiplication of *C. botulinum*. Toxin neutralization tests in mice, using monovalent antitoxins, can be used to identify the specific toxins involved and this method allowed the recent discovery of a new toxin, toxin H (Table 21.1).

Mildly affected animals may recover slowly without therapy. Polyvalent antiserum is effective in neutralizing unbound toxin but cost and availability limit this treatment. Vaccination of cattle with toxoid may be necessary in endemic regions in South Africa and Australia. Routine vaccination of farmed mink and foxes may be advisable.

Histotoxic clostridia

The histotoxic clostridia, through exotoxin production, cause both local tissue necrosis and systemic effects which may be lethal. Histotoxic clostridia and the diseases which they produce are presented in Table 21.2. Endospores of histotoxic clostridia

Table 21.2 Histotoxic clostridia, their major toxins and the diseases produced in domestic animals.

Clostridium species	Disease	Toxin Name	Toxin Biological activity
C. chauvoei	Blackleg in cattle and sheep	CCtA α β γ δ	Cytotoxin Lethal, haemolytic, necrotizing Deoxyribonuclease Hyaluronidase Oxygen-labile haemolysin
C. septicum	Malignant oedema in cattle, pigs and sheep. Abomasitis in sheep (braxy) and occasionally in calves	α β γ δ	Lethal, haemolytic, necrotizing Deoxyribonuclease Hyaluronidase Oxygen-labile haemolysin
C. novyi type A	'Big head' in young rams Wound infections	α	Necrotizing, lethal
C. perfringens type A	Necrotic enteritis in chickens Necrotizing enterocolitis in pigs Wound infections in several domestic animal species	α θ NetB	Haemolytic, necrotizing, lethal, lecithinase Cytolysin Possible role in necrotic enteritis
C. sordellii	Myositis in cattle, sheep and horses Abomasitis in lambs	α β	Lecithinase Oedema-producing lethal factor
C. novyi type B	Infectious necrotic hepatitis (black disease) in sheep and occasionally in cattle	α β	Necrotizing, lethal Necrotizing, haemolytic, lethal, lecithinase
C. haemolyticum	Bacillary haemoglobinuria in cattle and occasionally in sheep	β	Necrotizing, haemolytic, lethal, lecithinase

are widely distributed in soil. Although it is probable that the majority of ingested endospores are excreted in the faeces, some may be transported to the tissues in phagocytes. Tissue injury leading to reduced oxygen tension is required for spore germination. Endogenous infections, which include blackleg, infectious necrotic hepatitis and bacillary haemoglobinuria, result from the activation of dormant spores in muscle or liver. The exogenous infections – malignant oedema and gas gangrene – result from the introduction of clostridial organisms into wounds.

The clinical infections produced by histotoxic clostridia include blackleg, malignant oedema, gas gangrene, braxy, infectious necrotic hepatitis and bacillary haemoglobinuria. The pathogenesis of these diseases involves the induction of organism proliferation and toxin production through the action of some precipitating factor.

Blackleg, an acute disease of cattle and sheep caused by C. chauvoei and which is usually endogenous, occurs worldwide. The disease occurs in young thriving cattle from three months to two years of age. Latent spores in muscle become activated through traumatic injury. The large muscle masses of the limbs, back and neck are frequently affected. Skeletal muscle damage is manifest by lameness, swelling and crepitation due to gas accumulation.

Malignant oedema and gas gangrene are exogenous, necrotizing, soft-tissue infections. *Clostridium septicum* is often associated with malignant oedema and C. perfringens type A with gas gangrene. Malignant oedema manifests as cellulitis with minimal gangrene and gas formation. In gas gangrene, extensive bacterial invasion of damaged muscle tissue occurs. Gas production is detectable clinically as subcutaneous crepitation.

Braxy is an abomasitis of sheep caused by the exotoxins of C. septicum. The disease occurs in winter during periods of heavy frost or snow. Ingestion of frozen herbage may cause devitalization of abomasal tissue at its point of contact with the rumen, allowing invasion by C. septicum.

Infectious necrotic hepatitis (black disease) is an acute disease affecting sheep and occasionally cattle. Hepatic necrosis is caused by exotoxins of C. novyi type B replicating in liver tissue which has been damaged by immature *Fasciola hepatica* or other migrating parasites.

Bacillary haemoglobinuria, which occurs primarily in cattle, is an endogenous infection with C. haemolyticum. The clostridial endospores remain dormant in the liver, probably in Kupffer cells. Fluke migration facilitates spore germination and the vegetative cells produce β-toxin, a lecithinase, which causes intravascular haemolysis in addition to hepatic necrosis. Haemoglobinuria is a major clinical feature of the disease.

Fluorescent antibody techniques are used extensively for the diagnosis of diseases caused by histotoxic clostridia. *Clostridium perfringens* is cultured anaerobically on blood agar at 37°C for 48 hours. The Nagler reaction, a plate neutralization test, identifies the α-toxin of C. perfringens which has lecithinase activity. Multiplex PCR-based methods for the identification of histotoxic clostridia isolated from tissues or for their detection directly in clinical samples have been described.

Enteropathogenic clostridia

Clostridia which produce enterotoxaemia and enteropathy replicate in the intestinal tract and elaborate toxins that produce both localized and generalized tissue damage. *Clostridium*

Table 21.3 Types of *Clostridium perfringens*, their major toxins and associated diseases.

	Disease	Toxin Name	Toxin Biological activity
Type A	Necrotic enteritis in chickens	α (significant toxin)	Lecithinase
		NetB	Possible role in necrotic enteritis of chickens
	Necrotizing enterocolitis in pigs	α (significant toxin)	Lecithinase
	Canine haemorrhagic gastroenteritis	Enterotoxin	Cytotoxic
Type B	Lamb dysentery	α	Lecithinase
	Haemorrhagic enteritis in calves and foals	β (significant toxin)	Lethal, necrotizing
		ε (exists as a prototoxin and requires activation by proteolytic enzymes)	Increases intestinal and capillary permeability, lethal
Type C	'Struck' in adult sheep	TpeL	Cytotoxin
	Sudden death in goats and feedlot cattle	β2 (significant toxin)	Pore-forming toxin
	Haemorrhagic enteritis in neonatal farm animals	Enterotoxin	Pore-forming toxin
		θ	Cytolysin
		α	Lecithinase
		β	Lethal, necrotizing
Type D	Pulpy kidney in sheep	α	Lecithinase
	Enterotoxaemia in calves, adult goats and kids	ε (significant toxin, exists as a prototoxin and requires activation by proteolytic enzymes)	Increases intestinal and capillary permeability, lethal
Type E	Haemorrhagic enteritis in calves	α	Lecithinase
	Enteritis in rabbits	ι (significant toxin)	Lethal

perfringens types A–E produce a number of potent, immunologically distinct exotoxins which cause the local and systemic effects encountered in enterotoxaemias. The toxins produced by *C. perfringens* types A–E, their biological activities and associated diseases are presented in Table 21.3.

Lamb dysentery, caused by *C. perfringens* type B, can cause high mortality in lambs during the first week of life. Many animals die suddenly and the high susceptibility of this group is attributed to the absence of microbial competition and the low proteolytic activity in the neonatal intestine. Infection with *C. perfringens* type C causes 'struck', an acute enterotoxaemia in adult sheep in defined geograhical regions. The disease, which occurs in sheep at pasture, usually manifests as sudden death.

Pulpy kidney disease, caused by *C. perfringens* type D, occurs in sheep worldwide. Ingestion of excessive quantities of food may lead to the transfer of partially digested food from the rumen into the intestine and its high starch content is a suitable substrate for rapid clostridial proliferation. The ε-toxin, which exists as a prototoxin and requires activation by proteolytic enzymes, produces toxaemia and death shortly after clinical signs emerge. Focal symmetrical encephalomalacia, a manifestation of the subacute effects of the ε-toxin on the vasculature, is characterized by symmetrical haemorrhagic lesions in the basal ganglia and midbrain.

Direct smears from the mucosa or contents of the small intestine of recently dead animals which contain substantial numbers of large Gram-positive rods are consistent with enterotoxaemia. Toxin neutralization tests using mouse and guinea-pig inoculation can definitively identify the toxins of *C. perfringens* present in the contents of recently dead animals. ELISA can be used for demonstrating toxin in intestinal contents and are of comparable sensitivity to *in vivo* assays. Vaccination is the principal control method. Ewes should be vaccinated with toxoid six weeks before lambing to ensure passive protection for lambs. Sudden dietary changes and other factors predisposing to enterotoxaemias should be avoided.

Clostridium difficile is an enteropathogenic clostridium that is a major nosocomial pathogen in humans and which can cause diarrhoea in dogs, foals and young piglets. Antimicrobial treatment is an important predisposing factor in humans and animals, although disease in animals has been described in the absence of antimicrobial therapy. The organism produces three toxins, two of which are known to have a role in disease production and demonstration of their presence in intestinal contents by ELISA confirms diagnosis.

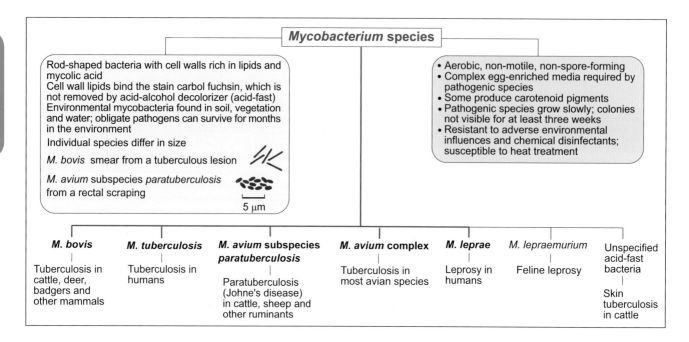

Mycobacterium species

Rod-shaped bacteria with cell walls rich in lipids and mycolic acid
Cell wall lipids bind the stain carbol fuchsin, which is not removed by acid-alcohol decolorizer (acid-fast)
Environmental mycobacteria found in soil, vegetation and water; obligate pathogens can survive for months in the environment
Individual species differ in size

M. bovis smear from a tuberculous lesion

M. avium subspecies *paratuberculosis* from a rectal scraping

5 μm

- Aerobic, non-motile, non-spore-forming
- Complex egg-enriched media required by pathogenic species
- Some produce carotenoid pigments
- Pathogenic species grow slowly; colonies not visible for at least three weeks
- Resistant to adverse environmental influences and chemical disinfectants; susceptible to heat treatment

M. bovis
Tuberculosis in cattle, deer, badgers and other mammals

M. tuberculosis
Tuberculosis in humans

M. avium subspecies *paratuberculosis*
Paratuberculosis (Johne's disease) in cattle, sheep and other ruminants

M. avium complex
Tuberculosis in most avian species

M. leprae
Leprosy in humans

M. lepraemurium
Feline leprosy

Unspecified acid-fast bacteria
Skin tuberculosis in cattle

Mycobacteria are aerobic, non-spore-forming, non-motile, rod-shaped acid-fast bacilli. Individual species differ in size; the rods of *Mycobacterium bovis* and *M. avium* subsp. *avium* are slender and up to 4 μm in length, whereas those of *M. avium* subsp. *paratuberculosis* are broad and are usually less than 2 μm long. Although mycobacteria are cytochemically Gram-positive, the high lipid and mycolic acid content of cell walls prevents uptake of the dyes employed in the Gram stain. The cell wall lipids bind carbol fuchsin which is not removed by the Ziehl–Neelsen (ZN) staining method. Bacilli which stain red by this method are described as acid-fast or ZN-positive.

The mycobacteria include diverse species ranging from environmental saprophytes and opportunistic invaders to obligate pathogens. Mycobacterial diseases in domestic animals are usually chronic and progressive. The *M. tuberculosis* complex includes a number of closely related species, including *M. tuberculosis*, *M. bovis* and *M. africanum* which cause tuberculosis in humans. Environmental mycobacteria are found in soil, on vegetation and in water. Obligate pathogens, shed by infected animals, can survive in the environment for extended periods.

The ZN staining method is used to differentiate mycobacteria from other bacteria. Differentation of pathogenic mycobacteria relies on cultural characteristics, biochemical tests, animal inoculation, chromatographic analysis and molecular techniques. Strict safety precautions must be observed when working with material containing mycobacteria. Pathogenic mycobacteria grow slowly at an optimal temperature of 37°C under aerobic

conditions and colonies are not evident until cultures have been incubated for at least three weeks. In contrast, colonies of rapidly growing saprophytes are visible within days. Pathogenic species of mycobacteria can be distinguished by their colonial appearance on egg-based media, the influence of added glycerol and sodium pyruvate on growth rate, and pigment production. Addition of glycerol enhances the growth of *M. tuberculosis* and the *M. avium* complex, while sodium pyruvate enhances the growth of *M. bovis*. Automated systems of culture in liquid media are available and growth, which is more rapid than on solid media, is detected using radiometric or fluorometric methods. Molecular techniques, including DNA probe detection of targets such as insertion sequences specific to particular members of the genus, are used for detection of *M. tuberculosis* complex and *M. paratuberculosis* in clinical specimens. These methods are much more rapid than culture and sensitivity can be further improved by combination with immunomagnetic separation methods. Spoligotyping, a system of identification of polymorphisms in spacer regions of the direct repeat regions of the chromosome, is a frequently employed method for epidemiological typing of *M. bovis*. Clinical and cultural characteristics of important pathogenic mycobacteria are presented in Table 22.1.

The diseases caused by pathogenic mycobacteria are presented in Table 22.2. The major pathogenic *Mycobacterium* species which affect domestic animals exhibit a considerable degree of host specificity, although they can produce sporadic disease in a number of other hosts. Diseases in domestic animals

Concise Review of Veterinary Microbiology, Second Edition. P.J. Quinn, B.K. Markey, F.C. Leonard, E.S. FitzPatrick and S. Fanning.
© 2016 John Wiley & Sons, Ltd. Published 2016 by John Wiley & Sons, Ltd.
Companion website: www.wiley.com/go/quinn/concise-veterinary-microbiology

Table 22.1 Clinical significance and growth characteristics of pathogenic mycobacteria.

	M. tuberculosis	*M. bovis*	*M. avium* complex	*M. avium* subsp. *paratuberculosis*
Significance of infection	Important in humans and occasionally in dogs	Important in cattle and occasionally in other domestic animals and humans	Important in free-range domestic poultry, opportunistic infections in humans and domestic animals	Important in cattle and other ruminants
Growth rate on solid media	Slow (3–8 weeks)	Slow (3–8 weeks)	Slow (2–6 weeks)	Exceptionally slow (up to 16 weeks)
Colonial features	Rough, buff, difficult to break apart	Cream-coloured, raised with central roughness, break apart easily	Sticky, off-white, break apart easily	Small, hemispherical; some pigmented colonies

caused by mycobacteria include tuberculosis in avian and mammalian species, paratuberculosis in ruminants and feline leprosy. Other clinical conditions, such as skin tuberculosis and bovine farcy in cattle and canine leproid granuloma in dogs, are associated with the presence of acid-fast bacteria in lesions. Avian tuberculosis, which occurs worldwide, is usually caused by members of the *M. avium* complex. The disease is encountered most often in free-range adult birds and transmission is usually by the faecal–oral route. Non-specific clinical signs, including dullness, anaemia, emaciation and lameness, develop in affected birds only when the disease is at an advanced stage. At postmortem examination, granulomatous lesions are characteristically present in the liver, spleen, bone marrow and intestines. Diagnosis is based on postmortem findings and on the demonstration of large numbers of ZN-positive bacilli in smears from lesions.

Tuberculosis in cattle

Bovine tuberculosis, caused by *M. bovis*, occurs worldwide. Because of the zoonotic implications of the disease and production losses due to its chronic progressive nature, eradication programmes have been introduced in many countries. Although *M. bovis* can survive for several months in the environment, transmission is mainly through aerosols generated by infected cattle. Dairy cattle in particular are at risk because husbandry methods allow close contact between animals at milking and when housed during winter months. Wildlife reservoirs of *M. bovis* are major sources of infection for grazing cattle in some countries. They include deer, wild boar and the badger in Europe, the brush-tailed possum in New Zealand and the Cape buffalo and other ruminants in Africa. These wildlife species may act as reservoir hosts which maintain infection within their own population or, in instances in which the disease does not

Table 22.2 Mycobacteria which are pathogenic for animals and humans.

Mycobacterium species	Main hosts	Species occasionally infected	Disease
Major animal pathogens			
M. bovis	Cattle	Deer, badgers, possums, humans, cats, other mammalian species	Tuberculosis
M. avium subsp. *paratuberculosis*	Cattle, sheep, goats, deer	Other ruminants	Paratuberculosis (Johne's disease)
M. avium complex	Most avian species except psittacines	Pigs, cattle	Tuberculosis
M. caprae	Goats, cattle	Wild boar, sheep, pigs	Tuberculosis
Major human pathogens			
M. tuberculosis	Humans, captive primates	Dogs, cattle, psittacine birds, canaries	Tuberculosis (worldwide)
M. africanum	Humans		Tuberculosis (regions in Africa)
M. leprae	Humans	Armadillos, chimpanzees	Leprosy
Other mycobacteria			
M. microti	Voles	Rarely other mammalian species	Tuberculosis
M. marinum	Fish	Humans, aquatic mammals, amphibians	Tuberculosis
M. pinnipedii	Seals	Humans, cattle, other mammalian species	Tuberculosis
M. lepraemurium	Rats, mice	Cats	Rat leprosy, feline leprosy
Unspecified acid-fast bacteria	Cattle		Associated with skin tuberculosis
M. senegalense, M. farcinogenes	Cattle		Implicated in bovine farcy

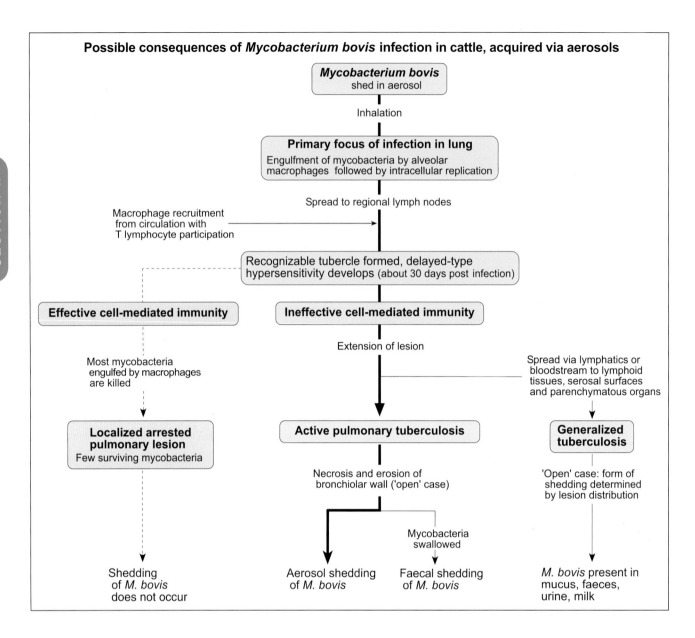

Possible consequences of *Mycobacterium bovis* infection in cattle, acquired via aerosols

Mycobacterium bovis
shed in aerosol

Inhalation

Primary focus of infection in lung
Engulfment of mycobacteria by alveolar macrophages followed by intracellular replication

Spread to regional lymph nodes

Macrophage recruitment from circulation with T lymphocyte participation

Recognizable tubercle formed, delayed-type hypersensitivity develops (about 30 days post infection)

Effective cell-mediated immunity

Ineffective cell-mediated immunity

Extension of lesion

Most mycobacteria engulfed by macrophages are killed

Spread via lymphatics or bloodstream to lymphoid tissues, serosal surfaces and parenchymatous organs

Localized arrested pulmonary lesion
Few surviving mycobacteria

Active pulmonary tuberculosis

Generalized tuberculosis

Necrosis and erosion of bronchiolar wall ('open' case)

'Open' case: form of shedding determined by lesion distribution

Mycobacteria swallowed

Shedding of *M. bovis* does not occur

Aerosol shedding of *M. bovis*

Faecal shedding of *M. bovis*

M. bovis present in mucus, faeces, urine, milk

persist in a population in the absence of contact with infected cattle, as spillover hosts.

The virulence of *M. bovis* relates to its ability to survive and multiply in host macrophages. Survival within the phagosome of macrophages is promoted by interference with phagosome–lysosome fusion and failure of lysosomal digestion. Clinical signs are evident only in advanced disease and cattle with extensive lesions can appear to be in good health. Loss of condition may become evident as the disease progresses. Tuberculous mastitis facilitates spread of infection to calves and cats, and is of major public health importance.

In the early stages of disease, lesions may be difficult to detect at postmortem examination. In older lesions, fibroplasia produces early capsule formation and there is central caseous necrosis, detectable grossly as yellowish cheesy material. The tuberculin test, based on a delayed-type hypersensitivity to mycobacterial tuberculoprotein, is the standard antemortem test in cattle. Reactivity in cattle is usually detectable 30–50 days after infection. Tuberculin, prepared from mycobacteria and called purified protein derivative (PPD), is injected intradermally to detect sensitization. In the single intradermal (caudal fold)

test, 0.1 mL of bovine PPD is injected into the caudal fold of the tail and the injection site is examined 72 hours later. A positive reaction is characterized by a hard or oedematous swelling. In the comparative intradermal test, 0.1 mL of avian PPD and 0.1 mL of bovine PPD are injected intradermally into separate clipped sites on the side of the neck about 12 cm apart. Skin thickness at the injection sites is measured with calipers before injection of tuberculins and after 72 hours. An increase in skin thickness at the injection site of bovine PPD which exceeds that at the avian PPD injection site by 4 mm or more is interpreted as evidence of infection and the animal is termed a reactor. False-positive reactions may be attributed to sensitization to mycobacteria other than *M. bovis*. False-negative results may be recorded if cattle are tested before delayed-type hypersensitivity to tuberculoproteins develops. In some cattle an unresponsive state, referred to as anergy, may accompany advanced tuberculosis. Cows may be unresponsive to the tuberculin test during the early postpartum period. Interferon-γ release assays can be used as an adjunct to the skin test in control programmes. Other blood-based tests which are being evaluated include ELISA for detecting circulating antibodies and lymphocyte transformation. Specimens

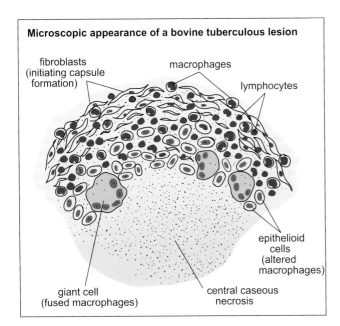

Microscopic appearance of a bovine tuberculous lesion

fibroblasts (initiating capsule formation)

macrophages

lymphocytes

epithelioid cells (altered macrophages)

giant cell (fused macrophages)

central caseous necrosis

suitable for laboratory demonstration or culture of *M. bovis* include lymph nodes, tissue lesions, aspirates and milk. Decontamination of specimens is required, to eliminate fast-growing contaminating bacteria, before inoculation of specialized liquid or solid culture media. Identification of isolates is usually carried out using molecular techniques. Tuberculin testing followed by isolation and slaughter of reactors is the basis of many national eradication schemes. Routine meat inspection forms part of the surveillance programme for bovine tuberculosis worldwide.

Paratuberculosis (Johne's disease)

This chronic, contagious, invariably fatal enteritis, which can affect domestic and wild ruminants, is caused by infection with *M. avium* subsp. *paratuberculosis*. Infection is acquired by calves at an early stage through ingestion of organisms shed in the faeces of infected animals. The organism is also shed in colostrum and milk and feeding of pooled colostrum is considered a risk factor for the acquisition of infection by calves in infected herds. Two main genotypes of *M. avium* subsp. *paratuberculosis* are recognized: S type or Type I in sheep and C type or Type II in cattle. Isolates can cross the species barrier,

although S type isolates appear to be less virulent for cattle. Under favourable conditions, *M. avium* subsp. *paratuberculosis* may remain viable in the environment for up to one year. Clinical disease is rarely encountered in cattle under two years of age. Ingested mycobacteria, engulfed by macrophages in which they survive and replicate, are found initially in Peyer's patches. Cell-mediated reactions are mainly responsible for the enteric lesions. As the disease progresses, an immune-mediated granulomatous reaction develops, with marked lymphocyte and macrophage accumulation in the lamina propria and submucosa. The resulting enteropathy leads to loss of plasma proteins and malabsorption of nutrients and water.

Affected cattle are usually more than two years of age when signs are first observed. The main clinical feature is diarrhoea, initially intermittent but becoming persistent and profuse. Progressive weight loss occurs in cattle despite an unaltered appetite. The mucosa of affected areas of the terminal small intestine and the large intestine of cattle is usually thickened and folded into transverse corrugations. The mesenteric and ileocaecal lymph nodes are enlarged and oedematous. Specimens for direct microscopy from live animals include scrapings or pinch biopsies from the rectum. Faeces may be submitted for culture or PCR procedures and serum for serological tests. ELISA is now the most commonly employed of the serological tests and several kit versions are commercially available. Although useful on a herd basis, sensitivity and specificity of these tests are highly variable when examining sera from individual animals. Postmortem specimens for histopathological examination from cattle include tissue from affected regions of the intestines and from regional lymph nodes. Isolation of *M. avium* subsp. *paratuberculosis* from faeces or tissues is difficult and time-consuming. Cell-mediated responses using johnin, the counterpart of tuberculin PPD, may be used as a field test. Real-time PCR methods, which are highly sensitive, are being used for rapid detection of the organism in faeces. Animals with clinical signs suggestive of paratuberculosis should be isolated. If the condition is confirmed, affected animals should be slaughtered promptly. Several countries are developing national control programmes for control of paratuberculosis in cattle, although these are hampered by the insidious nature of the disease and lack of sensitive, specific and inexpensive diagnostic tests.

23 *Enterobacteriaceae*

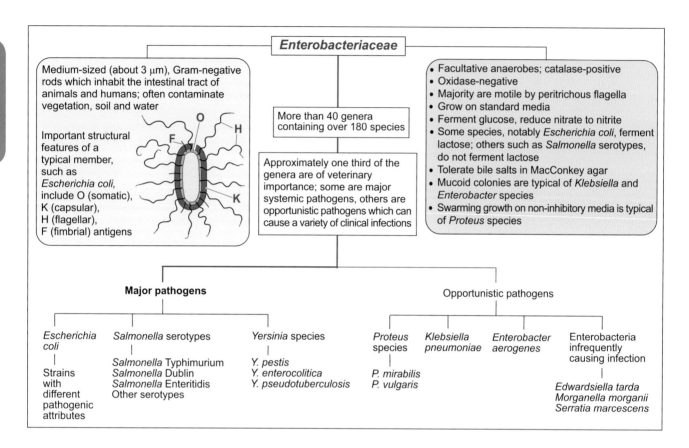

Enterobacteriaceae

Medium-sized (about 3 μm), Gram-negative rods which inhabit the intestinal tract of animals and humans; often contaminate vegetation, soil and water

Important structural features of a typical member, such as *Escherichia coli*, include O (somatic), K (capsular), H (flagellar), F (fimbrial) antigens

More than 40 genera containing over 180 species

Approximately one third of the genera are of veterinary importance; some are major systemic pathogens, others are opportunistic pathogens which can cause a variety of clinical infections

- Facultative anaerobes; catalase-positive
- Oxidase-negative
- Majority are motile by peritrichous flagella
- Grow on standard media
- Ferment glucose, reduce nitrate to nitrite
- Some species, notably *Escherichia coli*, ferment lactose; others such as *Salmonella* serotypes, do not ferment lactose
- Tolerate bile salts in MacConkey agar
- Mucoid colonies are typical of *Klebsiella* and *Enterobacter* species
- Swarming growth on non-inhibitory media is typical of *Proteus* species

Major pathogens

Escherichia coli
|
Strains with different pathogenic attributes

Salmonella serotypes
|
Salmonella Typhimurium
Salmonella Dublin
Salmonella Enteritidis
Other serotypes

Yersinia species
|
Y. pestis
Y. enterocolitica
Y. pseudotuberculosis

Opportunistic pathogens

Proteus species
|
P. mirabilis
P. vulgaris

Klebsiella pneumoniae

Enterobacter aerogenes

Enterobacteria infrequently causing infection
|
Edwardsiella tarda
Morganella morganii
Serratia marcescens

Bacteria belonging to the family *Enterobacteriaceae* are Gram-negative rods which ferment glucose and other sugars and are oxidase-negative. They are catalase-positive, non-spore-forming, facultative anaerobes which grow well on MacConkey agar. The family contains more than 40 genera and over 180 species. Less than one-third of the genera are of veterinary importance.

Enterobacteria inhabit the intestinal tract of animals and humans and contaminate vegetation, soil and water. They can be arbitrarily grouped in three categories: major pathogens, opportunistic pathogens and non-pathogens. Opportunistic pathogens such as *Proteus* species, *Klebsiella pneumoniae* and *Enterobacter aerogenes* occasionally cause clinical disease in locations other than the alimentary tract. The major animal pathogens *E. coli*, *Salmonella* species and *Yersinia* species can cause both enteric and systemic disease. Selected criteria for differentiating pathogenic members are presented in Table 23.1. Apart from some strains of *E. coli*, few enterobacteria produce haemoly-sis on blood agar. Lactose fermentation in MacConkey agar is an important identifying feature of *E. coli*, *Enterobacter aerogenes* and *Klebsiella pneumoniae*. Colonies of these organisms and the surrounding medium are pink, due to acid production from lactose. *Proteus* species produce characteristic swarming on non-inhibitory media such as blood agar. Mucoid colonies are typical of *Klebsiella* and *Enterobacter* species. A variety of biochemical tests can be used to differentiate members of the *Enterobacteriaceae* and miniaturized strips comprising many different tests are frequently employed. However, results generated in these systems are unreliable for detection of *Salmonella* serotypes and reactions in triple sugar iron (TSI) agar and lysine decarboxylase production are used for confirming the identity of suspect *Salmonella* isolates. Serotyping, using slide agglutination tests with antisera, are used to detect the somatic (O) and flagellar (H) antigens of *E. coli*, *Salmonella* and *Yersinia* species. This procedure allows identification of the organisms involved in disease outbreaks. Many molecular techniques for

Concise Review of Veterinary Microbiology, Second Edition. P.J. Quinn, B.K. Markey, F.C. Leonard, E.S. FitzPatrick and S. Fanning.
© 2016 John Wiley & Sons, Ltd. Published 2016 by John Wiley & Sons, Ltd.
Companion website: www.wiley.com/go/quinn/concise-veterinary-microbiology

Table 23.1 The clinical relevance and phenotypic characteristics of important members of the *Enterobacteriaceae*.

	Escherichia coli	*Salmonella* serotypes	*Yersinia* species	*Proteus* species	*Enterobacter aerogenes*	*Klebsiella pneumoniae*
Clinical importance	Major pathogen	Major pathogens	Major pathogens	Opportunistic pathogens	Opportunistic pathogen	Opportunistic pathogen
Cultural characteristics	Some strains haemolytic	Characteristic appearance on *Salmonella*-selective media	–	Swarming growth[a]	Mucoid	Mucoid
Motility at 30°C	Motile	Motile	Motile[b]	Motile	Motile	Non-motile
Lactose fermentation	+	–	–	–	+	+

[a]When cultured on non-inhibitory medium.
[b]Except *Y. pestis*.

identification and typing are available. PCR-based techniques, including multiplex and real-time PCR methods, are frequently employed for detection and identification of organisms. Typing methods include digestion with restriction enzymes followed by pulsed-field gel electrophoresis, multi-locus sequence typing and, in the case of *E. coli*, phylogenetic typing (see Chapter 4 for a description of these techniques).

Particular members of the *Enterobacteriaceae* are sometimes involved in localized opportunistic infections in diverse anatomical locations. Faecal contamination of the environment contributes to the occurrence of opportunistic infection. The clinical conditions arising from infection with these opportunistic members are presented in Table 23.2. *Klebsiella pneumoniae* and *Enterobacter aerogenes* are two opportunistic pathogens commonly encountered in coliform mastitis in dairy cattle. These organisms usually gain entry to the mammary gland from contaminated environmental sources. *Klebsiella pneumoniae* is also reported to be one of the commonest causes of metritis in mares. *Klebsiella* species and *Proteus* species cause infections of the lower urinary tract in dogs. *Proteus* species are often implicated in otitis externa in dogs and sometimes in cats.

Escherichia coli

Colonization of the mammalian intestinal tract by *E. coli* from environmental sources occurs shortly after birth and these organisms persist as important members of the normal flora of the intestine throughout life. Most strains of *E. coli* do not produce disease but may produce opportunistic infections in sites

Table 23.2 Opportunistic pathogens in the *Enterobacteriaceae* and their associated clinical conditions.

Bacterial species	Clinical conditions
Enterobacter aerogenes	Coliform mastitis in cows and sows
Klebsiella pneumoniae	Coliform mastitis in cows; endometritis in mares; pneumonia in calves and foals; urinary tract infections in dogs
Proteus mirabilis and *P. vulgaris*	Urinary tract infections in dogs and horses; associated with otitis externa in dogs

such as the mammary gland or in wounds. Predisposing factors which permit colonization include age, immune status, nature of diet and heavy exposure to pathogenic strains. As illustrated, pathogenic *E. coli* can be divided into strains causing intestinal and extraintestinal disease. Certain virulence factors are associated with particular pathotypes but the differentiation of *E. coli* strains is complex as many strains considered commensals also possess virulence determinants. Several pathotypes of intestinal *E. coli* are of importance in humans but a smaller number of types are responsible for disease in animals. In recent years, Shigatoxigenic *E. coli* have emerged as major food-borne zoonotic pathogens in humans, responsible for the haemorrhagic colitis and haemolytic uraemic syndrome.

Clinical infections in young animals may be limited to the intestines (enteric colibacillosis, neonatal diarrhoea), or may manifest as septicaemia or toxaemia. Extraintestinal localized infections in adult animals, many due to opportunistic invasion, can involve the urinary tract, mammary glands and uterus. The virulence factors of pathogenic strains of *E. coli* include capsules, endotoxin, structures responsible for colonization, enterotoxins and other secreted products. Capsular polysaccharides, which are produced by some strains of *E. coli*, interfere with the phagocytic uptake of these organisms. Endotoxin, a lipopolysaccharide (LPS) component of the cell wall of Gram-negative organisms, is released on death of the bacteria. The role of LPS in disease production includes pyrogenic activity, endothelial damage leading to disseminated intravascular coagulation and endotoxic shock. Fimbrial adhesins, which are present on many enterotoxigenic strains of *E. coli*, allow attachment to mucosal surfaces in the small intestine. The most significant adhesins in strains of *E. coli* producing disease in domestic animals are F4 (K88), F5 (K99), F6 (987P) and F41. The most common adhesin present in strains of *E. coli* infecting pigs is F4. The F5 and F41 adhesins occur in strains affecting calves and F5 in strains affecting lambs. The pathological effects of infection with pathogenic *E. coli*, other than those attributed to endotoxin, derive mainly from the production of enterotoxins, Shigatoxins or cytotoxic necrotizing factors. Unlike enterotoxins, which affect only the functional activity of enterocytes, Shigatoxins and cytotoxic necrotizing factors can produce demonstrable cell damage at their sites of action. To prevent enteric colibacillosis, neonatal diarrhoea and colisepticaemia, newborn animals should receive ample amounts of

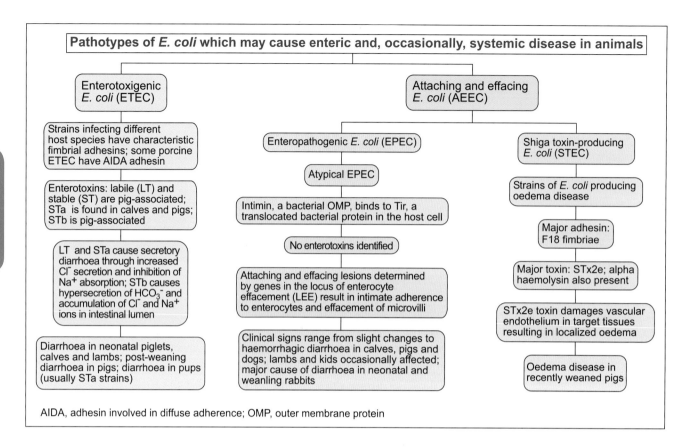

Pathotypes of *E. coli* which may cause enteric and, occasionally, systemic disease in animals

Enterotoxigenic *E. coli* (ETEC)

- Strains infecting different host species have characteristic fimbrial adhesins; some porcine ETEC have AIDA adhesin

- Enterotoxins: labile (LT) and stable (ST) are pig-associated; STa is found in calves and pigs; STb is pig-associated

- LT and STa cause secretory diarrhoea through increased Cl⁻ secretion and inhibition of Na⁺ absorption; STb causes hypersecretion of HCO_3^- and accumulation of Cl⁻ and Na⁺ ions in intestinal lumen

- Diarrhoea in neonatal piglets, calves and lambs; post-weaning diarrhoea in pigs; diarrhoea in pups (usually STa strains)

Attaching and effacing *E. coli* (AEEC)

Enteropathogenic *E. coli* (EPEC)

- Atypical EPEC

- Intimin, a bacterial OMP, binds to Tir, a translocated bacterial protein in the host cell

- No enterotoxins identified

- Attaching and effacing lesions determined by genes in the locus of enterocyte effacement (LEE) result in intimate adherence to enterocytes and effacement of microvilli

- Clinical signs range from slight changes to haemorrhagic diarrhoea in calves, pigs and dogs; lambs and kids occasionally affected; major cause of diarrhoea in neonatal and weanling rabbits

Shiga toxin-producing *E. coli* (STEC)

- Strains of *E. coli* producing oedema disease

- Major adhesin: F18 fimbriae

- Major toxin: STx2e; alpha haemolysin also present

- STx2e toxin damages vascular endothelium in target tissues resulting in localized oedema

- Oedema disease in recently weaned pigs

AIDA, adhesin involved in diffuse adherence; OMP, outer membrane protein

colostrum shortly after birth. Colostral antibodies can prevent colonization of the intestine by pathogenic *E. coli*. A clean, warm environment should be provided for newborn animals. Vaccination is of value for a limited number of diseases caused by *E. coli*.

Salmonella serotypes

The genus *Salmonella* contains more than 2,500 serotypes. Serotyping is based on the identification of somatic (O) and flagellar (H) antigens using specific antisera. These organisms occur worldwide and infect many mammals, birds and reptiles

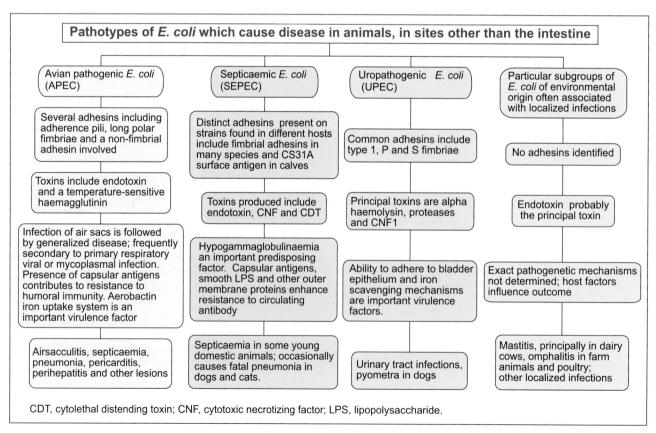

Pathotypes of *E. coli* which cause disease in animals, in sites other than the intestine

Avian pathogenic *E. coli* (APEC)

- Several adhesins including adherence pili, long polar fimbriae and a non-fimbrial adhesin involved

- Toxins include endotoxin and a temperature-sensitive haemagglutinin

- Infection of air sacs is followed by generalized disease; frequently secondary to primary respiratory viral or mycoplasmal infection. Presence of capsular antigens contributes to resistance to humoral immunity. Aerobactin iron uptake system is an important virulence factor

- Airsacculitis, septicaemia, pneumonia, pericarditis, perihepatitis and other lesions

Septicaemic *E. coli* (SEPEC)

- Distinct adhesins present on strains found in different hosts include fimbrial adhesins in many species and CS31A surface antigen in calves

- Toxins produced include endotoxin, CNF and CDT

- Hypogammaglobulinaemia an important predisposing factor. Capsular antigens, smooth LPS and other outer membrane proteins enhance resistance to circulating antibody

- Septicaemia in some young domestic animals; occasionally causes fatal pneumonia in dogs and cats.

Uropathogenic *E. coli* (UPEC)

- Common adhesins include type 1, P and S fimbriae

- Principal toxins are alpha haemolysin, proteases and CNF1

- Ability to adhere to bladder epithelium and iron scavenging mechanisms are important virulence factors.

- Urinary tract infections, pyometra in dogs

Particular subgroups of *E. coli* of environmental origin often associated with localized infections

- No adhesins identified

- Endotoxin probably the principal toxin

- Exact pathogenetic mechanisms not determined; host factors influence outcome

- Mastitis, principally in dairy cows, omphalitis in farm animals and poultry; other localized infections

CDT, cytolethal distending toxin; CNF, cytotoxic necrotizing factor; LPS, lipopolysaccharide.

and are mainly excreted in faeces. Ingestion is the main route of infection. Organisms may be present in water, soil, animal feeds, raw meat and offal, and in vegetable material. The source of environmental contamination is invariably faeces. In poultry, some species such as *Salmonella* Enteritidis infect the ovaries and vertical transmission occurs.

Salmonellosis is of common occurrence in domestic animals and the consequences of infection range from subclinical carrier status to acute fatal septicaemia. Some *Salmonella* serotypes, such as *Salmonella* Pullorum in poultry, *Salmonella* Choleraesuis in pigs and *Salmonella* Dublin in cattle, are relatively host-specific. In contrast, *Salmonella* Typhimurium has a comparatively wide host range. The *Salmonella* serotypes of importance in domestic animals and the consequences of infection are indicated in Table 23.3. *Salmonella* Dublin causes a variety of clinical effects in cattle of different ages including acute or chronic enteric disease, septicaemia and abortion. In calves, joint ill, osteomyelitis and terminal dry gangrene may follow septicaemia or enteric disease. The virulence of salmonellae relates to their ability to invade host cells, replicate in them and resist both digestion by phagocytes and destruction by the complement components of plasma. Many of the virulence factors are encoded by clusters of virulence genes termed Salmonella Pathogenicity Islands (SPI). Although there are many of these islands, SPI-1 and SPI-2 are well characterized as SPI-1 is responsible for local invasion of intestinal cells and SPI-2 is responsible for systemic invasion. Salmonellae often localize in the mucosae of the ileum, caecum and colon and in the mesenteric lymph nodes of infected animals. Latent infections, in which the organisms colonize organs such as the mesenteric lymph nodes but are not excreted, also occur. Clinical disease may develop from subclinical and latent infections if affected animals are stressed by overcrowding, transportation or adverse environmental conditions.

Table 23.3 Selected *Salmonella* serotypes of clinical importance and the consequences of infection.

Salmonella serotype	Hosts	Consequences of infection
Salmonella Typhimurium	Many animal species Humans	Enterocolitis and septicaemia Food poisoning
Salmonella Dublin	Cattle Sheep, horses, dogs	Many disease conditions Enterocolitis and septicaemia
Salmonella Choleraesuis	Pigs	Enterocolitis and septicaemia
Salmonella Pullorum	Chicks	Pullorum disease (bacillary white diarrhoea)
Salmonella Gallinarum	Adult birds	Fowl typhoid
Salmonella Arizonae	Turkeys	Arizona or paracolon infection
Salmonella Enteritidis	Poultry Many other species Humans	Often subclinical in poultry Clinical disease in mammals Food poisoning
Salmonella Brandenburg	Sheep	Abortion

Enterocolitis caused by salmonella organisms can affect most species of farm animals, irrespective of age. Acute disease is characterized by fever, depression, anorexia and profuse foul-smelling diarrhoea often containing blood, mucus and epithelial casts. Dehydration and weight loss follow and pregnant animals may abort. Severely affected young animals become recumbent and may die within a few days of acquiring infection. Septicaemic salmonellosis can occur in all age groups but is most common in calves, in neonatal foals and in young pigs. Onset of clinical disease is sudden with high fever, depression and recumbency. If treatment is delayed, many young animals with septicaemia die within 48 hours.

Laboratory confirmation is required for salmonellosis. Specimens for submission should include faeces and blood from live animals. Intestinal contents and samples from tissue lesions should be submitted from dead animals and abomasal contents from aborted foetuses. Specimens should be cultured directly onto brilliant green and XLD agars and also added to selenite F or tetrathionate broth for enrichment and subculture. Suspicious colonies can be subjected to further biochemical tests and confirmed as salmonellae using commercially available specific antisera. Many PCR-based procedures are available for rapid detection of the organism in clinical specimens and in food.

Control of salmonellosis is based on reducing the risk of exposure to infection by implementing a closed-herd policy, purchasing animals from reliable sources and preventing contamination of foodstuffs and water. Vaccination procedures for enhancing resistance and reducing the likelihood of clinical disease are used in cattle, sheep, pigs and poultry.

Yersinia species

Although there are 18 *Yersinia* species currently described, only *Y. pestis*, *Y. enterocolitica* and *Y. pseudotuberculosis* are pathogenic for animals and humans. All three species can survive within macrophages and produce *Yersinia* outer proteins (Yops) which are important for inhibition of both phagocytosis and proinflammatory cytokine production. *Yersinia pestis*, which causes bubonic and pneumonic plague ('black death'), is more invasive than *Y. pseudotuberculosis* and *Y. enterocolitica* and possesses additional virulence factors including an antiphagocytic protein capsule and a plasminogen activator which aids systemic spread. In endemic areas, wild rodents are important reservoirs of *Y. pestis*. Fleas, especially *Xenopsylla cheopis*, the oriental rat flea, transmit infection to humans and other animals. Feline plague, caused by *Y. pestis*, usually occurs when cats ingest infected rodents. Three clinical forms of the disease are recognized: bubonic, pneumonic and septicaemic. The most common form of the disease is characterized by enlarged lymph nodes (buboes) associated with lymphatic drainage from the site of infection. Septicaemia may occur without lymphadenopathy and is potentially fatal. In endemic areas, cats and dogs should be routinely treated for fleas and rodent control measures should be implemented. *Yersinia pseudotuberculosis* causes enteric infections in a wide variety of wild and domestic animals. A septicaemic form of the disease occurs in laboratory rodents and in caged birds.

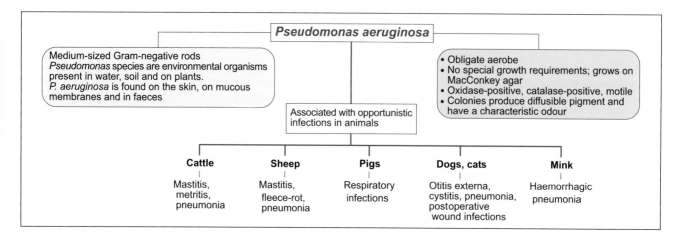

Pseudomonas species are environmental organisms which occur worldwide in water and soil, and on plants. *Pseudomonas aeruginosa* is a Gram-negative, obligate aerobe; it is motile and can produce up to four diffusible pigments. Pyocyanin (blue-green), unique to this organism, is produced by most strains and specifically identifies *P. aeruginosa*. Although *P. aeruginosa* is an environmental organism, it is also infrequently found on the skin, on mucous membranes and in faeces of some healthy animals.

Pseudomonas aeruginosa is an opportunistic pathogen and infection is preceded by a breach in host defences such as breaks in the skin, prolonged wetting or the presence of urinary or intravenous catheters. The organism produces a variety of toxins and enzymes which promote tissue invasion and damage. Attachment to host cells is mediated by fimbriae. Colonization and replication are aided by exoenzymes, extracellular slime and outer-membrane lipopolysaccharides. Tissue damage is caused by toxins such as exotoxin A, phospholipase C, proteases and cytotoxins delivered into host cells via a type III secretion system. The cytoplasmic membranes of neutrophils are damaged by a leukocidin. Host defence mechanisms against *P. aeruginosa* include opsonizing antibodies and phagocytosis by macrophages. Biofilm formation is an important virulence attribute which shields the organism from phagocytosis and from the action of antimicrobial agents.

Pseudomonas aeruginosa causes a wide range of opportunistic infections (Table 24.1). Although predisposing factors are associated with the occurrence of many of these infections, some species such as farmed mink appear to be particularly susceptible to the organism. Haemorrhagic pneumonia and septicaemia, caused by *P. aeruginosa*, occur sporadically in ranched mink with mortality rates up to 50% in some outbreaks. Bovine mastitis associated with this organism is often linked to udder washing with contaminated water, the insertion of contaminated intramammary antibiotic tubes or contaminated wipes. Fleece-rot of sheep, a condition associated with heavy or prolonged rainfall, has been reported from the UK and Australia. Maceration of the skin following water penetration of the fleece allows colonization by *P. aeruginosa*, resulting in suppurative dermatitis. Specimens suitable for laboratory examination include pus, respiratory aspirates, mid-stream urine, mastitic milk and ear swabs. Blood agar and MacConkey agar plates, inoculated with suspect material, are incubated aerobically at 37°C for 24–48 hours. On blood agar, the large flat colonies with a characteristic grape-like odour resemble those of some *Bacillus* species. Pyocyanin production is evident on both media. On MacConkey agar, lactose is not fermented.

Due to a number of diferent mechanisms, including low permeability of its outer membrane, efflux pumps and chromosomally encoded β-lactamases, *P. aeruginosa* is inherently resistant to many antimicrobial agents. Thus, susceptibility testing should always be carried out on clinical isolates.

Table 24.1 Clinical conditions in which *Pseudomonas aeruginosa* may be aetiologically involved.

Host	Disease condition
Cattle	Mastitis, metritis, pneumonia, dermatitis, enteritis (calves)
Sheep	Mastitis, fleece-rot, pneumonia, otitis media
Pigs	Respiratory infections, otitis
Horses	Genital tract infections, pneumonia, ulcerative keratitis
Dogs, cats	Otitis externa, cystitis, pneumonia, ulcerative keratitis
Mink	Haemorrhagic pneumonia, septicaemia
Chinchillas	Pneumonia, septicaemia
Reptiles (captive)	Necrotic stomatitis

Concise Review of Veterinary Microbiology, Second Edition. P.J. Quinn, B.K. Markey, F.C. Leonard, E.S. FitzPatrick and S. Fanning.
© 2016 John Wiley & Sons, Ltd. Published 2016 by John Wiley & Sons, Ltd.
Companion website: www.wiley.com/go/quinn/concise-veterinary-microbiology

Burkholderia mallei and *Burkholderia pseudomallei*

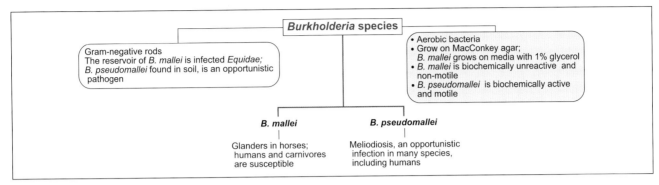

Burkholderia species, previously classified in the genus *Pseudomonas*, include *B. mallei*, the cause of glanders, and *B. pseudomallei*, the cause of melioidosis. Both diseases are zoonoses. *Burkholderia pseudomallei*, which is found in soil, occasionally infects animals and humans. Wild rodents can act as reservoirs for this organism. Although *B. mallei* can survive in the environment for up to six weeks, its reservoir is infected *Equidae*. These pathogens are Gram-negative rods which are obligate aerobes. Most isolates are oxidase-positive and catalase-positive. *Burkholderia pseudomallei* is motile but *B. mallei* is non-motile.

Glanders

This contagious disease of *Equidae*, caused by *B. mallei*, is characterized by the formation of nodules and ulcers in the respiratory tract or on the skin. Humans and carnivores are susceptible to infection. Glanders has been eradicated from most developed countries but sporadic cases of the disease occur in the Middle East, India, Pakistan, China and Mongolia with periodic outbreaks reported from Brazil in recent years also.

Transmission follows ingestion of food or water contaminated with the nasal discharges of infected *Equidae*. Less commonly, infection may be acquired by inhalation or through skin abrasions. An acute septicaemic form of the disease is characterized by fever, nasal discharge and respiratory signs. Death usually follows within weeks. Chronic disease is more common and presents as nasal, pulmonary and cutaneous forms, all of which may be observed in an affected animal. In the nasal form, ulcerative nodules develop on the mucosa of the nasal septum and turbinates. A purulent blood-stained nasal discharge is usually present. The respiratory form is characterized by respiratory distress and tubercle-like lesions in the lungs. The cutaneous form, termed farcy, is a lymphangitis in which nodules occur along the lymphatic vessels of the limbs. Ulcers develop and discharge a yellowish pus. Chronically affected horses may die after several months or may recover and continue to shed the organisms from the respiratory tract or skin. Virulence attributes include a type III secretion system, a capsule, possible antigenic variation and the ability to survive intracellularly. The presence of *B. mallei* in the host gives rise to a hypersensitivity reaction, the basis of the mallein test. The mallein intradermo-palpebral test for detection of infected animals is considered both sensitive and specific, although there are welfare concerns about its use. Serological tests such as CFT and ELISA are frequently employed for diagnostic reasons in individual animals and for surveillance purposes. The CFT is the prescribed test for international trade by the OIE (World Organization for Animal Health) but it is likely that a competitive ELISA will be approved for trade purposes once full validation is complete. A test and slaughter policy is enforced in countries where the disease is exotic.

In regions where the disease is endemic, clinical signs may be diagnostic. Specimens for laboratory diagnosis, such as discharges from lesions, must be processed in a biohazard cabinet. *Burkholderia mallei* grows on MacConkey agar without utilizing lactose; it is comparatively unreactive and non-motile.

Melioidosis

This disease, caused by *B. pseudomallei*, is endemic in tropical and subtropical regions of Asia and Australia where the organism is widely distributed in soil and water. Infection may follow ingestion, inhalation or skin contamination from environmental sources. Many animal species including humans are susceptible. Melioidosis is a chronic debilitating disease with a long incubation period. Abscesses may develop in many organs including the lungs, liver, spleen, joints and central nervous system. In horses, melioidosis can mimic glanders. *Burkholderia pseudomallei* is a facultative intracellular pathogen and is presumed to possess many virulence factors based on its genomic profile, including a type III secretion system, exoenzymes and a capsule.

Specimens for laboratory diagnosis should include pus from abscesses. A biohazard cabinet must be used for processing specimens. Identification criteria for isolates include colonial appearance on blood agar and MacConkey agar (lactose is utilized in MacConkey agar), biochemical characteristics and agglutination by specific antiserum. PCR-based tests have been developed for the identification of this pathogen and for distinguishing *B. mallei* from *B. pseudomallei*.

In countries where the disease is exotic, confirmation of infection is followed by slaughter of infected animals.

Concise Review of Veterinary Microbiology, Second Edition. P.J. Quinn, B.K. Markey, F.C. Leonard, E.S. FitzPatrick and S. Fanning.
© 2016 John Wiley & Sons, Ltd. Published 2016 by John Wiley & Sons, Ltd.
Companion website: www.wiley.com/go/quinn/concise-veterinary-microbiology

26 *Actinobacillus* species

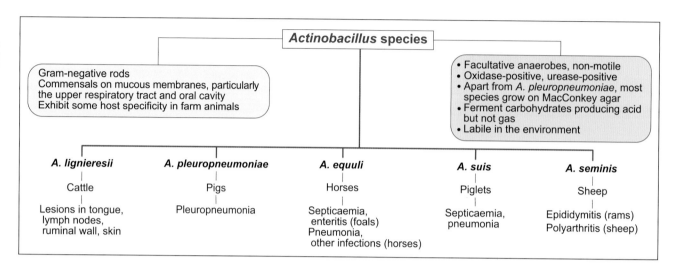

The bacteria which belong to the *Actinobacillus* species are non-motile, Gram-negative rods which occasionally have a coccobacillary appearence. Most species are urease-positive and oxidase-positive. Actinobacilli exhibit some host specificity and are mainly pathogens of farm animals. They are commensals on mucous membranes of animals, particularly in the upper respiratory tract and oral cavity; some species appear to be non-pathogenic and, in addition, virulence may differ between serotypes within species. Actinobacilli of veterinary importance are listed above. As these organisms survive for a short time in the environment, carrier animals play a major role in their transmission.

On primary isolation on blood agar, colonies of *A. lignieresii*, *A. equuli* and *A. suis* exhibit cohesive properties when touched with an inoculation loop. On MacConkey agar, *A. lignieresii*, *A. equuli* and *A. suis* grow well; *A. equuli* and *A. suis* ferment lactose, producing pink colonies (Table 26.1). Neither *A. pleuropneumoniae* nor *A. seminis* grow on MacConkey agar.

Actinobacilli can cause a variety of infections in farm animals including 'timber (wooden) tongue' in cattle, pleuropneumonia in pigs, systemic disease in foals and piglets and epididymitis in rams.

Actinobacillosis in cattle

Actinobacillosis, a chronic pyogranulomatous inflammation of soft tissues, is most often manifest clinically in cattle as induration of the tongue, referred to as 'timber tongue'. Lesions may also occur in the oesophageal groove and the retropharyngeal lymph nodes. The aetiological agent, *A. lignieresii*, is a commensal of the oral cavity and intestinal tract. The organisms enter tissues through erosions or lacerations in the mucosa and skin and consequently the disease is usually sporadic. Animals with timber tongue have difficulty in eating and drool saliva.

Involvement of the tissue of the oesophageal groove can lead to intermittent tympany. Localized pyogranulomatous lesions in the retropharyngeal lymph nodes are often found at slaughter.

Diagnosis is based on the history, induration of the tongue and a background of grazing rough pasture. Specimens for laboratory examination include pus, biopsy material and tissue from lesions at postmortem. Gram-negative rods are demonstrable in smears from exudates. Pyogranulomatous foci containing club colonies may be evident in tissue sections. Cultures incubated aerobically at 37°C for 72 hours, yield small, sticky, non-haemolytic colonies on blood agar and colonies which ferment lactose slowly in MacConkey agar. The identity of isolates can be confirmed by their biochemical profile and colonial appearance. Treatment with sodium iodide parenterally, potassium iodide orally, potentiated sulphonamides or a combination of penicillin and streptomycin is usually effective.

Pleuropneumonia of pigs

Pleuropneumonia, caused by *A. pleuropneumoniae*, can affect susceptible pigs of all ages and occurs worldwide. This highly contagious disease affects pigs under six months of age. Virulent strains of the organism possess capsules which are both antiphagocytic and immunogenic. Fimbriae and other adhesins allow organisms to attach to cells of the respiratory tract. In addition, *A. pleuropneumoniae* produces four RTX (repeat-in-toxin) toxins which damage cell membranes, iron uptake systems and, in common with other Gram-negative organisms, lipopolysaccharide.

Subclinical carrier pigs harbour the organism in their respiratory tracts and tonsils. Poor ventilation and a sudden fall in ambient temperature seem to precipitate disease outbreaks. Aerosol transmission occurs in confined groups. In outbreaks of acute disease, some pigs may be found dead while others show

Concise Review of Veterinary Microbiology, Second Edition. P.J. Quinn, B.K. Markey, F.C. Leonard, E.S. FitzPatrick and S. Fanning.
© 2016 John Wiley & Sons, Ltd. Published 2016 by John Wiley & Sons, Ltd.
Companion website: www.wiley.com/go/quinn/concise-veterinary-microbiology

Table 26.1 Differentiating features of *Actinobacillus* species.

Feature	*A. lignieresii*	*A. pleuropneumoniae*	*A. equuli*[a]	*A. suis*
Haemolysis on sheep blood agar	–	+	v	+
Colony type on blood agar	Cohesive	Not cohesive	Cohesive	Cohesive
Growth on MacConkey agar	+	–	+	+
Oxidase production	+	v	+	+
Catalase production	+	v	v	+
Urease production	+	+	+	+

[a] *A. equuli* subsp. *haemolyticus* is haemolytic on blood agar.
+, most isolates positive; v, variable reaction; –, most isolates negative.

dyspnoea, pyrexia and a disinclination to move. Blood-stained froth may be present around the nose and mouth and many pigs are cyanotic. Pregnant sows may abort. Morbidity rates may be up to 50%, with high mortality. Concurrent infections with *Pasteurella multocida* and mycoplasmas may exacerbate the condition. Areas of consolidation and necrosis are found in the lungs at postmortem examination along with fibrinous pleurisy. Blood-stained froth may be present in the trachea and bronchi. Specimens for laboratory examination should include tracheal washings or affected portions of lung tissue. Specimens, cultured on chocolate agar and blood agar, are incubated in an atmosphere of 5–10% CO_2 at 37°C for 72 hours. Identification criteria for isolates include small colonies surrounded by clear haemolysis and absence of growth on MacConkey agar. Biochemical tests may be used for identification of isolates but molecular methods are increasingly used for definitive typing of organisms. Fifteen serotypes and two biotypes are recognized; serotypes differ in virulence and geographical distribution. Serotypes within biotype 1 require factor V (nicotinamide adenine dinucleotide), supplied by chocolate agar, for growth. As cross-reactions occur between some serotypes, multiplex PCR-based methods have now been developed which are based on capsule loci and which will probably replace antibody-based testing in the future.

Chemotherapy should be based on the results of antibiotic susceptibility testing as antibiotic resistance is encountered in some strains. Polyvalent bacterins may induce protective immunity but do not prevent development of a carrier state. A subunit vaccine containing toxoids of three *A. pleuropneumoniae* toxins and capsular antigen has been developed. Predisposing factors such as poor ventilation, chilling and overcrowding should be avoided.

Sleepy foal disease

Two subspecies of *A. equuli* are recognized, subspecies *equuli* and subspecies *haemolyticus*. Subspecies *equuli* is associated with an acute, potentially fatal septicaemia of newborn foals, known as sleepy foal disease. Both subspecies may also be isolated from different clinical syndromes, such as respiratory disease, mastitis, metritis and arthritis, either as primary or secondary pathogens. *Actinobacillus equuli* is found in the reproductive and intestinal tract of mares. Foals can be infected *in utero* or after birth via the umbilicus. Affected foals are febrile and recumbent. Death usually occurs in one or two days. Foals which recover from the acute septicaemic phase may develop polyarthritis, nephritis, enteritis or pneumonia. Foals dying within 24 hours of birth have petechiation on serosal surfaces and enteritis. Those surviving for up to three days have typical pin-point suppurative foci in the kidneys. Although subspecies *haemolyticus* is known to produce an RTX toxin, other virulence factors for *A. equuli* have not been determined. Specimens should be cultured on blood agar and MacConkey agar. Identification criteria for isolates include sticky colonies on blood agar, lactose-fermenting colonies on MacConkey agar and biochemical profiles.

Other infections caused by actinobacilli

Actinobacillus suis can infect young pigs under three months of age. The disease is characterized by septicaemia and rapid death. Mortality may be up to 50% in some litters. Clinical signs include fever, respiratory distress and paddling of the forelimbs. *Actinobacillus seminis* is a common cause of epididymitis in young rams in New Zealand, Australia and South Africa. The organism is found in the prepuce, and epididymitis may follow an ascending opportunistic infection.

27 Pasteurella species, Mannheimia haemolytica and Bibersteinia trehalosi

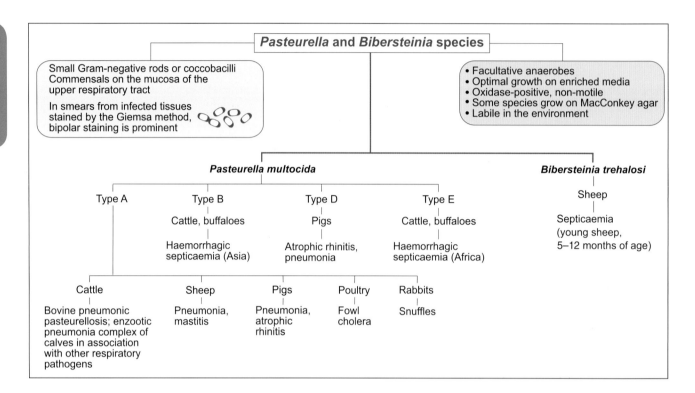

Pasteurella and Bibersteinia species

- Small Gram-negative rods or coccobacilli
  Commensals on the mucosa of the upper respiratory tract

  In smears from infected tissues stained by the Giemsa method, bipolar staining is prominent

- Facultative anaerobes
- Optimal growth on enriched media
- Oxidase-positive, non-motile
- Some species grow on MacConkey agar
- Labile in the environment

Pasteurella multocida

Type A	Type B	Type D	Type E
	Cattle, buffaloes	Pigs	Cattle, buffaloes
	Haemorrhagic septicaemia (Asia)	Atrophic rhinitis, pneumonia	Haemorrhagic septicaemia (Africa)

Cattle	Sheep	Pigs	Poultry	Rabbits
Bovine pneumonic pasteurellosis; enzootic pneumonia complex of calves in association with other respiratory pathogens	Pneumonia, mastitis	Pneumonia, atrophic rhinitis	Fowl cholera	Snuffles

Bibersteinia trehalosi

Sheep

Septicaemia (young sheep, 5–12 months of age)

Pasteurella, Bibersteinia and Mannheimia species are small, non-motile, Gram-negative rods or coccobacilli. They are oxidase-positive facultative anerobes, and most species are catalase-positive. These organisms grow best on media supplemented with blood or serum. Some species, such as Mannheimia haemolytica and Bibersteinia trehalosi, grow on MacConkey agar. In smears from infected tissues stained by the Giemsa method, pasteurellae exhibit bipolar staining. Most Pasteurella, Bibersteinia and Mannheimia species are commensals on the mucosae of the upper respiratory tracts of animals. Thus infections are frequently endogenous. Exogenous infections also occur, particularly during outbreaks of pasteurellosis in groups of animals and pathogen virulence is enhanced by animal-to-animal transmission.

Pasteurellae, Bibersteinia and Mannheimia species can be distinguished by colonial and growth characteristics and by biochemical reactions. Colonies of P. multocida are round, greyish, non-haemolytic and have a subtle characteristic odour. Colonies of M. haemolytica and B. trehalosi are haemolytic and odourless. Based on differences in their capsular polysaccharides, isolates of P. multocida are grouped into five serogroups. Twelve serotypes of M. haemolytica are recognized on the basis of extractable surface antigens. Four serotypes previously designated as T serotypes of M. haemolytica have been reclassified as B. trehalosi.

Many P. multocida infections are endogenous. The organisms may invade the tissues of immunosuppressed animals. Factors of importance in the development of disease include adhesion of the pasteurellae to the mucosa and avoidance of phagocytosis. Fimbriae may enhance mucosal attachment and the capsule, particularly in type A strains, has a major antiphagocytic role. PMT toxin, produced by serotypes A and D, is a cytotoxic protein which stimulates cell cytoskeletal rearrangements and is of importance in the pathogenesis of atrophic rhinitis in pigs. In septicaemic pasteurellosis, severe endotoxaemia and disseminated intravascular coagulation cause serious illness which can prove fatal. Four main virulence factors have been identified in strains of M. haemolytica and B. trehalosi: fimbriae, which may enhance colonization; a capsule, which enhances survival in serum; endotoxin, which can damage bovine leukocytes and endothelial cells; and leukotoxin, a pore-forming cytolysin that affects leukocyte and platelet function.

Although there are several species within the genera Pasteurella, Bibersteinia and Mannheimia, clinical infections in domestic animals are mainly attributed to P. multocida, M. haemolytica and B. trehalosi (Table 27.1). Pasteurella

Concise Review of Veterinary Microbiology, Second Edition. P.J. Quinn, B.K. Markey, F.C. Leonard, E.S. FitzPatrick and S. Fanning.
© 2016 John Wiley & Sons, Ltd. Published 2016 by John Wiley & Sons, Ltd.
Companion website: www.wiley.com/go/quinn/concise-veterinary-microbiology

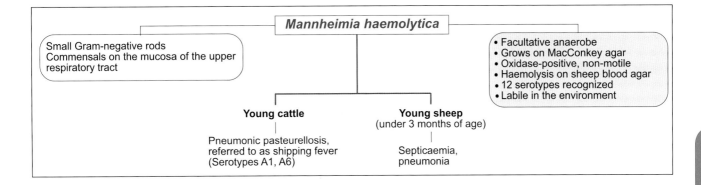

multocida has a wide host range, whereas *M. haemolytica* is largely restricted to ruminants, and *B. trehalosi* to sheep. The diseases associated with *P. multocida* infection include haemorrhagic septicaemia in ruminants, porcine atrophic rhinitis, fowl cholera and bovine pneumonic pasteurellosis. However, the main aetiological agent of bovine pneumonic pasteurellosis is *M. haemolytica* and this organism is also responsible for pneumonia in sheep and septicaemia in young lambs. Infection with *B. trehalosi* frequently results in septicaemia in older lambs.

Table 27.1 The major pathogenic *Pasteurella*, *Bibersteinia* and *Mannheimia* species, their principal hosts and associated diseases.

Hosts		Disease conditions
Pasteurella multocida		
Type A	Cattle	Associated with bovine pneumonic pasteurellosis (shipping fever); associated with enzootic pneumonia complex of calves; mastitis (rare)
	Sheep	Pneumonia, mastitis
	Pigs	Pneumonia, atrophic rhinitis
	Poultry	Fowl cholera
	Rabbits	Snuffles
	Other animal species	Pneumonia following stress
Type B	Cattle, buffaloes	Haemorrhagic septicaemia (Asia)
Type D	Pigs	Atrophic rhinitis, pneumonia
Type E	Cattle, buffaloes	Haemorrhagic septicaemia (Africa)
Type F	Poultry, especially turkeys	Fowl cholera
Mannheimia haemolytica	Cattle	Bovine pneumonic pasteurellosis (shipping fever)
	Sheep	Septicaemia (under 3 months of age); pneumonia; gangrenous mastitis
Bibersteinia trehalosi	Sheep	Septicaemia (5–12 months of age)

Bovine pneumonic pasteurellosis (shipping fever) occurs most commonly in young animals within weeks of being subjected to severe stress such as transportation, assembly in feedlots and close confinement. The condition is associated with *M. haemolytica*, principally serotype A1, although recent surveys have demonstrated the increasing importance of serotype A6 in Europe and elsewhere. Several respiratory viruses including parainfluenzavirus 3, bovine herpesvirus 1 and bovine respiratory syncytial virus may predispose to bacterial invasion. Clinical signs include sudden onset of fever, depression, anorexia, tachypnoea and serous nasal discharge. In mixed infections, there is usually a marked cough and ocular discharge. At postmortem, the cranial lobes of the lungs are red, swollen and consolidated. Isolation of *M. haemolytica*, often in association with other pathogens, from bronchoalveolar lavage fluid or affected lung tissue is confirmatory.

Outbreaks of ovine pneumonic pasteurellosis are usually caused by *M. haemolytica*, a commensal of the upper respiratory tract in a proportion of healthy sheep. Predisposing factors are poorly understood and flock outbreaks usually start with sudden deaths of some sheep and acute respiratory distress in others.

Septicaemic pasteurellosis in animals between 5 and 12 months of age is usually associated with *B. trehalosi* infection. *Bibersteinia trehalosi* is found in the tonsillar tissues of carrier sheep. As with most other pasteurella infections, clinical disease may be precipitated by a range of predisposing factors including transportation.

Toxigenic strains of *P. multocida* type D or A cause a severe progressive form of atrophic rhinitis in pigs. These toxigenic *P. multocida* isolates are designated AR+ (atrophic rhinitis-positive) strains. Early signs, usually encountered in pigs between three and eight weeks of age, include excessive lacrimation, sneezing and, occasionally, epistaxis. As the disease progresses, a distinct lateral deviation of the snout may develop. Affected pigs are usually underweight and damage to the turbinate bones may predispose to secondary bacterial infections of the lower respiratory tract.

Vaccines have been developed for the control of many of the diseases caused by the pasteurellae and *Mannheimia* species. The efficacy of some vaccines remains to be determined.

28 Histophilus, Haemophilus and Avibacterium species

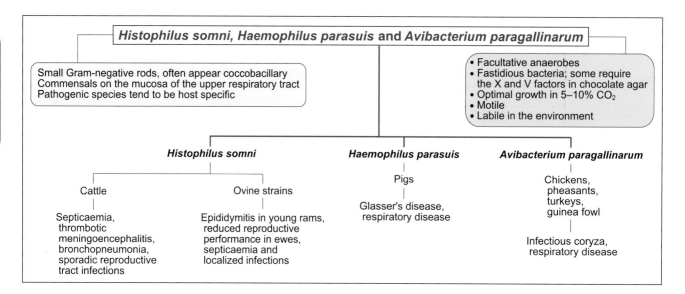

Bacteria which belong to the genera *Histophilus*, *Haemophilus* and *Avibacterium* are small Gram-negative rods which often appear coccobacillary. These motile facultative anaerobes do not grow on MacConkey agar. They are fastidious bacteria; *Haemophilus parasuis* and *Avibacterium paragallinarum* require growth factor V (nicotinamide adenine dinucleotide, NAD). Optimal growth for all these species occurs in an atmosphere of 5–10% CO_2 on chocolate agar, which supplies both X (haemin) and V factors although for *Histophilus somni*, X and V factors are not absolute requirements for growth. Small transparent colonies are formed after incubation for 48 hours. PCR-based tests have been developed for detection and identification of these pathogens and are of particular value when testing clinical specimens of poor quality or if laboratory expertise in culture of these fastidious bacteria is lacking. Organisms in these genera are commensals on the mucous membranes and survive for short periods away from their hosts.

In common with other members of the family *Pasteurellaceae*, a number of serotypes of each of these organisms has been identified. Although some serotypes appear less virulent than others, there is no clear correlation between serotype and pathogenicity.

Histophilus somni is part of the normal bacterial flora of the male and female bovine genital tracts and it can also colonize the upper respiratory tract. Environmental stress factors contribute to the development of clinical disease. This organism is more resistant in the environment than *Haemophilus* species. *Histophilus somni* can adhere firmly to several host cell types, although the exact mechanisms of adherence are not clear. The lipo-oligosaccharide (LOS) of *H. somni* is recognized as a major virulence factor for two reasons: its toxic lipid A component and the organism's ability to alter the structure of its LOS results in phase variation and evasion of the host immune response. Because septicaemia is commonly associated with *H. somni* infection, many organ systems may be involved. Thrombotic meningoencephalitis (TME), a common consequence of septicaemia, is encountered sporadically in young cattle within a short period of time following introduction into feedlots. Some animals may be found dead and others may present with high fever and depression. Sudden death

Table 28.1 Disease conditions caused by *Histophilus somni*, *Haemophilus parasuis* and *Avibacterium paragallinarum*.

Organism	Hosts	Disease conditions
Histophilus somni	Cattle	Septicaemia, thrombotic meningoencephalitis, bronchopneumonia (in association with other pathogens), sporadic reproductive tract infections
Histophilus somni (ovine strains)	Sheep	Epididymitis in young rams; vulvitis, mastitis and reduced reproductive performance in ewes; septicaemia, arthritis, meningitis and pneumonia in lambs
Haemophilus parasuis	Pigs	Glasser's disease, secondary invader in respiratory disease
Avibacterium paragallinarum	Chickens, pheasants, turkeys, guinea fowl	Infectious coryza Respiratory disease

Concise Review of Veterinary Microbiology, Second Edition. P.J. Quinn, B.K. Markey, F.C. Leonard, E.S. FitzPatrick and S. Fanning.
© 2016 John Wiley & Sons, Ltd. Published 2016 by John Wiley & Sons, Ltd.
Companion website: www.wiley.com/go/quinn/concise-veterinary-microbiology

due to myocarditis has also been described. Severe neurological signs in young feedlot cattle may be indicative of TME. *Histophilus somni* is one of the pathogens commonly isolated from the enzootic calf pneumonia complex. Definitive confirmation of the involvement of *H. somni* in bovine infections requires the isolation and identification of the pathogen from cerebrospinal fluid or postmortem lesion material.

Glasser's disease, caused by *H. parasuis*, manifests as polyserositis and leptomeningitis, usually affecting pigs from weaning up to 12 weeks of age. Some cases present as polyarthritis and some strains produce septicaemic disease. *Haemophilus parasuis* is part of the normal flora of the upper respiratory tract of pigs. The presence of maternally derived antibodies prevents the development of clinical signs. Previously, Glasser's disease was considered a sporadic disease of two- to four-week-old piglets subjected to stressful environmental conditions. However, modern, highly intensive pig production methods have resulted in this disease becoming an animal health problem of major economic importance worldwide. Virulence mechanisms of *H. parasuis* are poorly characterized but adhesion to host cells, LOS and capsule formation are considered important in disease development. Clinical signs develop two to seven days following exposure to stress factors such as weaning or transportation. Anorexia, pyrexia, lameness, recumbency and convulsions are features of the disease. Pigs may die suddenly without showing signs of illness. Postmortem findings may include fibrinous polyserositis, polyarthritis and meningitis. Isolation and identification of *H. parasuis* from joint fluid, heart blood, cerebrospinal fluid or postmortem tissues of a pig shortly after death are confirmatory. Commercially available bacterins or autogenous bacterins may stimulate serotype-specific protective immunity.

Avibacterium paragallinarum causes infectious coryza in chickens from approximately four weeks after hatching. In addition to swelling of the infraorbital sinuses, tracheitis, bronchitis and airsacculitis may be present. Isolation of the organism from clinical lesions is confirmatory and serology may be used to confirm the presence of *A. paragallinarum* in a flock. Vaccines are available for use in control programmes.

29 *Taylorella equigenitalis*

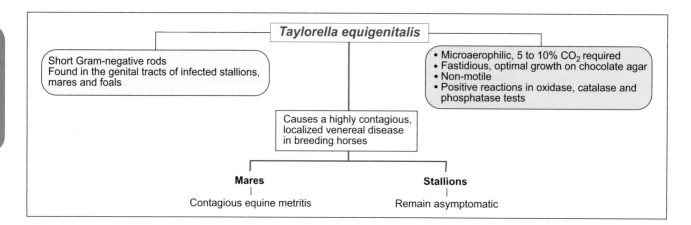

Taylorella equigenitalis

Short Gram-negative rods
Found in the genital tracts of infected stallions, mares and foals

- Microaerophilic, 5 to 10% CO_2 required
- Fastidious, optimal growth on chocolate agar
- Non-motile
- Positive reactions in oxidase, catalase and phosphatase tests

Causes a highly contagious, localized venereal disease in breeding horses

Mares
Contagious equine metritis

Stallions
Remain asymptomatic

This organism, *Taylorella equigenitalis*, is a short, non-motile, Gram-negative rod which gives positive reactions in catalase, oxidase and phosphatase tests. It is microaerophilic, slow-growing and highly fastidious, requiring chocolate agar and 5–10% CO_2 for optimal growth. Although the bacterium is not dependent on X or V factors, availability of factor X stimulates growth. *Taylorella equigenitalis*, the cause of contagious equine metritis (CEM), appears to infect only *Equidae*. The organism is found in the genital tract of stallions, mares and foals. Contagious equine metritis is a highly contagious, localized venereal disease characterized by mucopurulent vulval discharge and temporary infertility in mares. In the non-thoroughbred horse populations in parts of mainland Europe, CEM is thought to be endemic, with periodic spillover into the thoroughbred horse population. The condition is economically important because it disrupts breeding programmes on thoroughbred stud farms. Infected stallions and mares are the main reservoirs of infection. Transmission of the bacterium usually occurs during coitus, although infection may be transferred by contaminated instruments and is increasingly associated with the use of artificial insemination. Foals born to infected dams may acquire infection *in utero* or during parturition.

Infected stallions and a minority of infected mares remain asymptomatic. Most affected mares develop a copious mucopurulent vulval discharge without systemic disturbance within a few days of service by a carrier stallion. The discharge may continue for up to two weeks and infected mares remain infertile for several weeks. Although some mares recover without treatment, up to 25% of mares remain carriers. Infection does not confer protective immunity and reinfection can occur. After introduction into the uterus, the pathogenic organisms replicate and induce an acute endometritis.

Diagnosis is based on the history of individual animals and laboratory tests. A copious mucopurulent vulval discharge two to seven days after service may indicate the presence of CEM. Specimens for bacteriology should be collected before and during the breeding season. Swabs from mares should be taken from the clitoral fossa and sinuses, and from the endometrium at oestrus using a double-guarded swab. Swabs from stallions and teaser stallions are taken from the urethra, urethral fossa and penile sheath. Chocolate agar-based media are suitable for the isolation of *T. equigenitalis*. Inoculated plates are incubated in an atmosphere of 5 to 10% CO_2 for four to seven days. Identification criteria for isolates include small yellowish-grey colonies giving positive catalase, oxidase and phosphatase tests. A slide agglutination test and the fluorescent antibody technique may be used to confirm the identity of the isolate. A PCR technique has been developed for detecting *T. equigenitalis* in specimens. Strain typing techniques include pulsed-field gel electrophoresis-based methods and multi-locus sequence typing. If CEM is diagnosed on a stud farm, all breeding services should cease immediately.

Elimination of *T. equigenitalis* from both mares and stallions can be achieved by washing the external genitalia with a 2% solution of chlorhexidine, combined with local application of antimicrobial drugs. In many countries with an advanced thoroughbred industry, contagious equine metritis is a notifiable disease. A vaccine for the control of this disease is not available.

Concise Review of Veterinary Microbiology, Second Edition. P.J. Quinn, B.K. Markey, F.C. Leonard, E.S. FitzPatrick and S. Fanning.
© 2016 John Wiley & Sons, Ltd. Published 2016 by John Wiley & Sons, Ltd.
Companion website: www.wiley.com/go/quinn/concise-veterinary-microbiology

30 Moraxella bovis

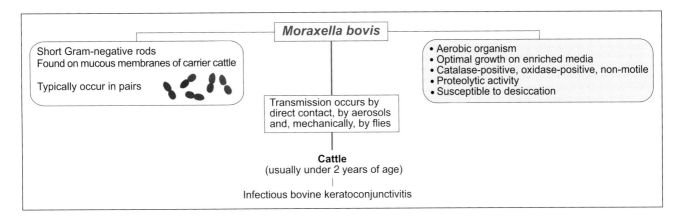

Moraxella bovis

Short Gram-negative rods
Found on mucous membranes of carrier cattle

Typically occur in pairs

Transmission occurs by direct contact, by aerosols and, mechanically, by flies

- Aerobic organism
- Optimal growth on enriched media
- Catalase-positive, oxidase-positive, non-motile
- Proteolytic activity
- Susceptible to desiccation

Cattle
(usually under 2 years of age)

Infectious bovine keratoconjunctivitis

Although there are a number of species within the genus *Moraxella*, the principal pathogenic species is *Moraxella bovis*. This organism occurs as short, plump, Gram-negative rods or cocci, typically in pairs. *Moraxella bovis* is non-motile, aerobic and usually catalase-positive and oxidase-positive. Growth of this proteolytic organism is enhanced by the addition of blood or serum to media. When isolated from cases of infectious bovine keratoconjunctivitis, virulent strains are fimbriate, haemolytic and grow into the agar. *Moraxella bovis* is found on mucous membranes of carrier animals. The organism, which is susceptible to desiccation, is short-lived in the environment.

Infectious bovine keratoconjunctivitis (IBK), sometimes referred to as 'pink eye', is a highly contagious condition, caused by *M. bovis*, affecting the superficial structures of the eyes. Factors which predispose to IBK include fly activity, ocular irritants such as dust, grass seeds, wind and UV light and concurrent infections. Affected animals are usually under two years of age and there appears to be an age-related immunity. Transmission can occur by direct contact, by aerosols and mechanically, by flies. The principal virulence factors of *M. bovis* are an RTX toxin and fimbriae; strains lacking either of these pathogenic attributes are avirulent. In spite of lacrimal secretions and blinking, fimbriae allow adherence of organisms to the cornea. The RTX toxin is a cytotoxin and is responsible for the haemolysis observed when the organism is cultured on blood agar.

Isolates from carrier animals are often non-haemolytic and non-fimbriate but reversion to virulence can occur. The disease initially manifests as blepharospasm, conjunctivitis and lacrimation. Progression of the condition through keratitis to corneal ulceration, opacity and abscessation may occasionally lead to panophthalmitis and permanent blindness. In most mild cases, the cornea heals within a few weeks, although there may be permanent scarring of the structure. The disease, which characteristically affects a number of animals in a herd, can be diagnosed by its clinical presentation and confirmed by isolation and identification of the pathogen in lacrimal discharges. The organism can also be detected using PCR-based methods and these methods can also be used to differentiate *M. bovis* from non-pathogenic moraxellae found on the eyes and mucous membranes of cattle.

Antimicrobial therapy should be administered subconjunctivally or topically early in the disease. Vaccines based on fimbrial antigens, which are available commercially in some countries, are of uncertain efficacy. Vaccines incorporating both cytotoxin and fimbriae have been developed and may provide enhanced protection. Management-related methods are important in the control of IBK. These include isolation of affected animals, reduction of exposure to mechanical irritants, the use of insecticidal ear tags and the control of concurrent diseases.

Concise Review of Veterinary Microbiology, Second Edition. P.J. Quinn, B.K. Markey, F.C. Leonard, E.S. FitzPatrick and S. Fanning.
© 2016 John Wiley & Sons, Ltd. Published 2016 by John Wiley & Sons, Ltd.
Companion website: www.wiley.com/go/quinn/concise-veterinary-microbiology

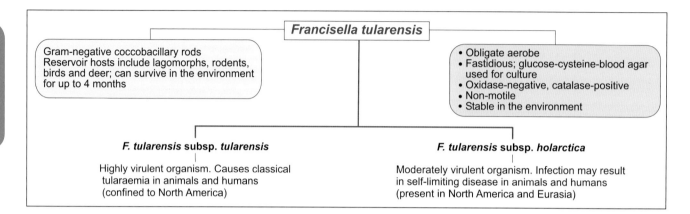

Francisella tularensis

Gram-negative coccobacillary rods
Reservoir hosts include lagomorphs, rodents, birds and deer; can survive in the environment for up to 4 months

- Obligate aerobe
- Fastidious; glucose-cysteine-blood agar used for culture
- Oxidase-negative, catalase-positive
- Non-motile
- Stable in the environment

F. tularensis subsp. tularensis

Highly virulent organism. Causes classical tularaemia in animals and humans (confined to North America)

F. tularensis subsp. holarctica

Moderately virulent organism. Infection may result in self-limiting disease in animals and humans (present in North America and Eurasia)

Bacteria within the genus *Francisella* are poorly staining Gram-negative rods with a coccobacillary appearance. These fastidious bacteria which are obligate aerobes, non-motile and oxidase-negative, require the addition of cysteine to blood agar for growth. There are a number of species within the genus *Francisella* but *F. tularensis* subsp. *tularensis* and *F. tularensis* subsp. *holarctica* are significant pathogens of animals and humans. The highly virulent *F. tularensis* subsp. *tularensis* occurs only in North America. *Francisella tularensis* subsp. *holarctica* is found in Asia and North America and is considerably less virulent than subspecies *tularensis*. Reservoir hosts of *F. tularensis* include lagomorphs, rodents, birds and deer. Many species of blood-sucking arthropods can transmit infection mechanically but ticks, in which transovarial transmission occurs, are also thought to act as reservoirs of infection. Infection can be acquired through biting arthropods, by inhalation or ingestion. Humans may acquire infection through handling infected lagomorphs and through bites or scratches inflicted by infected cats.

Outbreaks of tularaemia have been reported in sheep and infection of other domestic animals, notably cats, may also occur. *Francisella tularensis* is a facultative intracellular pathogen and invades a number of different cell types including phagocytes and endothelial and epithelial cells. The organism escapes from the phagosome and multiplies in the cytosol. When infected host cells reach the liver and spleen, fever, depression, inappetence and signs of septicaemia become evident. The onset of tularaemia in humans is typically sudden with a high temperature, fatigue and an indolent skin ulcer at the site of introduction of the organism. Enlargement of regional lymph nodes and septicaemia may follow. The pattern of disease in cats resembles that in humans. Infection with subspecies *holarctica* causes mild disease or subclinical infection. Isolation procedures for *F. tularensis* must be carried out in a biohazard cabinet. PCR procedures for detection of the organism have been described. A rising antibody titre in suspect animals is indicative of an active infection.

Care is required when handling suspect animals or materials from infected animals.

Concise Review of Veterinary Microbiology, Second Edition. P.J. Quinn, B.K. Markey, F.C. Leonard, E.S. FitzPatrick and S. Fanning.
© 2016 John Wiley & Sons, Ltd. Published 2016 by John Wiley & Sons, Ltd.
Companion website: www.wiley.com/go/quinn/concise-veterinary-microbiology

32 *Lawsonia intracellularis*

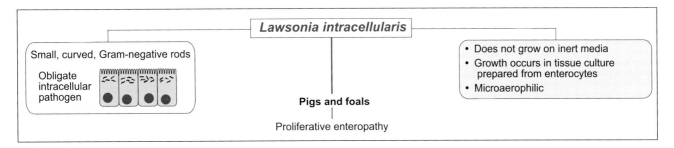

Lawsonia intracellularis, a slender, curved, Gram-negative rod, has not been grown in cell-free media. It is a microaerophilic, obligate, intracellular pathogen which is aetiologically implicated in proliferative enteropathy of pigs and foals and other animals. Some degree of host species adaptation occurs. *Lawsonia intracellularis* grows intracellularly in pig enterocytes and infected animals excrete small numbers in their faeces. It has been recovered from the tissues of foals and other animals affected with proliferative enteropathy. Subclinically affected pigs and foals and wildlife which share their environment with clinically affected animals may have a role in perpetuating infection on farms.

Infection of enterocytes with *L. intracellularis* induces proliferation of these cells with the development of adenomatous and inflammatory lesions in the terminal ileum, caecum and colon. The exact mechanism of infection has not been established but the organism apparently attaches and enters epithelial cells followed by release from the endosome with multiplication taking place in the cell cytoplasm. Gnotobiotic pigs, which are devoid of intestinal flora, do not develop the disease when dosed with *L. intracellularis* unless they are pre-dosed with porcine intestinal flora. Common intestinal organisms probably provide the appropriate microenvironmental conditions required for the colonization and proliferation of *L. intracellularis*. In addition, active proliferation and differentiation of crypt cells, as occurs at weaning, appears to be associated with lesion production.

Clinical signs, which occur most frequently in weaned pigs from 6 to 20 weeks of age, range from chronic intermittent diarrhoea with reduction in weight gain to acute haemorrhagic enteropathy; the latter syndrome is observed more commonly in young adult animals. Although sudden deaths may occur in severely affected pigs, most animals with the milder form of the disease recover without treatment. Lesions in the ileum, caecum and colon include thickening of the wall, mucosal necrosis and, in severe cases, clotted blood in the lumen. Enlargement of the mesenteric lymph nodes is a feature of the disease. In foals, clinical signs are observed after weaning and include rapid weight loss with diarrhoea and colic, depression, fever and subcutaneous ventral oedema.

Lawsonia intracellularis can be demonstrated in faeces or ileal mucosa by immunofluorescence or by PCR. Serological tests include indirect fluorescent antibody tests, ELISA and immunoperoxidase monolayer assays.

Antimicrobial agents such as tylosin or tiamulin may be used therapeutically in feed or water. A live attenuated vaccine for use in pigs is now available in many countries and is effective in reducing clinical signs of disease.

Concise Review of Veterinary Microbiology, Second Edition. P.J. Quinn, B.K. Markey, F.C. Leonard, E.S. FitzPatrick and S. Fanning.
© 2016 John Wiley & Sons, Ltd. Published 2016 by John Wiley & Sons, Ltd.
Companion website: www.wiley.com/go/quinn/concise-veterinary-microbiology

33 *Bordetella* species

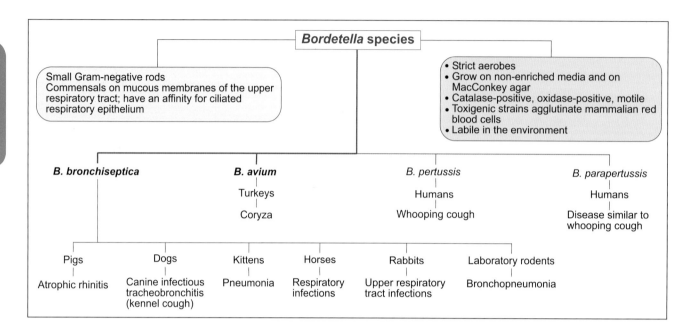

The genus *Bordetella* contains eight species, four of which, *B. pertussis*, *B. parapertussis*, *B. bronchiseptica* and *B. avium*, are significant human or animal pathogens. *Bordetella pertussis*, the type species, and *B. parapertussis* are human pathogens associated with whooping cough in children. *Bordetella bronchiseptica* infects a wide range of animal species, while *B. avium* is a pathogen of avian species. The bordetellae are occasional pathogens with an affinity for ciliated respiratory epithelium. *Bordetella bronchiseptica* and *B. avium* are small Gram-negative rods with a coccobacillary appearance. They are catalase-positive, oxidase-positive aerobes and are motile peritrichous bacteria. They derive their energy mainly from oxidation of amino acids. They are commensals on the mucous membranes of the upper respiratory tract of animals and their survival time in the environment is short.

Bordetellae can be identified by their growth characteristics, biochemical reactions and by their ability to agglutinate red blood cells (Table 33.1). *Bordetella avium* requires differentiation from *Alcaligenes faecalis*, which is non-pathogenic. Bordetellae exhibit phase changes, thought to be associated with loss of a capsule-like structure. These changes, which correlate with virulence, are identifiable by colonial appearance. Virulence is mediated by several factors including a filamentous haemagglutinin, pertactin and fimbriae which facilitate attachment to cilia of the upper respiratory tract. Bordetellae also produce a number of toxins, including an adenylate cyclase haemolysin with antiphagocytic activity, a tracheal cytotoxin and a dermonecrotic toxin responsible for nasal turbinate atrophy in infected pigs.

Clinical signs associated with bordetellae usually relate to upper respiratory tract infection. Young animals are more susceptible than adults and stress predisposes to outbreaks of disease. Canine infectious tracheobronchitis (kennel cough) is one of the most prevalent respiratory complexes of dogs. The microbial pathogens implicated in kennel cough include *B. bronchiseptica*, canine parainfluenzavirus 2 and canine adenovirus 2. Transmission occurs through respiratory secretions, either by direct contact or by aerosols. Indirect transmission via feed and water bowls can occur in kennels if hygiene is poor. Clinical signs, which include coughing, gagging or retching, develop within days of exposure. The disease, which may persist for up to 14 days, is usually self-limiting. Diagnosis is based on a history of recent exposure to carrier dogs and characteristic clinical signs. Detection of the associated pathogens can be performed by PCR-based techniques and, in the case of *B. bronchiseptica*, by culture. Selective media for the isolation of bordetellae have been developed. Carriage rates of *B. bronchiseptica* are high in healthy dogs and in the absence of clinical signs isolation of the organism may not be of diagnostic significance. Modified live vaccines decrease the severity of clinical signs but may not prevent infection.

In pigs, infection with *B. bronchiseptica* may facilitate colonization by toxigenic *Pasteurella multocida* type D, with the subsequent development of severe atrophic rhinitis and distortion of the snout. Infection is usually transmitted by direct contact, both from the sow to her piglets and through mixing of piglets at weaning. Overstocking and poor ventilation can contribute to the development of atrophic rhinitis. In addition to respiratory

Concise Review of Veterinary Microbiology, Second Edition. P.J. Quinn, B.K. Markey, F.C. Leonard, E.S. FitzPatrick and S. Fanning.
© 2016 John Wiley & Sons, Ltd. Published 2016 by John Wiley & Sons, Ltd.
Companion website: www.wiley.com/go/quinn/concise-veterinary-microbiology

Table 33.1 Differentiating features of *Bordetella bronchiseptica, B. avium* and *Alcaligenes faecalis.*

Feature	B. bronchiseptica	B. avium	Alcaligenes faecalis[a]
Colonial characteristics on:			
Sheep blood agar	Haemolysis	No haemolysis	No haemolysis
MacConkey agar	Pale, pinkish hue	Pale, pinkish hue	Pale
Oxidase production	+	+	+
Catalase production	+	+	+
Urease production	+	−	−
Utilization of carbon exclusively from:			
Citrate	+	+	+
Malonate	−	−	+
Nitrate reduction	+	−	−
Motility	+	+	+
Haemagglutinating activity of virulent strains	Agglutination of ovine and bovine red blood cells	Agglutination of guinea-pig red blood cells	−

[a]Not of veterinary significance, but may require differentiation from bordetellae.

signs, growth rates are affected and economic losses may be significant. Vaccines containing *B. bronchiseptica* bacterin and *P. multocida* toxoid are available for prevention of the disease in pigs. Atrophic rhinitis-free herds can be set up by depopulating and restocking with specific pathogen-free animals.

Bordetella avium causes coryza, rhinotracheitis and sinusitis in young turkey poults. Morbidity may be high but mortality is usually low in the absence of secondary infection by opportunistic pathogens such as *E. coli*. Buildings which have housed infected turkeys should be thoroughly cleaned and disinfected following a disease outbreak. If there are recurring outbreaks of disease in a turkey flock, vaccination should be considered.

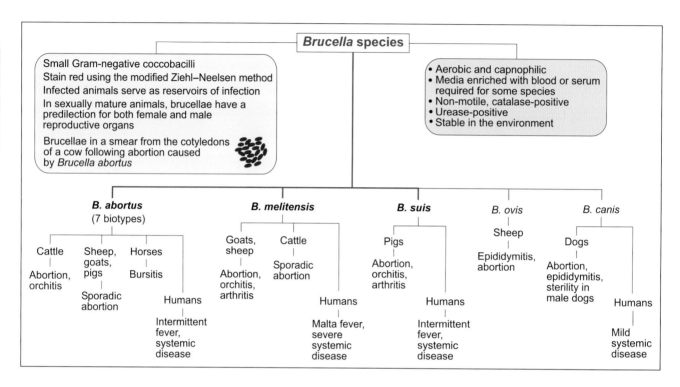

Brucella species are small, non-motile, coccobacillary, Gram-negative bacteria. As they are not decolorized by 0.5% acetic acid in the modified Ziehl–Neelsen (MZN) technique, they are classed as MZN-positive. Growth of brucellae is enhanced in an atmosphere of 5–10% CO_2. Media enriched with blood or serum are required for culturing *B. abortus* and *B. ovis*. Most brucellae have a tropism for both female and male reproductive organs in sexually mature animals and each *Brucella* species tends to infect a particular animal species. Infected animals serve as reservoirs of infection which often persists indefinitely. Organisms shed by infected animals can remain viable in a moist environment for many months. However, indirect transmission is not of major epidemiological importance; the primary route of transmission is through ingestion of organisms from aborted foetuses and post-abortion or post-calving discharges. Venereal transmission is significant with some *Brucella* species.

Brucella species are differentiated by colonial appearance, biochemical tests, specific cultural requirements and growth inhibition by dyes. In addition, agglutination with monospecific sera and susceptibility to bacteriophages are employed for definitive identification. Many of the species can be divided into a number of biovars or biotypes and there may be important epidemiological differences between them. Biovars of *B. suis*, in particular, infect a wide range of species and are found in well-defined geographical regions.

Virulent brucellae, when engulfed by phagocytes on mucous membranes, are transported to regional lymph nodes. Brucellae persist and multiply within macrophages but not within neutrophils and can also replicate in placental trophoblastic cells of pregnant animals. Both smooth and rough forms of the organism exist, the latter having defective LPS. The O-antigen of intact LPS has an important role in defence against intracellular killing; rough forms of brucellae cannot prevent fusion of lysosomes with vacuoles containing brucellae. Thus, inhibition of phagosome–lysosome function is a major mechanism for intracellular survival and an important determinant of bacterial virulence. Intermittent bacteraemia results in spread and localization in the reproductive organs and associated glands in sexually mature animals. Erythritol, a polyhydric alcohol which acts as a growth factor for brucellae, is present in high concentrations in the placentae of cattle, sheep, goats and pigs. This growth factor is also found in other organs such as the mammary gland and epididymis, which are targets for brucellae. Ten *Brucella* species are described, including species isolated from wildlife and marine mammals. Five of these species are of clinical significance in domestic animals and humans (Table 34.1). Although each *Brucella* species has its own natural host, *B. abortus*, *B. melitensis* and biotypes of *B. suis* can infect species of animals other than their preferred hosts.

The diagnosis of brucellosis depends on serological testing and on detection of the infecting *Brucella* species, either

Concise Review of Veterinary Microbiology, Second Edition. P.J. Quinn, B.K. Markey, F.C. Leonard, E.S. FitzPatrick and S. Fanning.
© 2016 John Wiley & Sons, Ltd. Published 2016 by John Wiley & Sons, Ltd.
Companion website: www.wiley.com/go/quinn/concise-veterinary-microbiology

Table 34.1 *Brucella* species of veterinary importance, their host range and the clinical significance of infection.

Brucella species	Usual host / Clinical significance	Species occasionally infected / Clinical significance
B. abortus	Cattle / Abortion, orchitis	Sheep, goats, pigs / Sporadic abortion Horses / Bursitis Humans / Intermittent fever, systemic disease
B. melitensis	Goats, sheep / Abortion, orchitis, arthritis; organisms present in milk	Humans / Malta fever, severe systemic disease Cattle / Sporadic abortion, brucellae in milk
B. suis, biovars 1, 2 and 3	Pigs / Abortion, orchitis, arthritis, spondylitis, infertility	Humans (biovars 1 or 3) / Intermittent fever, systemic disease
B. ovis	Sheep / Epididymitis in rams, sporadic abortion in ewes	
B. canis	Dogs / Abortion, epididymitis, discospondylitis, sterility in male dogs	Humans / Mild systemic disease

by culture or molecular methods. Care should be taken during collection and transportation of specimens, which should be processed in a biohazard cabinet. Specimens for laboratory examination should relate to the specific clinical condition encountered. MZN-stained smears from specimens, particularly cotyledons, foetal abomasal contents and uterine discharges, often reveal MZN-positive coccobacilli. In specimens containing cells, the organisms appear in clusters. A nutritious medium such as Columbia agar, supplemented with 5% serum and appropriate antimicrobial agents, is used for isolation. Most brucellae are capnophilic and accordingly plates are incubated at 37°C in 5–10% CO_2 for up to five days.

Molecular tests for identification and differentiation of *Brucella* species are available also. The genus is remarkably homogenous and thus identification of targets that vary between species can be more difficult than with other bacterial genera. Nevertheless, a number of PCR-based techniques are available.

Serological tests are used for regulating international trade in animals and for identifying infected herds, flocks or individual animals in national eradication schemes. ELISA, brucella complement fixation tests and fluorescence polarization assay are prescribed tests for international trade. Brucellae share antigens with some other Gram-negative bacteria such as *Yersinia enterocolitica* serotype O:9 and consequently cross-reactions can occur in agglutination tests.

With the exception of canine brucellosis, infections in animals are not treated with antimicrobial drugs. Control is based on serological testing for identification of infected animals, culling of positive reactors and vaccination. Antimicrobial therapy is employed in humans and antimicrobial resistance has not yet emerged as a problem with brucellae. Absence of plasmids and phages in these organisms may limit the opportunity for horizontal gene transfer.

Bovine brucellosis

Infection of cattle with *Brucella abortus* was formerly worldwide in distribution. National eradication programmes have reduced bovine brucellosis to low levels in many developed countries. Although acquired most often by ingestion, infection can occasionally follow venereal contact, penetration through skin abrasions, inhalation or transplacental transmission. Abortion storms may be encountered in herds with a high percentage of susceptible pregnant cows. Abortion usually occurs after the fifth month of gestation and subsequent pregnancies are usually carried to term. Large numbers of brucellae are excreted in foetal fluids for about two to four weeks following an abortion and at subsequent parturitions, although infected calves appear normal. Infection in calves is of limited duration, in contrast to cows, in which infection of the mammary glands and associated lymph nodes persists for many years. Brucellae may be excreted intermittently in milk for a number of years. In bulls, the structures targeted include seminal vesicles, ampullae, testicles and epididymides.

In affected herds, brucellosis can result in decreased fertility, reduced milk production, abortions in susceptible replacement animals and testicular degeneration in bulls. Abortion is a consequence of placentitis involving both cotyledons and intercotyledonary tissues. In bulls, necrotizing orchitis occasionally results in localized fibrotic lesions.

Although clinical signs are not specific for bovine brucellosis, abortions in first-calf heifers and replacement animals may suggest the presence of the disease. Clusters of MZN-positive coccobacilli may be evident in smears of cotyledons and MZN-positive organisms may also be detected in foetal abomasal contents and uterine discharges. Isolation and identification of *B. abortus* is confirmatory. Identification criteria for isolates include colonial appearance, MZN-positive organisms, bacterial cell agglutination with high-titre antiserum and rapid urease activity. A range of serological tests, varying in sensitivity and specificity, is available for the identification of infected animals (Table 34.2). Molecular methods such as PCR-based techniques for the detection of brucellae in tissues and fluids have been developed. National eradication schemes are based on the detection and slaughter of infected cattle. Three types of attenuated vaccines are used in cattle: strain 19 (S19) vaccine, adjuvanted 45/20 vaccine and RB51 vaccine. The S19 vaccine is administered to female calves up to five months of age. Vaccination of mature animals leads to persistent antibody titres. The 45/20 bacterin has been used in some national eradication schemes but, being a bacterin, is less effective in protecting

Table 34.2 Tests used for the diagnosis of bovine brucellosis using milk or serum.

Test	Comments
Brucella milk ring test	Conducted on bulk milk samples for monitoring infections in dairy herds. Sensitive but may not be reliable in large herds due to a dilution effect
Rose Bengal plate test	Useful screening test. Antigen suspension is adjusted to pH 3.6, allowing agglutination by IgG1 antibodies. Qualitative test only, positive results require confirmation by CFT or ELISA
Complement fixation test (CFT)	Widely accepted confirmatory test for individual animals
Indirect ELISA	Reliable screening and confirmatory test
Competitive ELISA (using monoclonal antibodies)	Highly specific test; capable of detecting all immunoglobulin classes and can be used to differentiate infected animals from S19-vaccinated cattle
Serum agglutination test (SAT)	A tube agglutination test which lacks specificity and sensitivity; IgG1 antibodies may not be detected, leading to false-negative results
Antiglobulin test	Sensitive test for detecting non-agglutinating antibodies not detected by the SAT
Fluorescence polarization assay	Rapid test (results within minutes) which can detect all immunoglobulin classes. The test is based on detection of antibody which, if present in test serum, binds to a fragment of the O polysaccharide of *Brucella* labelled with fluorescein isothiocyanate

against this intracellular pathogen. Even when administered to adult animals, this vaccine does not induce persistent antibody titres. The RB51 strain is a stable, rough mutant which induces good protection against abortion without stimulating serological responses detectable in conventional brucellosis surveillance programmes.

Caprine and ovine brucellosis

Brucellosis in goats and sheep, caused by *B. melitensis*, is most commonly encountered in countries around the Mediterranean littoral and in the Middle East, central Asia and parts of South America. Goats, in which the disease is more severe and protracted, tend to be more susceptible to infection than sheep.

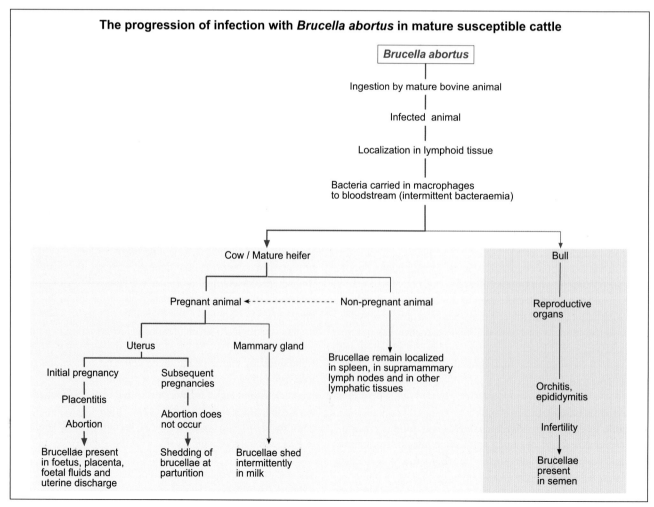

The progression of infection with *Brucella abortus* in mature susceptible cattle

The clinical disease resembles brucellosis in cattle in many respects. Clinical features include high abortion rates in susceptible populations, orchitis in male animals, arthritis and hygromas. Infection resulting in abortion may not induce protective immunity.

Diagnosis is based on clinical signs, direct examination of MZN-stained smears of fluids or tissues, isolation and identification of *B. melitensis* and serological testing. In countries where the disease is exotic, a test and slaughter policy is usually implemented. The Rose Bengal agglutination test and the complement fixation test are the most widely used serological methods for detecting infection with *B. melitensis*. The modified live *B. melitensis* Rev. 1 strain, administered by the subcutaneous or conjunctival routes, is used for vaccination of kids and lambs up to six months of age.

Porcine brucellosis

Porcine brucellosis, caused by *B. suis*, occurs occasionally in the USA but is more prevalent in Latin America and Asia. Biovar 2 infection occurs in Scandanavia and the Balkans and is prevalent in wild boars throughout Europe. Infection is acquired by ingestion or by coitus and may be self-limiting in some animals. Clinical signs in sows include abortion, stillbirths, neonatal mortality and temporary sterility. Boars excreting brucellae in semen may be either clinically normal or present with testicular abnormalities. Associated sterility may be temporary or permanent. Lesions may also be found in bones and joints. The Rose Bengal plate agglutination test and the indirect ELISA are the most reliable serological methods for the diagnosis of porcine brucellosis. A test and slaughter policy is the main control measure in countries where the disease is exotic.

Canine brucellosis

Infection with *Brucella canis* has been recorded in dogs in the USA, UK, Japan, and Central and South America. Because of difficulties with diagnosis, the distribution of the disease may be more extensive than is currently recognized. As *B. canis* is permanently in the rough form, it is of comparatively low virulence, causing relatively mild and asymptomatic infections. In breeding establishments, infection may manifest clinically as abortions, decreased fertility, reduced litter sizes and neonatal mortality. Most bitches which have aborted subsequently have normal gestations. In male dogs, the main clinical feature of the disease is infertility associated with orchitis and epididymitis.

Infertility may be permanent and dogs with chronic infections are often aspermic. Treatment should not be undertaken in animals intended for breeding as long-term resolution is difficult to achieve. A rapid slide agglutination test kit containing 2-mercaptoethanol is used as a screening test. Confirmatory tests include a tube agglutination test, ELISA and an agar gel immunodiffusion test. However, there are problems with the sensitivity and specificity of serological tests and definitive diagnosis can only be achieved by positive blood culture. Control is based on routine serological testing and removal of infected animals from breeding programmes.

Ovine epididymitis caused by B. ovis

Brucella ovis causes infection in sheep which is characterized by epididymitis in rams and placentitis in ewes. Infection with this pathogen, which was first recorded in New Zealand and Australia, is now present in many other countries. The consequences of infection include reduced fertility in rams, sporadic abortion in ewes and increased perinatal mortality. *Brucella ovis* may be present in semen about five weeks after infection and epididymal lesions can be detected by palpation at about nine weeks. In countries where the disease is endemic, pre-mating checks on rams include serological testing and scrotal palpation. The most efficient and widely used serological tests for *B. ovis* are the agar gel immunodiffusion test, the complement fixation test and the indirect ELISA. PCR-based tests for the detection of *B. ovis* in a range of clinical samples, including semen, preputial washes and urine, have been developed.

Brucellosis in humans

Humans are susceptible to infection with *B. abortus*, *B. suis*, *B. melitensis* and, rarely, *B. canis*. Transmission to humans occurs through contact with secretions or excretions of infected animals. Routes of entry include skin abrasions, inhalation and ingestion. Infection by inhalation can occur with as few as 10 organisms. Raw milk and dairy produce made with unpasteurized milk are important sources of infection. Brucellosis in humans, known as undulant fever, presents as fluctuating pyrexia, malaise, fatigue and muscle and joint pains. Abortion is not a feature of human infection. Osteomyelitis is the most common complication. Severe infection occurs with *B. melitensis* (Malta fever) and *B. suis* biovars 1 and 3. Human infections due to *B. abortus* are moderately severe, whereas those caused by *B. canis* are usually mild.

35 *Campylobacter* species

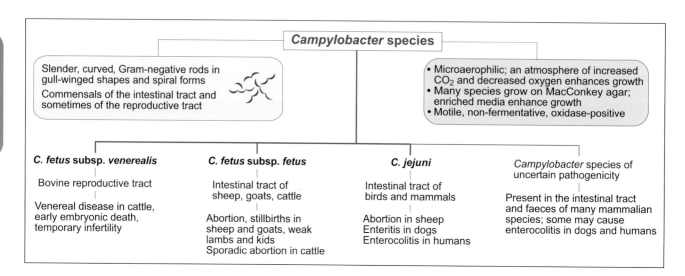

A number of morphological features distinguish *Campylobacter* species from other Gram-negative bacteria. They are slender, curved, motile, Gram-negative rods with polar flagella. Daughter cells which remain joined have a characteristic gull-winged appearance and long spirals formed by joined cells also occur. These microaerophilic organisms grow best on enriched media in an atmosphere of increased CO_2 and decreased oxygen tension. Many *Campylobacter* species grow on MacConkey agar. They are non-fermentative and oxidase-positive. *Campylobacter* species are found in the intestinal and genital tracts of domestic animals and are widely distributed geographically. *Campylobacter jejuni* subsp. *jejuni* (referred to as *C. jejuni*) and *C. lari* colonize the intestines of birds which can result in faecal contamination of watercourses and stored food. *Campylobacter fetus* subsp. *venerealis* appears to be adapted principally to bovine preputial mucosa. *Campylobacter* species are strictly microaerophilic, requiring an atmosphere of 5–10% CO_2 for growth. Some species such as *C. jejuni* grow optimally at 42°C. A selective enriched medium such as Skirrow agar is usually used for primary isolation. Because differentiation of isolates is difficult using conventional cultural and biochemical methods, molecular methods are increasingly used for definitive speciation and for strain typing. PCR-based methods are used for both identification of clinical isolates and for direct detection of *Campylobacter* species in clinical specimens. Pulsed-field gel electrophoresis is frequently employed for epidemiological investigation of clinical outbreaks of disease in animals and for food-borne infections caused by *C. jejuni* in humans.

The most important consequences of infections with organisms in this group are infertility in cattle due to *C. fetus* subsp. *venerealis* and abortion in ewes caused either by *C. fetus* subsp. *fetus* or by *C. jejuni*. In many developed countries, *C. jejuni* is the most frequent cause of bacterial food poisoning in humans.

Bovine genital campylobacteriosis

Campylobacter fetus subsp. *venerealis*, the principal cause of bovine genital campylobacteriosis, is transmitted during coitus to susceptible cows by asymptomatic carrier bulls. The disease is characterized by temporary infertility associated with early embryonic death, return to oestrus at irregular periods and, occasionally, by sporadic abortion. Information on virulence mechanisms is limited but the organism possesses a protein microcapsule or S layer, which confers resistance to serum-mediated destruction and phagocytosis. In addition, a number of different antigenic variants in the S layer may promote the organism's ability to evade the host immune response.

About one-third of infected animals become carriers, with the organisms persisting in the vagina of carrier cows. Extension of infection to the uterus with the development of endometritis and salpingitis can occur during the progestational phase of the oestrus cycle. The infertile period following uterine invasion can last for up to five months, after which specific immunity may develop. This protective immunity may last for up to four years. *Campylobacter fetus* subsp. *fetus*, an enteric organism acquired by ingestion, can cause sporadic abortions in cows.

Investigation of the breeding records and vaccination history of an affected herd may suggest campylobacteriosis. *Campylobacter* species can be detected by the fluorescent antibody technique in sheath washings from bulls or cervicovaginal mucus from cows. Isolation and identification or molecular detection of *C. fetus* subsp. *venerealis* from preputial or vaginal mucus is confirmatory. Dihydrostreptomycin, administered either systemically or topically, is used for treating bulls. Intrauterine administration of dihydrostreptomycin can be used therapeutically. Vaccination with bacterins in an oil emulsion adjuvant is used therapeutically and prophylactically in problem herds in some countries.

Concise Review of Veterinary Microbiology, Second Edition. P.J. Quinn, B.K. Markey, F.C. Leonard, E.S. FitzPatrick and S. Fanning.
© 2016 John Wiley & Sons, Ltd. Published 2016 by John Wiley & Sons, Ltd.
Companion website: www.wiley.com/go/quinn/concise-veterinary-microbiology

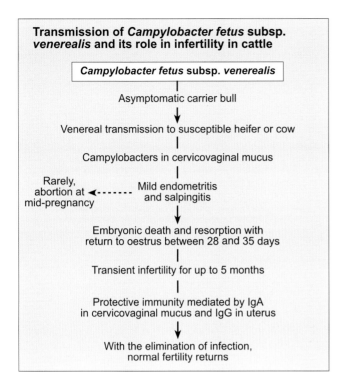

Transmission of *Campylobacter fetus* subsp. *venerealis* and its role in infertility in cattle

Campylobacter fetus subsp. *venerealis*
↓
Asymptomatic carrier bull
↓
Venereal transmission to susceptible heifer or cow
↓
Campylobacters in cervicovaginal mucus
↓
Rarely, abortion at mid-pregnancy ◄- - - - - - Mild endometritis and salpingitis
↓
Embryonic death and resorption with return to oestrus between 28 and 35 days
↓
Transient infertility for up to 5 months
↓
Protective immunity mediated by IgA in cervicovaginal mucus and IgG in uterus
↓
With the elimination of infection, normal fertility returns

Ovine genital campylobacteriosis

Campylobacteriosis in ewes may be caused by either *C. fetus* subsp. *fetus* or *C. jejuni*. The disease, which is worldwide in distribution, is one of the most common causes of ovine abortion in some countries. The relative importance of these two species differs in different geographical regions. Since the 1990s, *C. jejuni* has predominated as a cause of abortion in the USA and a new highly virulent tetracycline-resistant clone has emerged there in recent years. This change in tetracycline resistance may reflect the widespread use of tetracycline for control of ovine abortion in that country. Both *Campylobacter* species cause abortion in the UK whereas *C. fetus* subsp. *fetus* is more prevalent in New Zealand. *Campylobacter fetus* subsp. *fetus* is found in the faeces of cattle and sheep and *C. jejuni* may be present in the faeces of a wide range of birds and mammals. Transmission of both of these organisms is by the faecal–oral route. During pregnancy, localization in the uterus of susceptible ewes may follow bacter-

aemia. The subsequent necrotic placentitis may result in abortion late in pregnancy, stillborn lambs or weak lambs. Round, necrotic lesions up to 2 cm in diameter with pale raised rims and dark depressed centres are evident on the liver surface in some aborted lambs. Aborting ewes are major sources of infection for susceptible animals in a flock. Up to 20% of ewes in a susceptible flock may abort. Recovered ewes are immune for at least three years.

If present, typical hepatic lesions in aborted lambs are pathognomonic. Isolation and identification of *C. fetus* subsp. *fetus* or *C. jejuni* from foetal abomasal contents or birth fluids is confirmatory. Aborting ewes should be isolated and placentae and aborted foetuses promptly removed. The remainder of the flock should be moved to clean pasture. After confirmation of the disease in a flock, vaccination of ewes with a *C. fetus* subsp. *fetus* bacterin is reported to reduce the number of abortions.

Intestinal campylobacteriosis in dogs

Diarrhoea in dogs and other domestic animals has been attributed to infection with *Campylobacter* species, particularly *C. jejuni*. Confirmation is difficult because healthy animals may shed *Campylobacter* species in their faeces. However, the presence of large numbers of campylobacter-like organisms in dilute carbol fuchsin-stained faecal smears or rectal scrapings from dogs with diarrhoea may be indicative of infection. *Campylobacter* species may contribute to the severity of enteric disease in dogs infected with other enteropathogens such as enteric viruses, *Giardia* species and helminths. Dogs shedding *C. jejuni* are a potential source of human infection.

Intestinal campylobacteriosis in humans

Campylobacter jejuni is the main cause of human intestinal campylobacteriosis. *Campylobacter coli* and *C. lari* are sometimes implicated. These zoonotic infections are usually foodborne and poultry meat is the main source of human infection. Fever, abdominal pain and diarrhoea, sometimes with blood, are the most common manifestations of this enteric infection. The emergence of antimicrobial resistance in campylobacters, particularly to fluoroquinolones and macrolide antibiotics, is a major public health concern.

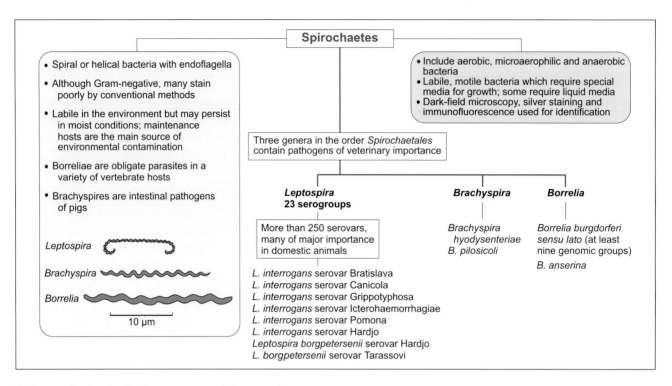

Spirochaetes

- Spiral or helical bacteria with endoflagella
- Although Gram-negative, many stain poorly by conventional methods
- Labile in the environment but may persist in moist conditions; maintenance hosts are the main source of environmental contamination
- Borreliae are obligate parasites in a variety of vertebrate hosts
- Brachyspires are intestinal pathogens of pigs

- Include aerobic, microaerophilic and anaerobic bacteria
- Labile, motile bacteria which require special media for growth; some require liquid media
- Dark-field microscopy, silver staining and immunofluorescence used for identification

Three genera in the order *Spirochaetales* contain pathogens of veterinary importance

Leptospira 23 serogroups

More than 250 serovars, many of major importance in domestic animals

L. interrogans serovar Bratislava
L. interrogans serovar Canicola
L. interrogans serovar Grippotyphosa
L. interrogans serovar Icterohaemorrhagiae
L. interrogans serovar Pomona
L. interrogans serovar Hardjo
Leptospira borgpetersenii serovar Hardjo
L. borgpetersenii serovar Tarassovi

Brachyspira

Brachyspira hyodysenteriae
B. pilosicoli

Borrelia

Borrelia burgdorferi sensu lato (at least nine genomic groups)

B. anserina

Leptospira

Brachyspira

Borrelia

10 μm

Pathogens in the family *Leptospiraceae* belong to the genus *Leptospira*. The genera *Borrelia* and *Treponema* in the family *Spirochaetaceae* and *Brachyspira* in the family *Brachyspiraceae* contain significant animal and human pathogens. Some non-pathogenic genera occur in each family. Pathogenic spirochaetes are difficult to culture and many require specialized media; some require liquid media.

Leptospira species

Members of this species (leptospires) are motile helical bacteria with hook-shaped ends. Although cytochemically Gram-negative, they do not stain well with conventional bacteriological dyes and dark-field microscopy is used for their detection in fluids or liquid media. Leptospirosis, which can affect all domestic animals and humans, ranges in severity from mild infections of the urinary or genital systems to serious systemic disease.

Leptospires can survive in ponds, rivers, surface waters, moist soil and mud when environmental temperatures are mild. Pathogenic leptospires can persist in the renal tubules or in the genital tract of carrier animals. These fragile organisms are transmitted most effectively by direct contact. Leptospiral species (genospecies) are classified by DNA homology. Within each species, serological reactions which identify surface antigens are employed to assign isolates to serogroups, Subsequently the organism can be further identifed to serovar level. At present, more than 250 serovars in 23 serogroups are defined, many of which may be associated with clinical disease.

Although leptospires are found worldwide, some serovars appear to have a limited geographical distribution. In addition, most serovars are associated with particular species, their maintenance hosts. The pathogenicity of leptospires relates to the

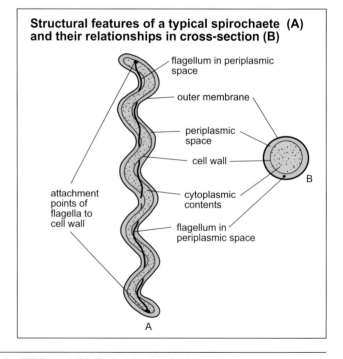

Structural features of a typical spirochaete (A) and their relationships in cross-section (B)

flagellum in periplasmic space

outer membrane

periplasmic space

cell wall

cytoplasmic contents

flagellum in periplasmic space

attachment points of flagella to cell wall

A

B

Concise Review of Veterinary Microbiology, Second Edition. P.J. Quinn, B.K. Markey, F.C. Leonard, E.S. FitzPatrick and S. Fanning.
© 2016 John Wiley & Sons, Ltd. Published 2016 by John Wiley & Sons, Ltd.
Companion website: www.wiley.com/go/quinn/concise-veterinary-microbiology

Table 36.1 Serovars of *Leptospira* which cause clinical infections in domestic animals and humans.

Serovar	Hosts	Clinical conditions
Leptospira borgpetersenii serovar Hardjo	Cattle, sheep	Abortions, stillbirths, agalactia
L. interrogans serovar Hardjo	Humans	Influenza-like illness; occasionally liver or kidney disease
L. borgpetersenii serovar Tarassovi	Pigs	Reproductive failure, abortions, stillbirths
L. interrogans serovar Bratislava	Pigs, horses, dogs	Reproductive failure, abortions, stillbirths
L. interrogans serovar Canicola	Dogs	Acute nephritis in pups. Chronic renal disease in adult animals
	Pigs	Abortions and stillbirths. Renal disease in young pigs
L. interrogans serovar Grippotyphosa	Cattle, pigs, dogs	Septicaemic disease in young animals; abortion
L. interrogans serovar Icterohaemorrhagiae	Cattle, sheep, pigs	Acute septicaemic disease in calves, piglets and lambs; abortions
	Dogs, humans	Peracute haemorrhagic disease; acute hepatitis with jaundice; human infection, Weil's disease
L. interrogans serovar Pomona	Cattle, sheep	Acute haemolytic disease in calves and lambs; abortions
	Pigs	Reproductive failure; septicaemia in piglets
	Horses	Abortions, periodic ophthalmia

virulence of the infecting serovar and the susceptibility of the host species. Maintenance hosts readily acquire infection; disease is frequently mild or subclinical and is often followed by prolonged excretion of leptospires in urine. In contrast, incidental host species are usually more resistant to infection, develop severe disease if successfully infected and are inefficient transmitters of leptospires to other animals. Leptospires invade tissues through moist softened skin or through mucous membranes. Motility and chemotaxis are essential for penetration of host tissues. The organisms spread through the body via the bloodstream but, following the appearance of antibodies about 10 days after infection, they are cleared from the circulation. Some organisms may evade the immune response and persist in the body, principally in the renal tubules and also in the uterus, eye or meninges. In susceptible animals, damage to red cell membranes and to endothelial cells, along with hepatocellular injury, produces haemoglobinuria and haemorrhage, associated with acute leptospirosis. Pulmonary haemorrhage is a significant lesion in peracute cases of disease in humans and has been documented in several animal species also.

Clinical signs, together with a history of probable exposure to contaminated urine, may indicate acute leptospirosis. Leptospires may be isolated from the blood during the first 10 days of infection and from the urine approximately two weeks after initial infection, by culture in liquid medium at 30°C but culture is a specialized technique used primarily in research. PCR-based procedures for detection and identification of organisms are now widely used in the diagnosis of disease. Fluorescent antibody procedures or silver impregnation techniques may be used for the demonstration of leptospires in tissues. The microscopic agglutination test, using live culture growth in a liquid medium, is the gold standard serological test for the diagnosis of leptospirosis. A number of ELISA tests have also been developed but none are commercially available for use in animals. The disease conditions associated with leptospiral infections in domestic animals and humans are presented in Table 36.1.

Leptospirosis in cattle and sheep

Cattle are maintenance hosts for *L. borgpetersenii* serovar Hardjo and this serovar may also be host-adapted for sheep. *Leptospira interrogans* serovar Hardjo is also host-adapted for cattle. Susceptible replacement heifers, reared separately and introduced into an infected dairy herd for the first time at calving, may develop acute disease with pyrexia and agalactia affecting all quarters. Infection may also result in abortion and stillbirths. Serovars incorporated into vaccines for use in a particular region should match leptospiral isolates from animals in that region.

Leptospirosis in horses

Leptospiral infection in horses is frequently subclinical. Clinical disease most often results from incidental infection with serovar Pomona. Signs include abortion in mares and renal disease in young horses. A recurring immune-mediated anterior uveitis (periodic ophthalmia, 'moon blindness') is associated with chronic leptospirosis in horses.

Leptospirosis in pigs

Acute leptospirosis in pigs is usually caused by rodent-adapted serovars such as Icterohaemorrhagiae and Copenhagenii. These serovars cause serious, sometimes fatal, disease in young pigs. In many parts of the world, the principal host-adapted serovar is Pomona. Infection can result in reproductive failure including abortions and stillbirths.

Leptospirosis in dogs and cats

Formerly, the serovars primarily associated with leptospirosis in dogs and cats were Canicola and Icterohaemorrhagiae. However, widespread vaccination against these serovars has resulted in the emergence of other serovars such as Grippotyphosa and Bratislava as causes of infection and disease. Serovar Canicola, which is host-adapted for dogs, causes severe renal disease in pups. Incidental canine infections are characterized by acute haemorrhagic disease or subacute hepatic and renal failure.

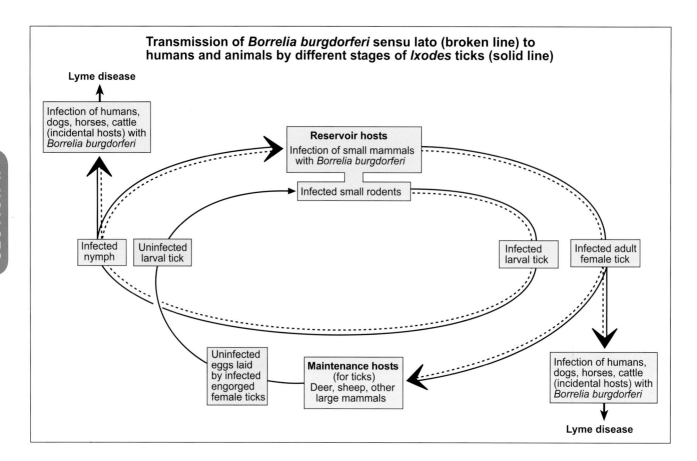

Transmission of *Borrelia burgdorferi* sensu lato (broken line) to humans and animals by different stages of *Ixodes* ticks (solid line)

Clinical leptospirosis is uncommon in cats although subclinical infection, usually acquired from rodents, occurs.

Borrelia species

Borreliae, which are longer and wider than other spirochaetes, have a similar helical shape. Although these spirochaetes can cause disease in animals and humans, subclinical infections are also common. Borreliae are transmitted by arthropod vectors. These spirochaetes are obligate parasites in a variety of vertebrate hosts and they depend on vetebrate reservoir hosts and arthropod vectors for long-term survival. Borreliae can be differentiated from other spirochaetes by their morphology, by the low guanine and cytosine content of their genomic DNA, and by ecological, cultural and biochemical features. Identification of *Borrelia* species depends mainly on genetic analysis. The species of particular veterinary importance are *B. burgdorferi sensu lato*, the cause of Lyme disease in animals and humans, and *B. anserina* which causes avian borreliosis (Table 36.2).

Lyme disease

This condition was first identified in 1975 following investigation of a cluster of arthritis cases in children near the town of Old Lyme, Connecticut. The causative agent, a spirochaete, was named *Borrelia burgdorferi*. Several genospecies of *B. burgdorferi* have subsequently been identified. In North America, *B. burgdorferi sensu stricto* is the only borrelia associated with Lyme disease, whereas at least five species are known to cause disease in Europe, the most important being *B. afzelii* and *B. garinii*. Lyme disease has been reported in humans, dogs, horses and cattle, and infection has been documented in sheep.

Ticks are the only competent vectors of *B. burgdorferi sensu lato*. Infection is usually acquired by larval stages of ticks feeding on small rodents. The spirochaetes persist through nymphal and adult stages of ticks, which transmit infection while feeding. The persistence of these pathogenic bacteria in a region is dependent on the presence of suitable reservoir hosts for borreliae and maintenance hosts for ticks. The most common tick vector for *B. burgdorferi sensu lato* in Europe is *Ixodes ricinus*. In the USA, different *Ixodes* species act as vectors: *I. scapularis* in central and eastern regions, *I. pacificus* on the west coast. After entering the bloodstream of a susceptible host, borreliae multiply and are disseminated throughout the body. Organisms can be demonstrated in joints, brain, nerves, eyes and heart.

Most infections are subclinical and serological surveys demonstrate that exposure is common in both animal and human populations in endemic areas. The clinical manifestations of Lyme disease relate mainly to the sites of localization of the organisms and are largely attributed to the host's inflammatory response to the pathogen. Clinical disease is reported frequently in dogs. Signs include fever, lethargy, arthritis and evidence of cardiac, renal or neurological disturbance. The clinical signs in horses are similar to those in dogs. In cattle and sheep, lameness has been reported. Laboratory confirmation of Lyme disease may prove difficult because the spirochaetes may be present in low numbers in specimens from clinically affected animals. A history of exposure to tick infestation in an endemic area in association with characteristic clinical signs may suggest Lyme disease. Rising antibody titres to *B. burgdorferi sensu lato* along with typical clinical signs are indicative of disease. ELISA and immunofluorescence assays are used for antibody detection. Culture of borreliae from clinically affected animals is confirmatory. Low numbers of borreliae can be detected in samples by PCR techniques.

Table 36.2 Tick vectors and natural hosts of *Borrelia* species and associated clinical conditions.

Species	Vector	Host	Clinical conditions
B. burgdorferi sensu lato	*Ixodes* species	Rodents, birds	Arthritic, neurological and cardiac disease in dogs and occasionally in horses, cattle, sheep. Lyme disease in humans
B. anserina	*Argas* species	Birds	Fever, weight loss and anaemia in domestic poultry
B. theileri	Many species of ticks	Cattle, sheep, horses	Mild, febrile disease with anaemia
B. coriaceae	*Ornithodoros* species	Cattle, deer	Associated with epizootic bovine abortion in USA

Acaricidal sprays, baths or dips should be used to control tick infestation. Where feasible, tick habitats such as rough brush and scrub should be cleared. A number of vaccines, including whole-cell bacterins and a recombinant subunit vaccine, are commercially available for use in dogs but their efficacy is questioned by some research workers.

Lyme disease is an important tick-borne infection of humans. Infection is often acquired by walking in endemic areas during periods of tick activity. Clinical signs include skin rash at site of tick attachment followed by arthritis, muscle pains, and cardiac and neurological complications.

Avian spirochaetosis

This acute disease of birds, caused by *Borrelia anserina*, can result in significant economic loss in flocks in tropical and subtropical regions. Chickens, turkeys, pheasants, ducks and geese are susceptible to infection. Soft ticks of the genus *Argas* frequently transmit the disease. The borreliae survive trans-stadial moulting in ticks and can be transmitted transovarially between tick generations. Outbreaks of avian spirochaetosis coincide with periods of peak tick activity during warm humid seasons. The disease is characterized by fever, marked anaemia and weight loss. Paralysis may develop as the disease progresses. Immunity, which follows recovery, is serotype-specific. Diagnosis can be confirmed by demonstration of the spirochaetes in buffy coat smears using dark-field microscopy. Giemsa-stained smears or silver impregnation techniques can be used to demonstrate the borreliae in tissues. Blood or tissue smears can be examined using immunofluorescence. Inactivated vaccines and tick eradication are the main control measures.

Brachyspira and *Treponema* species

Of the five genospecies of intestinal spirochaetes which have been isolated from pigs, two species, *Brachyspira hyodysenteriae* and *B. pilosicoli*, are the most pathogenic. These anaerobic spirochaetes can be differentiated by their pattern of haemolysis on blood agar, hippurate hydrolysis and by restriction endonuclease analysis. Pathogenic *Brachyspira* species are found in the intestinal tract of both clinically affected and normal pigs. *Brachyspira pilosicoli* is found in the intestines of pigs, chickens, wild birds, dogs, rodents and some non-human primates. Carrier pigs can shed *B. hyodysenteriae* for up to three months and are the principal source of infection for healthy pigs. Colonization is enhanced by factors in mucus with chemotactic activity for *B. hyodysenteriae*. Haemolytic activity, demonstrated *in vitro*, correlates with pathogenicity and motility is also an essential requirement for virulence.

Infections with *Brachyspira* species are of importance in pigs. *Brachyspira hyodysenteriae*, the cause of swine dysentery, and *B. pilosicoli*, the cause of porcine intestinal spirochaetosis, are recognized pathogens. Pigs acquire infection through exposure to contaminated faeces. Rodents and flies may act as transport hosts for the spirochaetes. *Brachyspira hyodysenteriae* can persist for several weeks in moist faeces. Infection with *B. hyodysenteriae* causes dysentery which is often encountered in weaned pigs from six to twelve weeks of age. Affected pigs lose condition and become emaciated. Appetite decreases and thirst may be evident. During recovery, there may be large amounts of mucus in the faeces. Although mortality is low, reduced weight gains due to poor food conversion causes major economic loss. The clinical signs of porcine intestinal spirochaetosis, caused by *B. pilosicoli*, are similar to those of swine dysentery but are less severe. Diarrhoea contains mucus rather than blood.

History, clinical signs and gross lesions may indicate swine dysentery. Blood agar incorporating antibiotics is used for the culture of *Brachyspira* species. Cultures are incubated anaerobically at 42°C for at least three days. Definitive identification can be made using immunofluorescence, PCR-based methods or biochemical tests. Medication of drinking water is a useful method of treatment although antimicrobial resistance is a problem in some countries. Depopulation, thorough cleaning, disinfection of premises and strict rodent control, are required for eradication of disease.

Treponemes are associated with digital dermatitis in cattle and contagious ovine digital dermatitis of sheep. *Treponema paraluiscuniculi* causes vent disease in rabbits.

37 Pathogenic, anaerobic, non-spore-forming Gram-negative bacteria

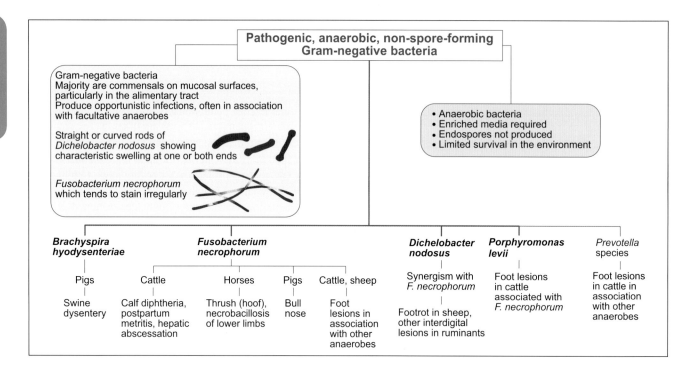

Many anaerobic, non-spore-forming, Gram-negative bacteria, often in association with facultative anaerobes, contribute to opportunistic mixed infections. Synergistic interactions between the organisms in these mixed infections are common. Non-spore-forming Gram-negative anaerobes are often found on mucous membranes, particularly in the digestive tract of animals and humans. Many non-spore-forming anaerobes are part of the normal flora of these sites and thus care in collection of clinical samples from these areas is essential to avoid contamination by these organisms. These bacteria are differentiated on the basis of bacterial morphology, colonial appearance, antibiotic susceptibility testing and fatty acid production. Anaerobic jars with an atmosphere of hydrogen and 10% CO_2 are used for incubating cultures at 37°C for up to seven days. Specimens should be processed promptly after collection. Due to volatile fatty acid production, colonies of Gram-negative anaerobes often have a foetid odour.

Non-spore-forming Gram-negative anaerobes usually exert their pathogenic effects when anatomical barriers are breached allowing invasion of underlying tissues. They replicate only at low or negative reduction potentials (E_h). Tissue trauma and necrosis, followed by multiplication of facultatively anaerobic bacteria, can lower E_h levels to a range suitable for the proliferation of non-spore-forming anaerobes. Most infections involving these organisms are mixed. Two or more bacterial species, interacting synergistically, may produce lesions which individual

organisms cannot. The synergism between *Trueperella pyogenes* and *Fusobacterium necrophorum* relates to growth factor production by the former. *Fusobacterium necrophorum* produces a number of potent virulence factors including a leukotoxin which is highly toxic for ruminant neutrophils, a haemagglutinin which promotes adherence to ruminant epithelium, a haemolysin and a dermonecrotic toxin. Synergism between *F. necrophorum* and *Dichelobacter nodosus* is also important in the pathogenesis of ruminant pedal lesions. *Fusobacterium necrophorum* is considered to be the primary pathogen in a number of disease conditions in farm animals (Table 37.1). Mixed bacterial infections are commonly implicated in the development of foot lesions in domestic ruminants and pigs (Table 37.2). Mixed infections with non-spore-forming anaerobes are also present in aspiration pneumonias and in bovine traumatic reticuloperitonitis and pericarditis.

Calf diphtheria

This condition usually presents as necrotic pharyngitis or laryngitis in calves under three months of age. *Fusobacterium necrophorum* can enter through abrasions in the mucosa of the pharynx or larynx often caused by ingestion of coarse feed. Clinical signs include fever, depression, anorexia, excessive salivation, respiratory distress and a foul smell from the mouth. Untreated calves may develop a fatal necrotizing pneumonia.

Concise Review of Veterinary Microbiology, Second Edition. P.J. Quinn, B.K. Markey, F.C. Leonard, E.S. FitzPatrick and S. Fanning.
© 2016 John Wiley & Sons, Ltd. Published 2016 by John Wiley & Sons, Ltd.
Companion website: www.wiley.com/go/quinn/concise-veterinary-microbiology

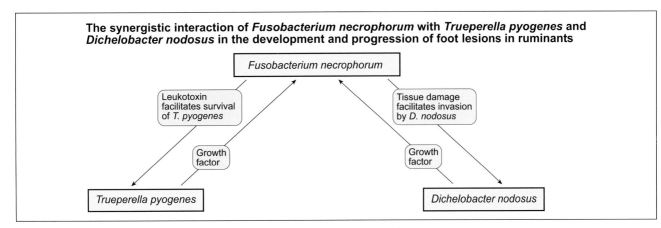

The synergistic interaction of *Fusobacterium necrophorum* with *Trueperella pyogenes* and *Dichelobacter nodosus* in the development and progression of foot lesions in ruminants

Bovine liver abscess

Hepatic abscessation in cattle, secondary to rumenitis, is encountered most commonly in feedlot animals. Feeding of rations high in carbohydrates and the resulting rapid intraruminal fermentation can lead to the development of ulcers in the ruminal mucosa. *Fusobacterium necrophorum* together with other anaerobes and *Trueperella pyogenes* invade the tissues, and occasional emboli may reach the liver via the portal vein and initiate abscess formation. Affected cattle rarely show clinical signs and lesions are usually detected at slaughter.

Footrot in sheep

Dichelobacter nodosus is the primary causal agent of footrot in sheep. *Fusobacterium necrophorum*, together with *T. pyogenes*, initiate the lesion in the interdigital space but the development of footrot is dependent on the presence of virulent strains of *D. nodosus*. Fimbriae on this pathogen promote adherence to host cells. The action of proteases is largely responsible for the severe tissue destruction, under-running of horn and clinical lameness characteristic of virulent footrot. Diagnosis of footrot can be based on clinical signs alone but definitive identification of virulent footrot relies on detection of *D. nodosus* and demonstration of virulence. This can be confirmed by isolation of the organism followed by protracted tests for demonstration of protease production or, more commonly, by PCR-based tests for virulence-associated genes. Carrier sheep are the principal reservoir of *D. nodosus* which survives less than seven days in the environment. Transmission occurs only in moist condi-

tions in temperatures of 10°C or greater. Eradication of footrot has been achieved in large parts of Australia through identification and culling of carrier sheep during the dry hot summers when conditions preclude transmission of *D. nodosus*. Control is difficult in more temperate climates; vaccines which have both prophylactic and therapeutic activity are available commercially.

Thrush of the hoof

This necrotic condition of the equine hoof is associated with poor hygiene, wet conditions and lack of regular cleaning of the hooves. Infection with *F. necrophorum*, secondary to hoof damage, results in localized inflammation. Thrush, which commonly affects the hind feet, is characterized by a foul-smelling discharge in the sulci, close to the frog. Dry clean stabling, regular attention to the hooves and exercise promote frog regeneration.

Table 37.2 Foot conditions in farm animals associated with mixed infections including anaerobic non-spore-forming bacteria.

Species	Disease condition	Bacteria implicated
Sheep	Interdigital dermatitis	*Fusobacterium necrophorum* *Dichelobacter nodosus* (benign strains)
	Heel abscess and lamellar suppuration	Mixed anaerobic flora including *Trueperella pyogenes*[a], *F. necrophorum*, and other opportunistic pathogens
	Footrot	*Dichelobacter nodosus* *Fusobacterium necrophorum* *Trueperella pyogenes*[a]
	Contagious ovine digital dermatitis	*Treponema* species
Cattle	Interdigital necrobacillosis (foul-in-the-foot)	*Fusobacterium necrophorum* *Porphyromonas levii*
	Interdigital dermatitis	*Dichelobacter nodosus* *Fusobacterium necrophorum* *Prevotella* species Spirochaetes may contribute to lesion development
	Bovine digital dermatitis (Mortellaro)	*Treponema* species
Pigs	Foot abscess in young pigs and bush foot (lamellar suppuration) in older animals	Mixed anaerobes

[a]Facultatively anaerobic.

Table 37.1 Disease conditions of farm animals in which *Fusobacterium necrophorum* plays a primary role.

Species	Disease condition	Predisposing factors
Cattle	Calf diphtheria	Rough feed producing mucosal damage
	Postpartum metritis	Dystocia
	Hepatic abscessation	Sudden dietary change, leading to acidosis and rumenitis
	Black spot of teat	Trauma to region adjacent to teat sphincter
Horses	Thrush (hoof)	Poor hygiene and wet housing conditions
	Necrobacillosis of lower limbs	Poor hygiene
Pigs	Bull nose	Trauma to nasal mucosa

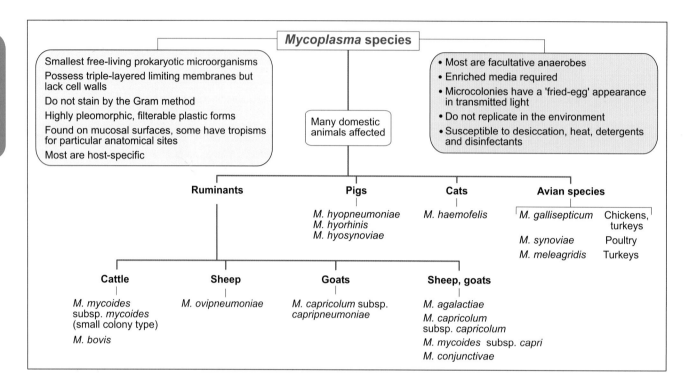

***Mycoplasma* species**

- Smallest free-living prokaryotic microorganisms
- Possess triple-layered limiting membranes but lack cell walls
- Do not stain by the Gram method
- Highly pleomorphic, filterable plastic forms
- Found on mucosal surfaces, some have tropisms for particular anatomical sites
- Most are host-specific

- Most are facultative anaerobes
- Enriched media required
- Microcolonies have a 'fried-egg' appearance in transmitted light
- Do not replicate in the environment
- Susceptible to desiccation, heat, detergents and disinfectants

Many domestic animals affected

Ruminants

Pigs
M. hyopneumoniae
M. hyorhinis
M. hyosynoviae

Cats
M. haemofelis

Avian species
M. gallisepticum — Chickens, turkeys
M. synoviae — Poultry
M. meleagridis — Turkeys

Cattle
M. mycoides subsp. *mycoides* (small colony type)
M. bovis

Sheep
M. ovipneumoniae

Goats
M. capricolum subsp. *capripneumoniae*

Sheep, goats
M. agalactiae
M. capricolum subsp. *capricolum*
M. mycoides subsp. *capri*
M. conjunctivae

Microorganisms in the class *Mollicutes*, including mycoplasmas, are the smallest prokaryotic cells capable of self-replication. Because these pleomorphic organisms cannot synthesize peptidoglycan or its precursors, they do not possess rigid cell walls but have flexible triple-layered outer membranes. They are resistant to antibiotics such as penicillin which interfere with the synthesis of bacterial cell walls. They require enriched media for growth and although most mycoplasmas are facultative anaerobes, some grow optimally in an atmosphere of 5 to 10% CO_2. Characteristically, microcolonies have an umbonate appearance when illuminated obliquely and a 'fried-egg' appearance in transmitted light.

Mycoplasmas are found on mucosal surfaces of the conjunctiva, nasal cavity, oropharynx, and intestinal and genital tracts of animals and humans. The haemotropic mycoplasmas are found on the surface of red blood cells. In general, they are

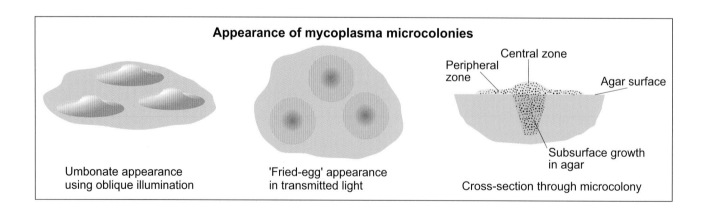

Appearance of mycoplasma microcolonies

Umbonate appearance using oblique illumination

'Fried-egg' appearance in transmitted light

Peripheral zone
Central zone
Agar surface
Subsurface growth in agar
Cross-section through microcolony

Concise Review of Veterinary Microbiology, Second Edition. P.J. Quinn, B.K. Markey, F.C. Leonard, E.S. FitzPatrick and S. Fanning.
© 2016 John Wiley & Sons, Ltd. Published 2016 by John Wiley & Sons, Ltd.
Companion website: www.wiley.com/go/quinn/concise-veterinary-microbiology

Table 38.1 *Mycoplasma* species of veterinary significance, the disease conditions which they cause and their geographical distribution.

Mycoplasma species	Hosts	Disease conditions	Geographical distribution
M. mycoides subsp. *mycoides* (small colony type)	Cattle	Contagious bovine pleuropneumonia	Endemic in parts of Africa; not currently reported from other continents
M. bovis	Cattle	Mastitis, pneumonia, arthritis	Worldwide
M. agalactiae	Sheep, goats	Contagious agalactia	Parts of Europe, northern Africa, western Asia
M. capricolum subsp. *capripneumoniae*	Goats	Contagious caprine pleuropneumonia	Northern and eastern Africa, Turkey, parts of Asia
M. capricolum subsp. *capricolum*	Sheep, goats	Septicaemia, mastitis, polyarthritis, pneumonia	Africa, Europe, Australia, USA
M. mycoides subsp. *capri*	Goats	Septicaemia, pleuropneumonia, arthritis, mastitis	Parts of Asia, Africa, Europe, Australia
M. hyopneumoniae	Pigs	Enzootic pneumonia	Worldwide
M. hyorhinis	Pigs (3–10 weeks of age)	Polyserositis	Worldwide
M. hyosynoviae	Pigs (10–30 weeks of age)	Polyarthritis	Worldwide
M. gallisepticum	Chickens	Chronic respiratory disease	Worldwide
	Turkeys	Infectious sinusitis	Worldwide
M. synoviae	Chickens, turkeys	Infectious synovitis	Worldwide
M. meleagridis	Turkeys	Airsacculitis, bone deformities, reduced hatchability and growth rate	Worldwide
M. haemofelis	Cats	Feline infectious anaemia	Worldwide

host-specific and survive for short periods in the environment. The genera *Mycoplasma* and *Ureaplasma* contain animal pathogens. The major diseases associated with infection by *Mycoplasma* species are summarized in Table 38.1. *Mycoplasma* and *Ureaplasma* species increasingly associated with disease in animals are listed in Table 38.2.

Mycoplasmas are differentiated by their host specificity, colonial morphology, requirement for cholesterol and biochemical reactivity. For growth, these organisms require enriched media containing animal protein, a sterol component or adenine dinucleotide. Immunological tests, using specific antisera produced against each pathogenic species, are required for definitive identification. Growth inhibition tests in which filter paper discs impregnated with specific antisera are placed on an agar plate seeded with the mycoplasma are used for species identification. Fluorescent antibody staining of individual microcolonies can also be used for identification. Rapid plate agglutination tests are employed for screening poultry flocks and for the field diagnosis of contagious bovine pleuropneumonia. Many of the difficulties associated with culture and identification of mycoplasmas have been resolved with the advent of molecular techniques. PCR-based procedures can be used for the detection of organisms in clinical samples and for specific identification of cultured mycoplasmas.

Mycoplasmas adhere to host cells, an attribute essential for pathogenicity. This close contact, which facilitates toxic damage to host cells by soluble factors such as hydrogen peroxide produced by the pathogen, often occurs on mucosal surfaces. Variation in surface proteins is an important virulence attribute of *Mycoplasma* species as it allows the organism to rapidly adapt to the host environment and to evade the developing immune response. Mechanisms facilitating horizontal gene transfer, together with a high mutation rate, also contribute to the ability of mycoplasmas to rapidly evolve and adapt to their host environment. Some *Mycoplasma* species have the ability to produce biofilm, which may contribute to their persistence in some animals despite treatment with antimicrobial agents. In addition, the recently demonstrated ability of some mycoplasmas to survive intracellularly may account for their persistence in particular tissues. Factors such as extremes of age, stress and intercurrent infections may predispose to tissue invasion. In some instances, mycoplasmas may exacerbate disease initiated by other pathogens, particularly in the respiratory tract. Mycoplasmal infections cause respiratory diseases of major economic importance in farm animals, especially in ruminants, pigs and poultry.

Contagious bovine pleuropneumonia, a severe contagious disease of cattle, is caused by *M. mycoides* subsp. *mycoides*.

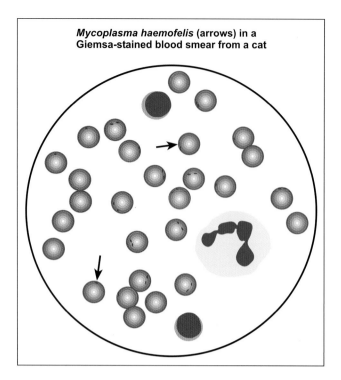

Mycoplasma haemofelis (arrows) in a
Giemsa-stained blood smear from a cat

The disease, which is transmitted by aerosols, requires close contact with clinically affected animals or asymptomatic carriers. Although spread of infection may be slow, the mortality rate may be high. The acute form of the disease is characterized by sudden onset of high fever, anorexia, depression, accelerated respiration and coughing. At postmortem, pneumonic lungs have a marbled appearance. The disease can be confirmed by isola-

tion and definitive identification of the pathogen by serology and by molecular techniques. In countries where the disease is exotic, slaughter of affected and in-contact cattle is mandatory. In endemic regions, control strategies are based on prohibiting movement of suspect animals, mandatory quarantine and the elimination of carrier animals by serological testing and slaughter. Annual vaccination with attenuated vaccines is carried out in endemic areas but although it decreases the severity of clinical signs, it does not prevent infection.

Contagious caprine pleuropneumonia, caused by *M. capricolum* subsp. *capripneumoniae*, is a disease in goats similar to contagious bovine pleuropneumonia of cattle. The disease, which is highly contagious, is transmitted by aerosols. Pleuropneumonia in goats can also be caused by *M. mycoides* subsp. *capri* and differentiation of isolates from those of *M. capricolum* subsp. *capripneumoniae* can be carried out using PCR-based procedures. Vaccination gives good protection against *M. capricolum* subsp. *capripneumoniae*.

Strains of *M. bovis*, which is worldwide in distribution, can cause severe pneumonia in calves in the absence of other respiratory pathogens and can exacerbate respiratory disease caused by *Pasteurella* and *Mannheimia* species. *Mycoplasma bovis* is associated with chronic respiratory disease and there is convincing evidence that the organism plays a central role in the development of lesions in caseonecrotic bronchopneumonia frequently observed in natural outbreaks of *M. bovis* infection and disease. This organism is also associated with mastitis and polyarthritis. Treatment and control of respiratory disease is based on management practices and antimicrobial therapy, although response to treatment is frequently poor in chronic disease.

Table 38.2 *Mycoplasma* and *Ureaplasma* species which are being increasingly associated with clinical conditions in domestic animals.

Hosts	Pathogen	Clinical conditions
Cattle	Mycoplasma alkalescens	Mastitis
	M. bovigenitalium	Seminal vesiculitis, vaginitis, mastitis
	M. bovirhinis	Mastitis
	M. bovoculi	Role in keratoconjunctivitis
	M. californicum	Mastitis
	M. canadense	Mastitis
	M. dispar	Pneumonia in calves
	M. leachii	Mastitis, polyarthritis, pneumonia
	Ureaplasma diversum	Vulvitis, infertility, abortion
	M. wenyonii	Mild anaemia
Sheep, goats	M. conjunctivae	Keratoconjunctivitis
	M. ovipneumoniae	Pneumonia
	M. ovis	Haemolytic anaemia, varying in severity
Goats	M. putrefaciens	Mastitis, arthritis
Turkeys	M. iowae	Embryo mortality
Horses	M. felis	Pleuritis
	M. equigenitalium	Implicated in abortion
Cats	M. felis	Conjunctivitis, respiratory disease
	M. gateae	Arthritis, tenosynovitis
Dogs	M. cynos	Implicated in the kennel cough complex
	M. haemocanis	Mild or subclinical anaemia; more severe signs in splenectomised animals
Pigs	M. suis	Mild anaemia, poor growth rates

Enzootic pneumonia of pigs, caused by *M. hyopneumoniae*, is an economically important disease which occurs worldwide in intensively reared pigs. Poor ventilation, overcrowding and temperature fluctuations may precipitate an outbreak. Clinical, epidemiological and pathological findings are usually indicative of the presence of the condition. Although antimicrobial drugs such as tylosin or tiamulin are used therapeutically, prevention and control are primarily based on the development of specific-pathogen-free herds. Vaccines are also available.

Mycoplasmas are important pathogens of poultry and with some mycoplasma species, such as *M. gallisepticum* and *M. meleagridis*, egg transmission is an important means of spread. Aerosol transmission also occurs and is the principal means of spread for *M. synoviae*. Disease control measures include vaccination, antimicrobial prophylaxis and development of specific-pathogen-free flocks.

Haemotropic mycoplasmas cause infections in a wide variety of hosts. Although disease is usually mild or subclinical, reduced productivity in farm animals can cause significant economic loss. Pathogenicity appears to be associated with direct damage to erythrocytes through adhesion and invasion by the organism and through immune-mediated lysis of red blood cells. Some haemotropic mycoplasmas also target vascular endothelium and may contribute to vascular thrombosis and haemorrhagic diathesis. Feline infectious anaemia, which is caused by *M. haemofelis*, occurs worldwide and is considered to be one of the most clinically significant diseases caused by haemotropic mycoplasmas. Disease is comparatively common in free-roaming tom cats between one and three years of age and transmission through bite-wounds or by biting arthropods has been suggested. Recovered cats may remain asymptomatic carriers. The acute form of the disease presents with fever, anaemia, depression, weakness and, occasionally, jaundice. *Mycoplasma haemofelis* may be demonstrated on the surface of erythrocytes in Giemsa-stained blood smears but PCR analysis is currently the preferred method for diagnosis of infection with haemotropic mycoplasmas. Doxycycline therapy initiated early and continued for up to 21 days is effective for treatment of clinical signs but may not eliminate infection.

39 Chlamydiae

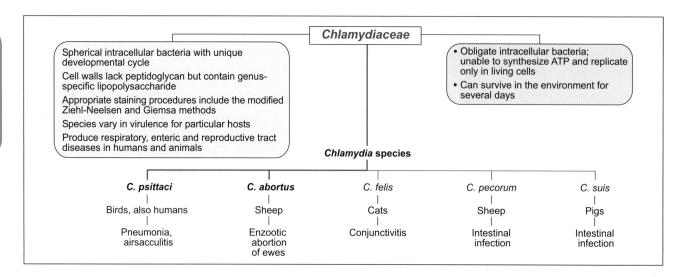

Chlamydiae are obligate intracellular bacteria with an unusual developmental cycle during which unique infectious forms are produced. They replicate within cytoplasmic vacuoles in host cells. On account of their apparent inability to generate ATP, with resultant dependence on host cell metabolism, they have been termed 'energy parasites'. The order *Chlamydiales* consists of eight families including *Chlamydiaceae*, *Parachlamydiaceae*, *Simkaniaceae* and *Waddliaceae*. *Waddlia chondrophila* and *Parachlamydia* species have been implicated in bovine abortion, while *Neochlamydia hartmannellae*, an amoebic endosymbiont, has been associated with ocular disease in cats. However, by far the most significant species from a veterinary and medical point of view are found in the family *Chlamydiaceae*. Based on differences demonstrated by nucleic acid sequencing studies of the 16S and 23S rRNA genes, two genera, *Chlamydia* and *Chlamydophila*, have been validly published. However, it has been formally proposed to combine these two genera into the single genus *Chlamydia*, comprising 11 species. Two species, *C. trachomatis* and *C. pneumoniae*, are important human pathogens responsible for a range of conditions including trachoma, non-specific urethritis, lymphogranuloma venereum and respiratory disease.

In the developmental cycle of chlamydiae, infectious and reproductive forms are morphologically distinct. Infectious extracellular forms, called elementary bodies (EBs), are small (200–300 nm), metabolically inert and osmotically stable. Each EB is surrounded by a conventional bacterial cytoplasmic membrane, a periplasmic space and an outer envelope containing LPS. The periplasmic space does not contain a detectable peptidoglycan layer, although peptidoglycan has been detected in the septum of dividing reticulate bodies (RBs). Rather, the EB relies on disulphide cross-linked envelope proteins for osmotic stability. Elementary bodies enter host cells by receptor-mediated

Table 39.1 Chlamydial infections of veterinary and zoonotic importance.

Pathogen	Hosts	Clinical conditions
Chlamydia psittaci	Birds	Pneumonia and airsacculitis, intestinal infection and diarrhoea, conjunctivitis, pericarditis, encephalitis
	Humans	Psittacosis/ornithosis
C. avium	Birds	Typically isolated from asymptomatic chickens and pigeons. Respiratory outbreaks in psittacine species described
C. gallinacea	Birds	Isolated from asymptomatic domestic poultry. Possible zoonosis
C. abortus	Sheep	Enzootic abortion of ewes (EAE)
	Goats	Chlamydial abortion
	Cattle	Chlamydial abortion
	Pigs	Chlamydial abortion
	Humans	Abortion
C. felis	Cats	Conjunctivitis (feline pneumonitis)
	Humans	Conjunctivitis
C. caviae	Guinea-pigs	Guinea-pig inclusion conjunctivitis
C. pecorum	Sheep	Intestinal infection, conjunctivitis, polyarthritis
	Cattle	Sporadic bovine encephalomyelitis, polyarthritis, metritis
C. suis	Pigs	Intestinal infection
C. muridarum	Mice	Respiratory infection

Concise Review of Veterinary Microbiology, Second Edition. P.J. Quinn, B.K. Markey, F.C. Leonard, E.S. FitzPatrick and S. Fanning.
© 2016 John Wiley & Sons, Ltd. Published 2016 by John Wiley & Sons, Ltd.
Companion website: www.wiley.com/go/quinn/concise-veterinary-microbiology

Development of chlamydial forms in host cells

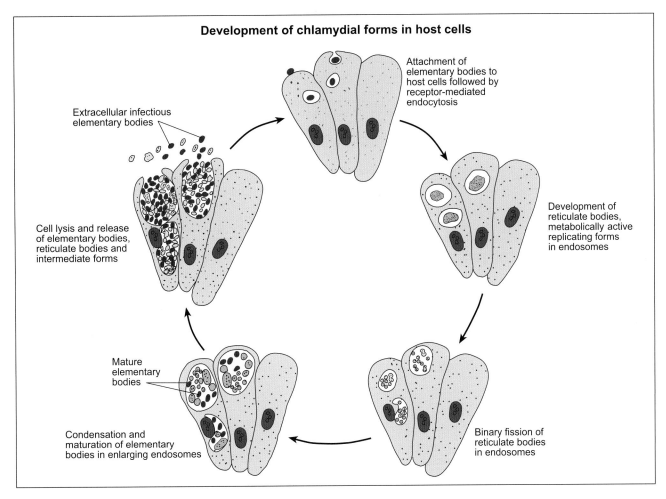

Extracellular infectious elementary bodies

Attachment of elementary bodies to host cells followed by receptor-mediated endocytosis

Development of reticulate bodies, metabolically active replicating forms in endosomes

Cell lysis and release of elementary bodies, reticulate bodies and intermediate forms

Binary fission of reticulate bodies in endosomes

Mature elementary bodies

Condensation and maturation of elementary bodies in enlarging endosomes

endocytosis. Acidification of the endosome and fusion with lysosomes are prevented by mechanisms which are not fully understood. A process of structural reorganization within the pathogen, of several hours duration, results in the conversion of an EB into an RB. The RB, about 1 μm in diameter, is metabolically active, osmotically fragile and replicates by binary fission within the endosome. When stained, the endosome and its contents are called an inclusion. About 20 hours after infection, the developmental cycle becomes asynchronous, with some RBs continuing to divide while others condense and mature, forming EBs. In general, replication continues for up to 72 hours after infection when the host cell lyses, releasing several hundred bodies which include EBs, RBs and intermediate forms. Chlamydial replication may be delayed in the presence of interferon γ or penicillin or when the availability of tryptophan or cysteine is limited, resulting in persistent infection.

Chlamydiae infect over 450 species of birds and a large number of mammalian species including humans (Table 39.1). In recent years, isolations have also been reported from invertebrate species. Chlamydial species are usually associated with specific diseases in particular hosts. Both the severity and the type of disease produced by chlamydiae are highly variable, ranging from clinically inapparent infections and local infections of epithelial surfaces to severe systemic infections. Diseases associated with chlamydial infections include conjunctivitis, arthritis, abortion, urethritis, enteritis, pneumonia and encephalomyelitis. Clinical signs and their severity are influenced by factors related to both host and pathogen, and one type of clinical presentation usually predominates in outbreaks of disease. Infection with

C. pecorum is associated with conjunctivitis, arthritis and inapparent intestinal infection. The type of clinical presentation relates to the route of infection and the degree of exposure. Environmental factors and management practices can influence the prevalence of some chlamydial infections such as enzootic abortion in ewes, which tends to be more prevalent in intensively managed lowland flocks.

The gastrointestinal tract appears to be the usual site of infection with *Chlamydia* species in animals. Intestinal infections are often subclinical and persistent. Faecal shedding of the organisms, which is typically prolonged, becomes intermittent with time. The EBs can survive in the environment for several days. In sheep, *C. abortus* is an important cause of abortion whereas infections with *C. pecorum* are frequently inapparent. Interspecies transmission is uncommon. When it occurs, the outcome of infection in the secondary host may be either similar to that in the primary host, as in transmission from sheep to cattle, or severe, as in transmission from sheep to pregnant women.

Methods used for the diagnosis of chlamydial infections include demonstration of organisms in stained impression smears, immunohistochemistry, detection of chlamydial DNA by PCR and isolation in susceptible cell culture or embryonated eggs. Animal infections can be confirmed by serology. However, interpretation of results is complicated by the fact that many of the available serological procedures detect antibodies against chlamydial LPS and therefore do not distinguish the chlamydial species involved in a particular infection. An additional limitation of serology is that cross-reactions occur between the LPS of chlamydiae and some Gram-negative bacteria.

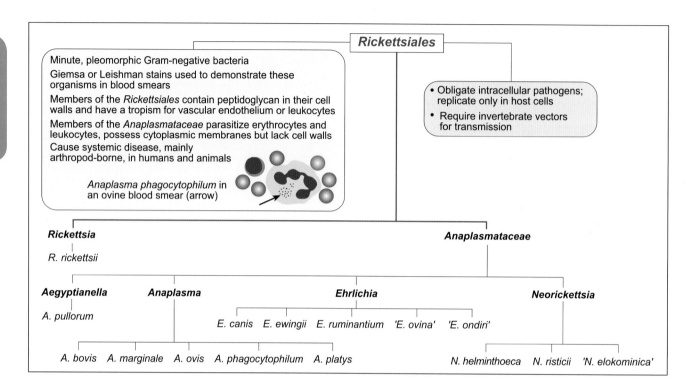

Organisms in the order *Rickettsiales* form a diverse group of non-motile Gram-negative bacteria which replicate only in host cells. In addition to host-cell dependence and poor affinity for basic dyes, a requirement for an invertebrate vector distinguishes them from most conventional bacteria.

At present, two families, *Rickettsiaceae* and *Anaplasmataceae*, comprise the *Rickettsiales*. The genera *Rickettsia* and *Orienta* belong to the family *Rickettsiaceae*, with *Rickettsia rickettsii* the principal pathogen of veterinary importance. Members of the *Anaplasmataceae* parasitize cells of the haematopoietic system and possess cytoplasmic membranes but lack cell walls (Table 40.1). The genera *Haemobartonella* and *Eperythrozoon*, previously classified in the *Anaplasmataceae*, have been transferred to the genus *Mycoplasma*. *Coxiella burnetii* is now classified within the order *Legionellales* and is dealt with in a separate section of this chapter.

Animal hosts and arthropod vectors, frequently ticks, are the reservoirs of most rickettsias. In arthropods, rickettsias replicate in epithelial cells of the gut before spreading to the salivary glands and ovaries where further replication may occur. Organisms are transmitted when the arthropod feeds on the animal host. Some organisms are maintained in tick populations by transovarial transmission; trans-stadial but not transovarial transmission of *Ehrlichia canis* and *Anaplasma phagocytophilum* occurs in ticks. Transmission by flukes has been confirmed for *Neorickettsia* species.

Rickettsial organisms are relatively host-specific. Because definitive arthropod or fluke vectors are involved in the transmission of most rickettsias, diseases associated with these organisms tend to occur in defined geographical regions. The clinical signs frequently reflect the targeting of a particular cell type by the causal rickettsial agent.

Rocky Mountain spotted fever, caused by *Rickettsia rickettsii*, is a common rickettsial disease of humans in the Americas, and also affects dogs. These highly pathogenic organisms have a predilection for endothelial cells of small blood vessels. *Ehrlichia* species have a predilection for leukocytes. Members of the *Anaplasmataceae* have an affinity for erythrocytes and neutrophils. Tick-borne fever, caused by *Anaplasma phagocytophilum*, affects domestic and wild ruminants in many European countries. The organism can presist for months or years in a proportion of infected animals. Wildlife may constitute an important reservoir of infection also. Fever, inappetence and a reduced growth rate may be evident in young animals, while abortions or stillbirths may occur in susceptible, pregnant animals. Transient immunosuppression is a feature of the disease. Variants of *A. phagocytophilum* infecting different species of animals are reported, but the epidemiological significance of these variants is not determined.

Members of the *Rickettsiales* can be recognized and differentiated by the species of animals affected, cell predilection, microscopic appearance and molecular techniques. Blood or tissue

Concise Review of Veterinary Microbiology, Second Edition. P.J. Quinn, B.K. Markey, F.C. Leonard, E.S. FitzPatrick and S. Fanning.
© 2016 John Wiley & Sons, Ltd. Published 2016 by John Wiley & Sons, Ltd.

Companion website: www.wiley.com/go/quinn/concise-veterinary-microbiology

Table 40.1 Rickettsial pathogens of veterinary importance.

Pathogen	Hosts / Vectors	Disease	Geographical distribution
Rickettsia rickettsii	Humans, dogs / Ticks	Rocky Mountain spotted fever	Western hemisphere, principally the Americas
Aegyptianella pullorum	Poultry / Ticks	Aegyptianellosis	Africa, Asia, Mediterranean region
Anaplasma bovis	Cattle / Ticks	Bovine ehrlichiosis	Africa, Middle East, Asia, South America
A. marginale	Ruminants / Ticks	Anaplasmosis	Tropical and subtropical regions
A. ovis	Sheep, goats / Ticks	Anaplasmosis	Asia, Africa, Europe, USA
A. phagocytophilum	Ruminants, horses, humans / Ticks	Tick-borne fever, equine and human granulocytotropic anaplasmosis	Worldwide
A. platys	Dogs / Ticks suspected	Canine cyclic thrombocytopenia	Americas, Middle East, Mediterranean
Ehrlichia canis	Dogs / Ticks	Canine monocytic ehrlichiosis	Tropical and subtropical regions
E. ewingii	Dogs / Ticks	Canine granulocytic ehrlichiosis	USA
E. ruminantium	Ruminants / Ticks	Heartwater	Sub-Saharan Africa, Caribbean islands
'E. ondiri'[a]	Cattle / Ticks suspected	Bovine petechial fever	Highlands of East Africa
'E. ovina'[a]	Sheep / Ticks	Ovine ehrlichiosis	Africa, Asia, Middle East
'Neorickettsia elokominica'[a]	Dogs, bears, racoons / Flukes	Elokomin fluke fever	West coast of North America
N. helminthoeca	Dogs, bears / Flukes	Salmon poisoning disease	West coast of North America
N. risticii	Horses / Flukes	Potomac horse fever	North America, Europe

[a]These organisms do not have fully approved taxonomic status.

smears stained by the Giemsa technique can be used to demonstrate the morphology of many rickettsial organisms. They occur as purplish-blue, small individual organisms, sometimes in clusters. Fluorescent antibody techniques can be used to identify specific rickettsial organisms in smears. Some rickettsias can be isolated in the yolk sac of embryonated eggs or in defined tissue culture cell lines. However, *Ehrlichia* and *Anaplasma* species which target granulocytes and *Anaplasma* species which affect erythrocytes have not been cultured *in vitro*. Molecular methods, including nucleic acid probes and PCR techniques, have been developed to detect most rickettsial pathogens.

A limited number of vaccines are available for rickettsial pathogens. In many instances, arthropod vectors such as ticks are involved in pathogen transmission. For diseases transmitted in this manner, tick control is an essential part of disease prevention. Tetracyclines administered early in the disease, may be effective. For some rickettsial diseases, such as Rocky Mountain spotted fever, treatment should be continued for up to two weeks.

Coxiella burnetii

Although the biological features and reproductive strategies of this unusual organism are similar to those of rickettsial organisms, analysis of the 16S rRNA gene has resulted in its reclassification within the *Legionellales* order. This obligate intracellular pathogen produces endospore-like forms, which can survive for long periods in the environment. Aerosol transmission of *C. burnetii* commonly occurs in domestic animals and humans. *Coxiella burnetii* localizes in cells of the female reproductive tract and mammary glands of ruminants and replicates in the acidic environment of the phagolysosome. Infection may cause abortion in many species of ruminants, including small ruminants. Q fever, caused by *C. burnetii*, is an influenza-like occupational disease of humans in contact with farm animals and their contaminated products. Most infections are acquired by inhalation of aerosols from parturient sheep, goats or cattle. The largest outbreak of Q fever recorded to date occurred in humans in the Netherlands between 2007 and 2010, with more than 4000 cases documented. Infection can be diagnosed using serology, isolation in embryonated eggs or tissue culture, or by PCR-based methods. Control measures include careful disposal of birth products from ruminants to prevent aerosol transmission of the organisms and attention to disinfection procedures. Vaccines are available for use in ruminants. A vaccine has also been developed for use in humans at high risk of infection.

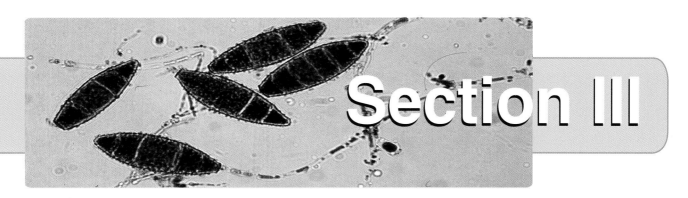

Section III

Mycology

41 General features of fungi associated with disease in animals

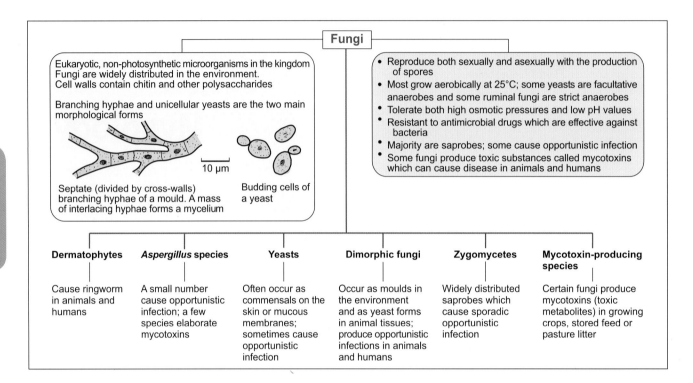

Fungi

- Eukaryotic, non-photosynthetic microorganisms in the kingdom Fungi are widely distributed in the environment. Cell walls contain chitin and other polysaccharides
- Branching hyphae and unicellular yeasts are the two main morphological forms

10 μm

Septate (divided by cross-walls) branching hyphae of a mould. A mass of interlacing hyphae forms a mycelium

Budding cells of a yeast

- Reproduce both sexually and asexually with the production of spores
- Most grow aerobically at 25°C; some yeasts are facultative anaerobes and some ruminal fungi are strict anaerobes
- Tolerate both high osmotic pressures and low pH values
- Resistant to antimicrobial drugs which are effective against bacteria
- Majority are saprobes; some cause opportunistic infection
- Some fungi produce toxic substances called mycotoxins which can cause disease in animals and humans

Dermatophytes
Cause ringworm in animals and humans

***Aspergillus* species**
A small number cause opportunistic infection; a few species elaborate mycotoxins

Yeasts
Often occur as commensals on the skin or mucous membranes; sometimes cause opportunistic infection

Dimorphic fungi
Occur as moulds in the environment and as yeast forms in animal tissues; produce opportunistic infections in animals and humans

Zygomycetes
Widely distributed saprobes which cause sporadic opportunistic infection

Mycotoxin-producing species
Certain fungi produce mycotoxins (toxic metabolites) in growing crops, stored feed or pasture litter

Fungi are eukaryotic, non-photosynthetic heterotrophs which produce exoenzymes and obtain nutrients by absorption. Of the approximately 100,000 fungal species that have been described to date, only a few hundred are known to be pathogenic for animals and humans. The two main morphological fungal forms are moulds and yeasts. Moulds grow as branching filaments called hyphae, whereas the unicellular yeasts have an oval or spherical appearance. Although most fungi grow aerobically, some yeasts are facultatively anaerobic and fungi found in the rumen of cattle are strict anaerobes. Incubation temperatures and time required for development of distinctive colonial morphology are indicated in Table 41.1. Dimorphic fungi occur in both mould and yeast forms. Environmental temperature and other factors usually determine the form in which a dimorphic fungus occurs.

Classification of fungi has traditionally relied heavily on morphology and sexual reproduction. The form of a fungal species during its sexually reproductive life cycle is termed its

Table 41.1 Incubation conditions appropriate for fungal cultures.

Fungal group	Incubation conditions	
	Temperature (°C)	Time
Dermatophytes	25	2–4 weeks
Aspergillus species	35–37	1–4 days
Yeasts (pathogenic)	37	1–4 days
Dimorphic fungi		
Mould phase	25	1–4 weeks
Yeast phase	37	1–4 weeks
Zygomycetes	34	1–4 days

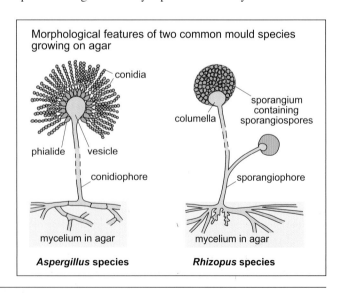

Morphological features of two common mould species growing on agar

conidia

phialide   vesicle

conidiophore

mycelium in agar

***Aspergillus* species**

sporangium containing sporangiospores

columella

sporangiophore

mycelium in agar

***Rhizopus* species**

Concise Review of Veterinary Microbiology, Second Edition. P.J. Quinn, B.K. Markey, F.C. Leonard, E.S. FitzPatrick and S. Fanning.
© 2016 John Wiley & Sons, Ltd. Published 2016 by John Wiley & Sons, Ltd.
Companion website: www.wiley.com/go/quinn/concise-veterinary-microbiology

Asexual spores produced by fungi of veterinary importance

Arthroconidia (arthrospores)
Spores which are formed and subsequently released during the process of hyphal fragmentation. Spores may be formed successively as in dermatophytes (A), or with intervening empty cells as in *Coccidioides immitis* (B)

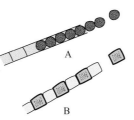

Blastoconidia (blastospores)
Conidia (arrows) which are produced by budding, as in *Candida albicans*, from a mother cell (A), from hyphae (B) or from pseudohyphae (C)

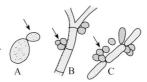

Chlamydoconidia (chlamydospores)
Thick-walled, resistant spores which contain storage products. These structures are formed by some fungi in unfavourable environmental conditions

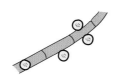

Macroconidia
Large multi-celled conidia which are produced by dermatophytes in culture

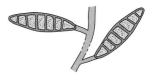

Microconidia
Small conidia which are produced by certain dermatophytes

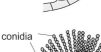

Phialoconidia
Conidia produced from phialides. The phialides of *Aspergillus* species arise from a vesicle

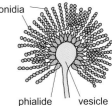

conidia

phialide   vesicle

Sporangiospores
Spores (arrow), formed by zygomycetes such as *Rhizopus* species, are released when a mature sporangium ruptures

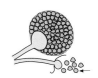

teleomorph, while its asexual form is referred to as its anamorph. Fungi that lack a meiotic stage are referred to as mitosporic fungi. Formerly, fungi with no known sexual stage were placed in a heterogeneous group called the *Deuteromycota* or Fungi Imperfecti. Molecular methods are increasingly being used to assign fungal species to their appropriate grouping. A dual naming system has been in use for many years with separate teleomorphic and anamorphic names used; as an example the teleomorphic name of the dermatophyte *Microsporum canis* is *Arthroderma otae*. Advances in diagnostic molecular methods should eventually replace this dual naming system. Seven phyla are recognized within the kingdom Fungi: *Glomeromycota, Microsporidia, Blastocladiomycota, Chytridiomycota, Ascomycota, Basidiomycota* and *Neocallimastigomycota*. Fungi of veterinary importance are found in three phyla: *Ascomycota, Basidiomycota* and *Zygomycota*. The status of the phylum *Zygomycota* is uncertain and it may be broken up, with species of veterinary importance assigned to the subphyla *Mucoromycotina* and *Entomophthoromycotina* currently listed as *incertae sedis* (Latin for 'of uncertain placement'). However, the term 'zygomycetes' is still in use, encompassing species of interest previously recognized within the phylum.

Fungal species may be saprobes, symbionts, commensals or parasites. Saprobic fungi, which are widespread in the environment and are involved in the decomposition of organic matter, occasionally cause sporadic, opportunistic infections in animals. The parasitic dermatophytes cause ringworm in animals. Overgrowth of yeasts, which are often commensals on skin and mucous membranes, sometimes causes localized lesions.

Hyphal cell walls are composed mainly of carbohydrate components including chitin macromolecules with cellulose cross-linkages. In yeasts, cell walls contain protein complexed with polysaccharides. Both moulds and yeasts have nuclei with well-defined nuclear membranes, mitochondria and networks of microtubules.

Moulds tend to form large colonies with growth and extension of hyphae at their periphery. Several types of asexual spores are produced by fungi. Conidia are formed on conidiophores while sporangiospores are formed within a sac-like sporangium. In most yeasts, asexual division is by budding. Colonies of yeast-like fungi are soft, smooth and round. The pathogenic mechanisms whereby fungi produce disease are listed in Box 41.1. Factors which predispose to infection with fungi are outlined in Box 41.2.

Methods of differentiating fungal species include examination of sporing heads for conidial arrangement or the presence of a sporangium. Features of vegetative hyphae used for differentiation include the presence or absence of septa and pigment. The size, appearance and colour of fungal colonies are useful for species differentiation. Yeasts can be differentiated by colonial appearance and by the size and shape of individual cells.

Box 41.1 Mechanisms involved in fungal diseases

- Tissue invasion (mycosis)
- Toxin production (mycotoxicosis)
- Induction of hypersensitivity

Box 41.2 Factors which may predispose to fungal invasion of tissues

- Immunosuppression
- Prolonged antibiotic therapy
- Immunological defects
- Immaturity, ageing and malnutrition
- Exposure to heavy challenge of fungal spores
- Traumatized tissues
- Persistent moisture on skin surface
- Some neoplastic conditions

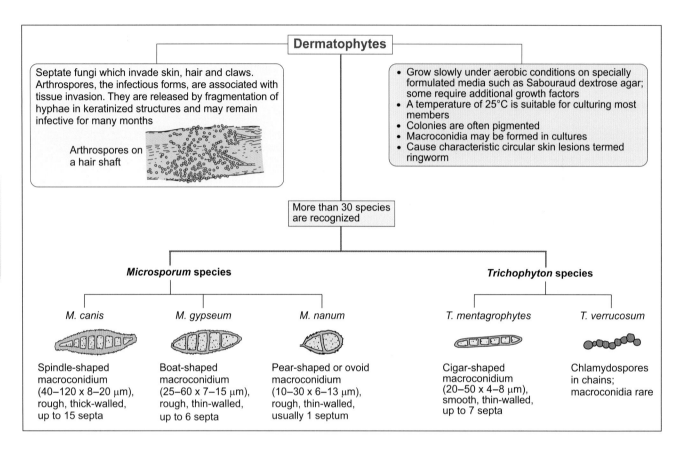

The dermatophytes are a group of septate fungi which occur worldwide and invade superficial keratinized structures such as skin, hair and claws. More than 30 species of dermatophytes are recognized, classified in three anamorphic genera: *Microsporum*, *Trichophyton* and *Epidermophyton*. When a sexual stage of a species is identified, that species is placed in the teleomorphic genus *Arthroderma* (phylum *Ascomycota*). Arthrospores (arthroconidia), the infectious forms associated with tissue invasion by this group of fungi, are released by fragmentation of hyphae in keratinized structures. These resistant forms can remain viable for more than 12 months in suitable environments. Macroconidia and microconidia are produced in culture. The colonies of many dermatophytes are pigmented with a characteristic appearance.

Dermatophytosis (ringworm) affects many animal species (Table 42.1). The disease is a zoonosis and many human infections are caused by *Microsporum canis*. Dermatophytes can be grouped on the basis of their habitats and host preferences as geophilic, zoophilic or anthropophilic (Table 42.2). Zoophilic and anthropophilic dermatophytes are obligate pathogens of animals and humans respectively. Geophilic dermatophytes inhabit and replicate in soil. Animals can acquire infection with geophilic dermatophytes from soil or through contact with infected animals. Dermatophytes invade keratinized structures such as the stratum corneum of the epidermis, hair follicles, hair shafts and feathers. The hyphae grow centrifugally from the initial lesion towards normal skin, producing typical ringworm lesions. The metabolic products of hyphal growth may provoke a local inflammatory response. Alopecia, tissue repair and non-viable hyphae occur at the centre of developing lesions. Young, aged, debilitated and immunosuppressed animals are particularly susceptible to infection. Clinical features of the disease include classical ringworm lesions, miliary dermatitis and, rarely, generalized lesions in immunosuppressed animals. Secondary bacterial infection sometimes follows mycotic folliculitis.

Microsporum canis is the most common cause of dermatophytosis in dogs and cats in most countries. Inapparent infections are known to occur in cats. Dogs may also become infected with *M. gypseum* and *Trichophyton mentagrophytes*. The disease usually presents as areas of alopecia, scaling and broken hairs surrounded by inflammatory zones. Generalized infections may be associated with conditions such as hyperadrenocorticism and immunosuppression. *Trichophyton verrucosum* is the usual

Concise Review of Veterinary Microbiology, Second Edition. P.J. Quinn, B.K. Markey, F.C. Leonard, E.S. FitzPatrick and S. Fanning.
© 2016 John Wiley & Sons, Ltd. Published 2016 by John Wiley & Sons, Ltd.
Companion website: www.wiley.com/go/quinn/concise-veterinary-microbiology

Table 42.1 Dermatophytes of animals, their main hosts and reported geographical distribution.

Dermatophyte	Hosts	Geographical distribution
Microsporum canis var. *canis*	Cats, dogs	Worldwide
M. canis var. *distortum*	Dogs	New Zealand, Australia, North America
M. equinum (considered to be identical to *M. canis*)	Horses	Africa, Australasia, Europe, North and South America
M. gallinae	Chickens, turkeys	Worldwide
M. gypseum	Horses, dogs, rodents	Worldwide
M. nanum	Pigs	North and South America, Europe, Australasia
Trichophyton equinum	Horses	Worldwide
T. equinum var. *autotrophicum*	Horses	Australia and New Zealand
T. mentagrophytes var. *mentagrophytes*	Rodents, dogs, horses and many other animal species	Worldwide
T. mentagrophytes var. *erinacei*	European hedgehogs, dogs	Europe, New Zealand
T. verrucosum	Cattle	Worldwide

Table 42.2 Dermatophytes grouped according to host preference or habitat.

Zoophilic group	Geophilic group	Anthropophilic group[a]
Microsporum canis	*Microsporum cookei*	*Epidermophyton floccosum*
M. gallinae	*M. gypseum*	*M. audouinii*
Trichophyton equinum	*M. nanum*	*M. ferrugineum*
T. mentagrophytes	*M. persicolor*	*T. rubrum*
T. verrucosum	*T. simii*	*T. schoenleinii*

[a] Anthropophilic dermatophytes rarely infect animals.

cence may be evident when infected hairs are exposed to UV light in up to 50% of infected animals. Specimens suitable for laboratory examination include plucked hair, deep skin scrapings from the edge of lesions, scrapings from affected claws and biopsy material. Hair and skin scrapings treated with 10% potassium hydroxide should be examined microscopically for the presence of arthrospores. Histological sections of skin can be stained by the PAS or methenamine silver techniques to demonstrate fungal structures. Specimens are cultured on Sabouraud dextrose agar, usually with the addition of yeast extract, chloramphenicol and cycloheximide. Inoculated plates are incubated aerobically at 25°C and examined twice weekly for up to five weeks. Identification is based on colonial morphology and the microscopic appearance of macroconidia or other structures. Molecular detection of dermatophytes in dogs and cats using real-time PCR is available commercially.

Treatment and control are particularly important in domestic carnivores because dermatophytoses are zoonoses. Owners of animals with ringworm and veterinary staff dealing with suspect animals should wear gloves. Animals with suspicious lesions should be isolated and early laboratory confirmation is essential. Removal of the hair coat by clipping may be necessary around affected areas, followed by topical treatment with miconazole shampoo. A solution of 0.2% enilconazole is approved in most countries for use in dogs, cats, horses and cattle. Clippings should be disposed of carefully. Oral treatment with itraconazole or other suitable antifungal drugs may be necessary if lesions are extensive. Contaminated bedding should be burned and grooming equipment should be disinfected with 0.5% sodium hypochlorite.

Topical treatment with captan or natamycin may be effective in cattle. Affected horses should be treated topically and contaminated harness and grooming gear should be disinfected with 0.5% sodium hypochlorite.

cause of ringworm in cattle. Calves are most commonly affected and often develop characteristic lesions on the face and around the eyes. Oval areas of affected skin are alopecic with greyish-white crusts. Infection is most common in winter and a number of animals are usually involved. A vaccine composed of an attenuated strain of *T. verrucosum* has been used for the control of bovine dermatophytosis. In horses, *Trichophyton equinum* is the main cause of ringworm. Transmission occurs by direct contact or from contaminated harness or grooming gear. Horses under four years of age are particularly susceptible to dermatophytosis.

Definitive diagnosis based on clinical signs is usually difficult and laboratory investigation of dermatophytosis is often necessary. As dermatophytes tend to parasitize particular hosts, the animal species affected may indicate the dermatophyte likely to be involved (Table 42.1). In cats and dogs with suspicious lesions, examination with a Wood's lamp should be carried out to detect infection with *M. canis*. A characteristic green fluores-

43 *Aspergillus* species

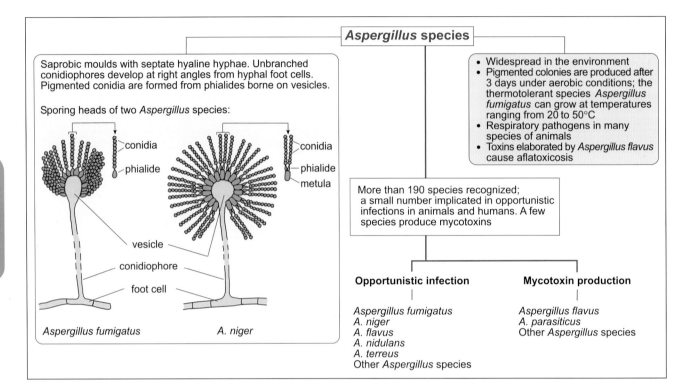

Aspergillus species

Saprobic moulds with septate hyaline hyphae. Unbranched conidiophores develop at right angles from hyphal foot cells. Pigmented conidia are formed from phialides borne on vesicles.

Sporing heads of two *Aspergillus* species:

conidia
phialide

conidia
phialide
metula

vesicle
conidiophore
foot cell

Aspergillus fumigatus   *A. niger*

- Widespread in the environment
- Pigmented colonies are produced after 3 days under aerobic conditions; the thermotolerant species *Aspergillus fumigatus* can grow at temperatures ranging from 20 to 50°C
- Respiratory pathogens in many species of animals
- Toxins elaborated by *Aspergillus flavus* cause aflatoxicosis

More than 190 species recognized; a small number implicated in opportunistic infections in animals and humans. A few species produce mycotoxins

Opportunistic infection

Aspergillus fumigatus
A. niger
A. flavus
A. nidulans
A. terreus
Other *Aspergillus* species

Mycotoxin production

Aspergillus flavus
A. parasiticus
Other *Aspergillus* species

Although the genus *Aspergillus* contains more than 190 species, only a limited number have been implicated in opportunistic infections in animals and humans. *Aspergillus* species are saprobes which are widely distributed in the environment. *Aspergillus fumigatus* is the species most often involved in tissue invasion; other potentially invasive species include *A. niger*, *A. flavus, A. nidulans, A. flavipes, A. deflectus* and *A. terreus*. Although the teleomorph or sexual stage is not known for many *Aspergillus* species, the sexual reproductive cycle of *Aspergillus fumigatus* has been demonstrated and its teleomorph *Neosartorya fumigata* has been described.

Aspergilli are aerobic and grow rapidly, forming distinct colonies after incubation for two to three days. The colour of the obverse side of colonies, which may be bluish-green, black, brown or yellow, varies with individual species and cultural conditions. *Aspergillus fumigatus*, a thermotolerant species, grows at temperatures ranging from 20 to 50°C.

The hyphae are septate, hyaline and up to 8 μm in diameter. Unbranched conidiophores develop at right angles from specialized hyphal foot cells. The tip of the conidiophore enlarges forming a vesicle which becomes partially or completely covered with flask-shaped phialides. The phialides produce chains of round pigmented conidia which are up to 5 μm in diameter. Respiratory infection may occur following inhalation of spores. Occasionally, infection can result from ingestion of spores or

following the introduction of spores into tissues by trauma. Systemic infection is invariably associated with immunosuppression. Species such as *A. flavus*, which elaborate potent toxins when growing on cereals and other crops, cause mycotoxicoses.

Aspergillus species grow on standard laboratory media such as Sabouraud dextrose agar. Because the genus contains a large number of species, differentiation is difficult. Colonies can be up to 5 cm in diameter after incubation for five days. The colonies of *A. fumigatus* become velvety or granular and bluish-green with narrow white peripheries. Colonies of *A. niger* are black and granular, features imparted by the large pigmented sporing heads. *Aspergillus flavus* colonies are yellowish-green with a fluffy texture.

Infection with *Aspergillus* species, mainly *A. fumigatus*, has been recorded in many species of animals. Aspergillosis, which is primarily a respiratory infection, follows spore inhalation. Immune competence of the host largely determines the outcome of infection. Factors which modify immune competence such as corticosteroid therapy, cytotoxic drugs and immunosuppressive viral infections may predispose to tissue invasion. Hyphal invasion of blood vessels leads to vasculitis and thrombus formation. Mycotic granulomas may develop in the lungs and occasionally in other internal organs.

Clinical cases of aspergillosis are comparatively uncommon and usually sporadic. The clinical conditions caused by

SECTION III

Concise Review of Veterinary Microbiology, Second Edition. P.J. Quinn, B.K. Markey, F.C. Leonard, E.S. FitzPatrick and S. Fanning.
© 2016 John Wiley & Sons, Ltd. Published 2016 by John Wiley & Sons, Ltd.
Companion website: www.wiley.com/go/quinn/concise-veterinary-microbiology

Table 43.1 Clinical conditions caused by *Aspergillus* species in domestic animals.

Hosts	Condition	Comments
Birds	Brooder pneumonia	Occurs in newly hatched chickens in incubators
	Pneumonia and airsacculitis	Chickens and poults up to 6 weeks of age are most susceptible; older birds sometimes affected
	Generalized aspergillosis	Dissemination of infection usually from the respiratory tract
Horses	Guttural pouch mycosis	Confined to guttural pouch, often unilateral
	Nasal granuloma	Produces a nasal discharge and interferes with breathing. Fungi other than *Aspergillus* species may initiate this condition
	Keratitis	Localized infection following ocular trauma
Cattle	Mycotic abortion	Occurs sporadically; produces thickened placenta and plaques on skin of aborted foetus
	Mycotic pneumonia	Uncommon condition of housed calves
	Mycotic mastitis	May result from the use of contaminated intramammary antibiotic tubes
	Intestinal aspergillosis	May cause acute or chronic diarrhoea in calves
Dogs	Nasal aspergillosis	Invasion of nasal mucosa and turbinate bones; occurs periodically
	Otitis externa	*Aspergillus* species may constitute part of a mixed infection
	Disseminated aspergillosis	Uncommon; may result in osteomyelitis or discospondylitis
Cats	Systemic aspergillosis	Rarely encountered; immunosuppressed animals are at risk

Aspergillus species in domestic animals are summarized in Table 43.1. Brooder pneumonia affects newly hatched chickens which are exposed to high numbers of *A. fumigatus* spores. Affected chickens develop somnolence and inappetence and many may die. Yellowish nodules are present in the lungs, air sacs and, occasionally, in other organs. Histopathological evidence of tissue invasion by fungi and culture of *A. fumigatus* from lesions are required for confirmation. Strict hygiene and routine fumigation of incubators are effective control measures. Aspergillosis in mature birds frequently follows inhalation of spore-laden dust derived from contaminated litter or feed. Poultry, captive penguins, raptors and psittacine birds may be affected. Clinical signs, which are variable, include dyspnoea and emaciation. Yellowish nodules resembling lesions of avian tuberculosis can be observed in lungs and air sacs. Diagnosis is confirmed by histopathology and culture.

In horses, guttural pouch mycosis, which is frequently associated with *A. fumigatus* infection, is usually unilateral. Plaque-like lesions develop in the mucosa of the pouch wall. When fungal hyphae penetrate to deeper tissues they cause tissue necrosis, thrombosis, erosion of blood vessel walls and neural damage. Clinical signs include epistaxis, dysphagia and laryngeal hemiplegia. Diagnosis is based on clinical signs, radiographic evidence of fluid accumulation in the pouch and demonstration of characteristic lesions by endoscopy. Confirmation is based on the demonstration of fungal hyphae in biopsy specimens and isolation of *A. fumigatus* from lesions. Therapeutic options include infusion of antifungal agents such as itraconazole into the pouch and surgical intervention to deal with serious haemorrhage. The spores of *A. fumigatus* are among the allergens reported to be capable of inducing the allergic condition recurrent airway obstruction in horses, also known as chronic obstructive pulmonary disease and 'heaves'.

Nasal aspergillosis in dogs is encountered predominantly in young to middle-aged dolichocephalic breeds. Clinical signs, which are often unilateral, include persistent profuse sanguinopurulent nasal discharge with sneezing and bouts of epistaxis. Radiography may reveal an increased radiolucency of turbinate bones and computerized tomography scans are of high diagnostic value. Rhinoscopy is also useful for clinical examination. Culture and histopathological examination of biopsy material are essential for confirmation. Flushing of the frontal sinuses and nasal chambers with clotrimazole may be used together with systemic treatment with itraconazole, fluconazole or voriconazole. Treatment for six to eight weeks may be required.

Mycotic abortion in cows occurs sporadically and its prevalence may be influenced by poor-quality contaminated fodder harvested in wet seasons. *Aspergillus fumigatus* can proliferate in damp hay, in poor-quality silage and in brewer's grains. Infection, which reaches the uterus haematogenously, causes placentitis, leading to abortion late in gestation. Affected cows usually show no signs of systemic illness. Intercotyledonary areas of the placenta are thickened and leathery and the cotyledons are necrotic. Aborted foetuses may have raised cutaneous plaques, resembling ringworm lesions. Diagnosis is based on culture of *A. fumigatus* from foetal abomasal contents and histopathological evidence of mycotic placentitis.

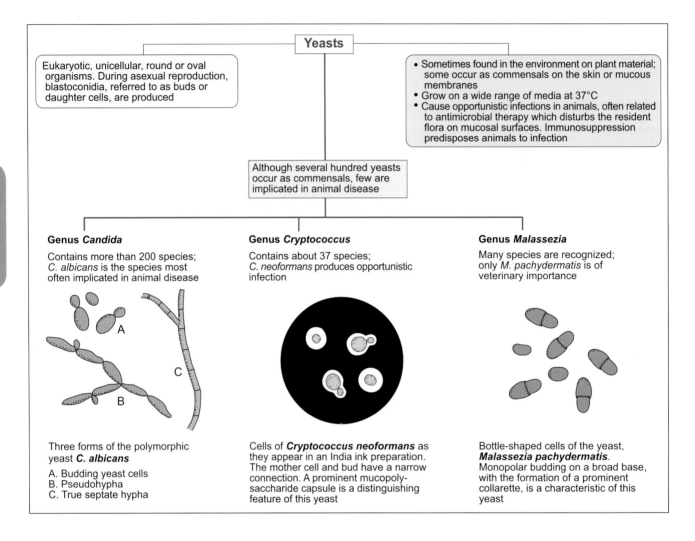

Yeasts

Eukaryotic, unicellular, round or oval organisms. During asexual reproduction, blastoconidia, referred to as buds or daughter cells, are produced

- Sometimes found in the environment on plant material; some occur as commensals on the skin or mucous membranes
- Grow on a wide range of media at 37°C
- Cause opportunistic infections in animals, often related to antimicrobial therapy which disturbs the resident flora on mucosal surfaces. Immunosuppression predisposes animals to infection

Although several hundred yeasts occur as commensals, few are implicated in animal disease

Genus *Candida*

Contains more than 200 species; *C. albicans* is the species most often implicated in animal disease

Genus *Cryptococcus*

Contains about 37 species; *C. neoformans* produces opportunistic infection

Genus *Malassezia*

Many species are recognized; only *M. pachydermatis* is of veterinary importance

Three forms of the polymorphic yeast *C. albicans*

A. Budding yeast cells
B. Pseudohypha
C. True septate hypha

Cells of ***Cryptococcus neoformans*** as they appear in an India ink preparation. The mother cell and bud have a narrow connection. A prominent mucopoly-saccharide capsule is a distinguishing feature of this yeast

Bottle-shaped cells of the yeast, ***Malassezia pachydermatis***. Monopolar budding on a broad base, with the formation of a prominent collarette, is a characteristic of this yeast

Yeasts are eukaryotic, unicellular, round or oval, single-celled organisms. During asexual reproduction, blastoconidia, also referred to as buds or daughter cells, develop. Yeasts grow aerobically on Sabouraud dextrose agar and species capable of tissue invasion grow well at 37°C. Colonies, which are usually moist and creamy in texture, resemble large bacterial colonies. In addition to their environmental habitat on plants or plant material, yeasts also occur as commensals on the skin or mucous membranes of animals. Immunosuppression or factors such as antimicrobial therapy which disturb the resident flora on mucosal surfaces may facilitate yeast overgrowth leading to tissue invasion. Yeasts of importance in animal disease are *Candida* species (particularly *C. albicans*), *Cryptococcus neoformans* and *Malassezia pachydermatis*. *Macrorhabdus ornithogaster* (formerly referred to as 'megabacteria') is a yeast found in the proventriculus of several avian species. It is associated with

'going light' in budgerigars, a fatal disease characterized by progressive weight loss.

Candida species

Although there are more than 200 species in the genus *Candida*, the species most often implicated in animal disease is *Candida albicans*. It grows aerobically at 37°C on a wide range of media, including Sabouraud dextrose agar. Colonies are composed of budding oval cells approximately $5.0 \times 8.0\,\mu m$. In animal tissues, *C. albicans* may exhibit polymorphism in the form of pseudo-hyphae or hyphae. The transition from budding to hyphal forms probably facilitates tissue penetration and increases resistance to phagocytosis due to the larger size of the hyphae.

Opportunistic infections with *Candida* species occur sporadically. Localized mucocutaneous tissue invasion referred to as thrush can occur in the oral cavity or in the gastrointestinal

Concise Review of Veterinary Microbiology, Second Edition. P.J. Quinn, B.K. Markey, F.C. Leonard, E.S. FitzPatrick and S. Fanning.
© 2016 John Wiley & Sons, Ltd. Published 2016 by John Wiley & Sons, Ltd.
Companion website: www.wiley.com/go/quinn/concise-veterinary-microbiology

Table 44.1 Clinical conditions associated with *Candida albicans*.

Hosts	Clinical conditions
Pups, kittens, foals	Mycotic stomatitis
Pigs, foals, calves	Gastro-oesophageal ulcers
Calves	Rumenitis
Dogs	Enteritis, cutaneous lesions
Chickens	Thrush of the oesophagus or crop
Geese, turkeys	Cloacal and vent infections
Cows	Reduced fertility, abortion, mastitis
Mares	Pyometra
Cats	Urocystitis, pyothorax
Cats, horses	Ocular lesions
Dogs, cats, pigs, calves	Disseminated disease

and urogenital tracts. Predisposing factors include defects in cell-mediated immunity, concurrent disease, disturbance of the normal flora by prolonged use of antimicrobial drugs and damage to the mucosal surface from indwelling catheters. The clinical conditions attributed to *C. albicans* are presented in Table 44.1. Suitable specimens for culture and histopathology include biopsy or postmortem tissue samples and milk samples. Tissue sections, stained by the PAS or methenamine silver methods, may reveal budding yeast cells or hyphae. Culture is carried out aerobically at 37°C for up to five days on Sabouraud dextrose agar. Criteria used for identification of *C. albicans* isolates include characteristic colonies yielding budding yeast cells, growth on media containing cycloheximide, biochemical profile, germ tube production when incubated for two hours in serum at 37°C and chlamydospore production in cornmeal agar.

Cryptococcus neoformans

Although the genus *Cryptococcus* contains more than 30 species, only *C. neoformans* produces opportunistic infections. The yeast cells are round to oval and 3.5–8 μm in diameter. A daughter cell is formed as a bud from the mother cell on a narrow neck. When recovered directly from affected animals, the yeasts have thick mucopolysaccharide capsules. *Cryptococcus* species are aerobic and form mucoid colonies on a variety of media, including Sabouraud dextrose agar.

Cryptococcus neoformans is considered to be a species complex consisting of *C. neoformans* var. *grubii* (serotype A), *C. neoformans* var. *neoformans* (serotype D) and subspecies *C.*

gatii (serotypes B, C). Infection with *C. neoformans* occurs through inhalation of yeast cells in contaminated dust. Virulence factors of *C. neoformans* include the capsule, which is antiphagocytic, the ability to grow at mammalian body temperature and the production of phenol oxidase. Infection with *C. neoformans* is usually associated with defective cell-mediated immunity.

Nasal, cutaneous, neural and ocular forms of cryptococcosis are recognized in cats. The disease in dogs, which is less common than in cats, is often disseminated with neurological and ocular signs. Surgical removal combined with parenteral antifungal drugs is the usual method for treating cutaneous cryptococcosis. Therapy should continue for at least two months.

When first isolated, colonies of *Cryptococcus* species are mucoid due to the presence of capsular material. They may have a cream, tan or yellowish appearance. Budding yeasts with wide capsules can be demonstrated in India ink preparations. Identification criteria for *C. neoformans* include the ability to grow at 37°C, brown colonies on birdseed agar, and melanin demonstrable in cell walls using the Fontana–Masson stain on tissue sections.

Malassezia pachydermatis

Malassezia species, commensals on the skin of animals and humans, are aerobic, non-fermentative, urease-positive yeasts which grow at 35–37°C. One species, *Malassezia pachydermatis*, is of veterinary importance. The cells of *M. pachydermatis*, which are bottle-shaped, thick-walled and up to 6.5 μm in length, reproduce by monopolar budding on a broad base.

Malassezia pachydermatis is an opportunistic pathogen associated with two clinical conditions, otitis externa and dermatitis in dogs. Colonization and growth of the organism in these locations may be associated with immunosuppression and other predisposing factors such as persistently moist skin folds, poor ear conformation and excessive use of antibiotics. When the yeast cells are present in high numbers on the skin, they apparently induce excessive sebaceous secretion, a feature of seborrhoeic dermatitis. Treatment with miconazole–chlorhexidine shampoo or a combination of topical and oral ketoconazole may be effective. In otitis externa, the production of proteolytic enzymes by *M. pachydermatis* results in damage to the epithelial lining of the ear canal. The condition is characterized by a dark pungent discharge from the ear canal and intense pruritis.

Numerous, characteristic yeast cells may be demonstrable in exudates or impression smears stained with methylene blue. *Malassezia pachydermatis* can be cultured aerobically at 37°C for four days on Sabouraud dextrose agar containing chloramphenicol. Identification criteria include colonial appearance, growth without the need for lipid supplementation and characteristic microscopic appearance.

45 Dimorphic fungi

Dimorphic fungi

Dimorphic fungi occur in two distinct forms, a mould form and a yeast form. They exist as moulds in the environment and when cultured on Sabouraud dextrose agar at 25°C. In animal tissues and when cultured at 37°C on suitable media, most grow as yeasts.

- Saprobes in soil and in decaying vegetation; some dimorphic fungi grow on wet timber fittings
- Some have defined geographical distribution; others occur worldwide
- Produce opportunistic infections in animals and humans

Blastomyces dermatitidis

Mould form

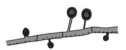

Oval or pear-shaped conidia on septate hyphae when cultured at 25°C

Yeast form

Thick-walled yeast cells form when cultured at 37°C; also found in tissues

Coccidioides immitis

Mould form

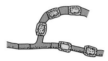

Septate hyphae with barrel-shaped arthrospores separated by empty cells when cultured at 25°C

Spherule

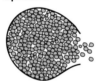

Mature spherules (30 to 100 μm) containing endospores are found in tissues

Histoplasma capsulatum

Mould form

Septate hyphae bearing conidia; later, sunflower-like macroconidia form when cultured at 25°C

Yeast form

Small oval budding yeast cells in cultures at 37°C. Found also in mammalian host cells

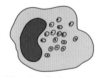

Yeast cells in a macrophage

Sporothrix schenckii

Mould form

Thin septate hyphae with tapering conidiophores bearing conidia in rosette-like clusters. Conidia also occur singly along the hyphae. These forms are found in cultures at 25°C

Yeast form

Cigar-shaped pleomorphic budding yeast cells when cultured at 37°C. Found also in exudates

---

Some fungi, referred to as dimorphic fungi, occur in two distinct forms, a mould form and a yeast form. They exist as moulds in the environment and when cultured on Sabouraud dextrose agar at 25 to 30°C. In animal tissues, and when cultured at 37°C on brain–heart infusion agar with the addition of 5% blood, most grow as yeasts after conversion from the more stable mould form. The dimorphic fungi most often associated with disease in domestic animals are *Blastomyces dermatitidis*, *Histoplasma capsulatum* and *Coccidioides immitis*. The spores of these dimorphic fungi usually enter hosts by the respiratory route. A variant of *H. capsulatum*, referred to as *H. farciminosum*, generally enters through skin abrasions and produces lymphocutaneous lesions in horses. *Sporothrix schenckii* also produces opportunistic lymphocutaneous infections in animals. Table 45.1 summarizes important features of dimorphic fungi associated with disease in animals and humans.

Blastomyces dermatitidis

Blastomycosis, caused by *B. dermatitidis*, most commonly affects dogs and humans. The teleomorph of *B. dermatitidis* is a member of the phylum *Ascomycota* designated *Ajellomyces dermatitidis*. The disease is encountered in North America, Africa, the Middle East and India. Infection usually occurs by inhalation and pulmonary blastomycosis is the usual form of the disease. Presenting signs include coughing, exercise intolerance and dyspnoea. Amphotericin B, which may be combined with ketoconazole, is effective if administered early in the course of the disease.

When incubated at 25 to 30°C on Sabouraud dextrose agar, mould colonies are white and cottony, usually becoming brown with age. When incubated at 37°C on brain–heart infusion agar with added cysteine and 5% blood, yeast colonies are cream to tan, wrinkled and waxy. Yeast cells may be demonstrated

Concise Review of Veterinary Microbiology, Second Edition. P.J. Quinn, B.K. Markey, F.C. Leonard, E.S. FitzPatrick and S. Fanning.
© 2016 John Wiley & Sons, Ltd. Published 2016 by John Wiley & Sons, Ltd.
Companion website: www.wiley.com/go/quinn/concise-veterinary-microbiology

SECTION III

Table 45.1 Dimorphic fungi which are associated with disease in animals and humans.

	Blastomyces dermatitidis	Histoplasma capsulatum	Histoplasma farciminosum	Coccidioides immitis and C. posadasii	Sporothrix schenckii
Disease	Blastomycosis	Histoplasmosis	Epizootic lymphangitis	Coccidioidomycosis	Sporotrichosis
Geographical distribution	Eastern regions of North America, sporadic cases in India and the Middle East	Endemic in the Mississippi and Ohio river valleys, sporadic cases in some countries	Africa, Middle East, Asia	Semi-arid regions of south-western USA, Central and South America	Worldwide, most common in subtropical and tropical regions
Usual habitat	Acid soil rich in organic matter	Soil enriched with bat or bird faeces	Soil	Desert soils at low elevation	Dead vegetation, rose thorns, wooden posts, sphagnum moss
Main hosts	Dogs, humans	Dogs, cats, humans	Horses, other Equidae	Dogs, horses, cats, humans	Horses, cats, dogs, humans
Site of lesions	Lungs, dissemination to skin and other tissues	Lungs, dissemination to other organs	Skin, lymphatic vessels, lymph nodes	Lungs, dissemination to bones, skin and other tissues	Skin, lymphatic vessels

in cytological and histopathological preparations from affected tissues. Serological assays are available.

Histoplasma capsulatum

Although histoplasmosis, caused by *H. capsulatum*, occurs in many countries, it is endemic in the Mississippi and Ohio river valleys and in other areas of the USA. Disseminated disease in dogs and cats is probably associated with impaired cell-mediated immunity. Granulomatous lesions may be found in the lungs of both dogs and cats. Clinical signs in affected dogs include a chronic cough, persistent diarrhoea and emaciation. Ketoconazole and amphotericin B can be used for treatment.

Epizootic lymphangitis, caused by *H. capsulatum* var. *farciminosum*, occurs in *Equidae* in Africa, the Middle East and Asia. Horses usually acquire infection from environmental sources through minor skin abrasions on the limbs. Characteristic lymphocutaneous lesions consist of ulcerated discharging nodules, usually located along the course of thickened, hard, lymphatic vessels. Yeast cells of *H. farciminosum* are found in large numbers in lesions, mainly in macrophages. When cultured at 25 to 30°C on Sabouraud dextrose agar, the mould form of *H. capsulatum* grows as white to buff colonies with aerial hyphae. Septate hyphae bear small conidia and in mature colonies sunflower-like macroconidia may be present. When cultured at 37°C on brain–heart infusion agar with added cysteine and 5% blood, yeast colonies are round, mucoid and cream-coloured. Budding yeast cells are oval to spherical. Histopathological examination of affected tissues reveals pyogranulomatous foci containing yeast forms.

Coccidioides immitis

The geophilic fungus *C. immitis* can infect many animal species including humans. Although grouped with the dimorphic fungi, *C. immitis* is biphasic rather than dimorphic because typical yeast forms are not produced. Large spherules containing endospores develop in tissues. Respiratory infections may follow inhalation of arthrospores.

Clinical infections caused by *Coccidioides* species are limited to defined arid regions of south-western USA, Mexico, and Central and South America. Isolates from outside the endemic region of the San Joaquin Valley in California (formerly referred to as 'non-California' *C. immitis*) have been found to be sufficiently different to be given separate species status with the name *C. posadasii*. The domestic species most often affected is the dog. Canine coccidioidomycosis may present with non-specific signs including coughing, fever and inappetence. Dissemination from pulmonary lesions often results in osteomyelitis and lameness. Treatment with azole drugs for at least six months may be effective.

Diagnosis is usually based on clinical findings and histopathology. Spherules of *C. immitis* may be demonstrated in exudates or aspirates cleared with 10% KOH and also in stained tissue sections. Culturing of *Coccidioides* species is hazardous due to the production of thick-walled, barrel-shaped arthroconidia which are readily aerosolized.

Sporothrix schenckii

This saprobic fungus, which is widely distributed in the environment, grows on dead or senescent vegetation and on wet timber fittings. Infections caused by *S. schenckii* occur sporadically in horses, cats, dogs and humans.

Sporotrichosis is a chronic cutaneous or lymphocutaneous disease which rarely becomes generalized. Lymphocutaneous sporotrichosis is the most common form of the disease in horses. Fungal spores usually enter through abrasions in the lower limbs, and nodules, which ulcerate and discharge a yellowish exudate, develop along the course of superficial lymphatic vessels. Subcutaneous oedema in the affected limb may result from lymphatic obstruction. In feline sporotrichosis, nodular skin lesions occur most often on limb extremities, head and tail. Nodules ulcerate and discharge a seropurulent exudate. Sporotrichosis in dogs often manifests as multiple, ulcerated and crusted alopecic cutaneous lesions over the head and trunk.

Direct microscopic examination of exudates from feline lesions usually reveals large numbers of cigar-shaped yeast cells. Infected cats carry the organism in their nose and mouth and on their nails, facilitating transmission through biting and scratching. In exudates from other animals, yeast cells are sparse. Sporotrichosis may be treated with itraconazole, fluconazole or voriconazole.

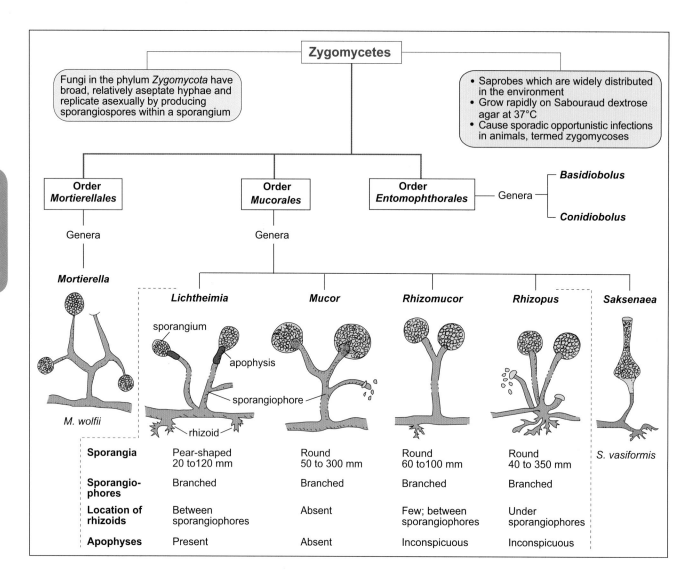

	Lichtheimia	*Mucor*	*Rhizomucor*	*Rhizopus*
Sporangia	Pear-shaped 20 to 120 mm	Round 50 to 300 mm	Round 60 to 100 mm	Round 40 to 350 mm
Sporangiophores	Branched	Branched	Branched	Branched
Location of rhizoids	Between sporangiophores	Absent	Few; between sporangiophores	Under sporangiophores
Apophyses	Present	Absent	Inconspicuous	Inconspicuous

Fungi in the phylum *Zygomycota* usually have broad (up to 15 μm in diameter), coenocytic (relatively aseptate) hyphae and replicate asexually by producing sporangiospores within a sporangium. Sexual reproduction involves fusion of gametangia from two different strains, resulting in the production of a thick-walled zygospore.

Three orders in the class *Zygomycetes* – *Mucorales*, *Mortierellales* and *Entomophthorales* – are of veterinary significance. Genera in these orders contain potentially pathogenic species. These rapidly growing fungi, which are widely distributed saprobes, can cause sporadic opportunistic infections in animals.

Infection with these fungi is uncommon in healthy immunocompetent animals. Factors which may predispose to infection are listed in Box 46.1. Following ingestion or inhalation of spores from a contaminated environment, hyphae invade the mucosa, submucosa and local vessel walls, producing an acute necrotizing thrombotic vasculitis. Chronic lesions are usually localized and granulomatous.

Box 46.1 **Factors which may predispose to zygomycoses**

- Immunodeficiency
- Corticosteroid therapy
- Prolonged administration of broad-spectrum antibiotics
- Immunosuppressive viral diseases

Concise Review of Veterinary Microbiology, Second Edition. P.J. Quinn, B.K. Markey, F.C. Leonard, E.S. FitzPatrick and S. Fanning.
© 2016 John Wiley & Sons, Ltd. Published 2016 by John Wiley & Sons, Ltd.
Companion website: www.wiley.com/go/quinn/concise-veterinary-microbiology

Table 46.1 Zygomycoses of domestic animals.

Fungal disease	Hosts	Clinical conditions
Mucormycosis (fungi belonging to the sub-phylum *Mucoromycotina*, orders *Mucorales* and *Mortierellales*)	Cattle	Mesenteric and mediastinal lymphadenitis
		Abortion
		Pneumonia, following abortion caused by *Mortierella wolfii*
		Oesophagitis and enteritis in calves
		Rumenitis, abomasal ulceration
		Cerebral mucormycosis
	Pigs	Enteritis in piglets
		Mesenteric and mandibular lymphadenitis
		Gastrointestinal ulcers
	Cats	Focal necrotizing pneumonia
		Necrotic enteritis
	Dogs	Enteritis
Entomophthomycosis (fungi belonging to the order *Entomophthorales*)	Horses	Cutaneous granulomas caused by *Basidiobolus* species
		Nasal granulomas caused by *Conidiobolus* species
	Dogs	Subcutaneous, gastrointestinal and pulmonary granulomas caused by *Basidiobolus* species
		Subcutaneous granulomas caused by *Conidiobolus* species
	Sheep	Nasal granulomas caused by *Conidiobolus* species

Clinical infections

The zygomycoses of domestic animals are presented in Table 46.1. Apart from *Mortierella wolfii*, which may produce abortion followed by acute pneumonia, members of the *Mucorales* rarely cause recognizable disease syndromes in animals. Mycotic lesions caused by members of the *Mucorales* are less commonly encountered than those caused by *Aspergillus* species. Laboratory procedures, including isolation of the fungus and demonstration of hyphae in affected tissues, are essential for the diagnosis of zygomycoses.

Although *Aspergillus* species account for the majority of mycotic abortion cases in cattle, *M. wolfii*, *Lichtheimia* (*Absidia*) species, *Mucor* species and *Rhizopus* species have been implicated. Mycotic abortion, which usually occurs late in gestation, is often linked to the feeding of mouldy hay or silage. The location of lesions on cotyledons suggests haematogenous infection of the uterus. The cotyledons are enlarged and necrotic and the intercotyledonary placental tissue is thickened and leathery. Occasionally, lesions may be observed grossly on the skin of aborted foetuses.

Mycotic rumenitis in cattle may follow mucosal damage associated with ruminal lactic acidosis. The microscopic appearance of the causal fungi in ruminal lesions suggests that, in most cases, zygomycetes are involved. Infarction due to thrombotic arteritis, necrosis and haemorrhage are major features of the mycotic lesions. Extension of the inflammatory process through the ruminal wall results in fibrinous peritonitis. Zygomycotic abomasitis in calves, which may follow neonatal infection, can also produce perforation and peritonitis.

Two genera in the *Entomophthorales*, *Basidiobolus* and *Conidiobolus*, are sometimes associated with opportunistic infections in animals. *Basidiobolus* species and *Conidiobolus* species are saprobes in soil and in decaying vegetation. The route of entry of these fungi is probably through minor abrasions in the skin or nasal mucous membranes, giving rise to granulomatous lesions. *Basidiobolus* species cause cutaneous lesions in the horse, while *Conidiobolus* species cause nasal granulomas in horses, sheep and llamas.

Specimens for laboratory examination should include biopsy or postmortem tissues for histopathology and culture. Staining of tissue sections by the PAS or methenamine silver techniques facilitates detection of hyphae. Isolation is carried out on Sabouraud dextrose agar without cycloheximide. Cultures are incubated aerobically at 34°C for up to five days. Growth of *Lichtheimia* (*Absidia*), *Mucor*, *Rhizomucor* and *Rhizopus* species is rapid, filling the Petri dish with greyish or brownish-grey fluffy colonies within a few days. *Mortierella wolfii* has characteristic white velvety colonies with lobulated outlines after incubation for four days. Differentiation to species level is carried out in mycological reference laboratories.

47 Mycotoxins and mycotoxicoses

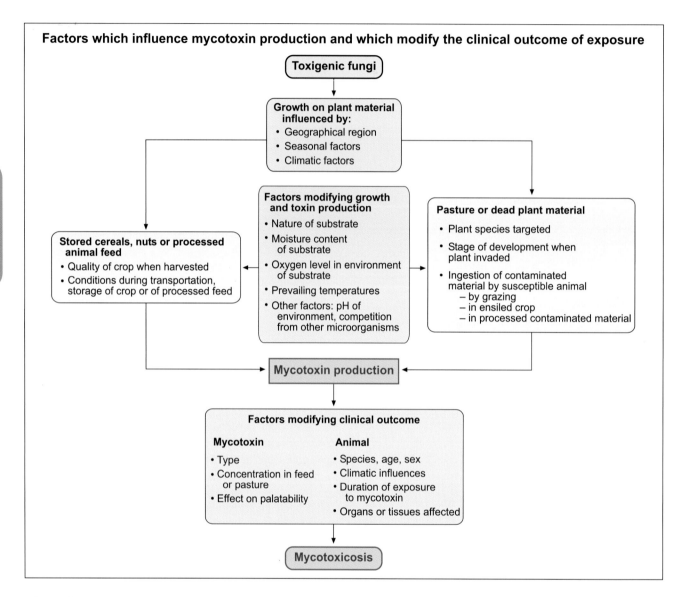

Factors which influence mycotoxin production and which modify the clinical outcome of exposure

Toxigenic fungi

Growth on plant material influenced by:
- Geographical region
- Seasonal factors
- Climatic factors

Factors modifying growth and toxin production
- Nature of substrate
- Moisture content of substrate
- Oxygen level in environment of substrate
- Prevailing temperatures
- Other factors: pH of environment, competition from other microorganisms

Stored cereals, nuts or processed animal feed
- Quality of crop when harvested
- Conditions during transportation, storage of crop or of processed feed

Pasture or dead plant material
- Plant species targeted
- Stage of development when plant invaded
- Ingestion of contaminated material by susceptible animal
   – by grazing
   – in ensiled crop
   – in processed contaminated material

Mycotoxin production

Factors modifying clinical outcome

Mycotoxin
- Type
- Concentration in feed or pasture
- Effect on palatability

Animal
- Species, age, sex
- Climatic influences
- Duration of exposure to mycotoxin
- Organs or tissues affected

Mycotoxicosis

Mycotoxins, secondary metabolites of certain fungal species, are produced when toxigenic strains of fungi grow under defined conditions on crops, pasture or stored feed. The acute or chronic intoxication following ingestion of contaminated plant material is termed mycotoxicosis. More than 100 fungal species, many of them belonging to the genera *Penicillium*, *Aspergillus* and *Fusarium* are known to elaborate mycotoxins. For fungal growth and toxin production, a suitable substrate must be available, along with moisture and optimal temperature and oxygen levels.

Mycotoxins are non-antigenic, low-molecular-weight compounds. Many are heat-stable, retaining toxicity following exposure to the processing temperatures used for pelleting and other procedures (Box 47.1). Some mycotoxins produce clinical signs

Box 47.1 Characteristics of mycotoxins

- Low-molecular-weight, heat-stable substances
- Unlike many bacterial toxins, non-antigenic; exposure does not induce a protective immune response
- Many are active at low dietary levels
- Specific target organs or tissues affected
- Toxic effects include immunosuppression, mutagenesis, teratogenesis and carcinogenesis
- Accumulation in tissues of food-producing animals or excretion in milk may result in human exposure

Concise Review of Veterinary Microbiology, Second Edition. P.J. Quinn, B.K. Markey, F.C. Leonard, E.S. FitzPatrick and S. Fanning.
© 2016 John Wiley & Sons, Ltd. Published 2016 by John Wiley & Sons, Ltd.
Companion website: www.wiley.com/go/quinn/concise-veterinary-microbiology

relating to alterations in functioning of the CNS. Immunosuppression, mutagenesis, neoplasia or teratogenesis may also result from exposure. Epidemiological and clinical features of mycotoxicoses are summarized in Box 47.2.

Mycotoxicoses of defined veterinary importance are presented in Table 47.1. The severity of clinical signs is influenced by the duration of exposure to contaminated feed or pasture, the effect of the mycotoxin on palatability, the amount of mycotoxin ingested and the organs or tissues affected.

Aflatoxicosis

Ingestion of aflatoxins, a large group of difuranocoumarins produced by toxigenic strains of *Aspergillus flavus*, *A. parasiticus* and some other *Aspergillus* species, can cause aflatoxicosis. Aflatoxins B_1, B_2, G_1 and G_2 are particularly important in disease production. After absorption from the gastrointestinal tract, aflatoxins are metabolized in the liver to a range of toxic and non-toxic products. Toxicity relates to binding of metabolites to macromolecules, especially nucleic acid and nucleoproteins. Toxic effects include reduced protein synthesis, hepatotoxicity, carcinogenesis, teratogenesis and depressed cell-mediated immunity.

Clinical signs of disease are usually vague. Epidemiological features and postmortem findings may be of diagnostic value. Aflatoxin may be demonstrated in tissues obtained postmortem. Procedures for aflatoxin detection include thin-layer chromatography, high performance liquid chromatography, immunoassay techniques and biological assays.

Ergotism

Ingestion of toxic levels of certain ergopeptide alkaloids found in the sclerotia of *Claviceps purpurea* can cause ergotism. This disease occurs worldwide in many domestic animal species and in humans. The fungus colonizes the seed-heads of ryegrasses, rye and other cereals. The most important ergopeptide alkaloids in the sclerotia are ergotamine and ergometrine. These alkaloids have a number of pharmacological effects including direct stimulation of adrenergic nerves supplying arteriolar smooth muscle.

Convulsive ergotism, an acute form of the disease following ingestion of a large amount of mycotoxins, is occasionally observed in ruminants. Small amounts of mycotoxins absorbed over relatively long periods result in persistent arteriolar constriction and endothelial damage. Swelling and redness of body extremities accompanied by lameness is followed by terminal gangrene. Ergotism can often be diagnosed clinically and the presence of ergots in pasture grasses or grain provides supporting evidence. The presence of alkaloids can be confirmed by chromatography.

Facial eczema

This economically important disease of sheep and cattle occurs in Australia, New Zealand and South Africa. The skin lesions develop as a result of photosensitization following exposure to the hepatotoxin sporidesmin in the spores of the saprobic fungus *Pithomyces chartarum*.

During warm, humid conditions in late summer or early autumn, the fungus sporulates prolifically on pasture litter. Hepatobiliary lesions develop as a result of the accumulation and concentration of sporidesmin in the bile. Necrosis of biliary epithelium results in obstruction of intrahepatic ducts. The reduced capacity of the liver to excrete phylloerythrin, a potent photodynamic compound formed from chlorophyll by enteric organisms, results in photosensitization. In sheep, lesions develop in non-pigmented areas not covered by wool. Jaundice is usually present. In cattle, lesions are limited to areas of non-pigmented skin. Milk production may be seriously affected. In ruminants, photosensitization accompanied by jaundice is suggestive of the disease. Elevated liver enzymes are found in affected animals. Using competitive ELISA techniques, sporidesmin can be detected in many body fluids.

Mycotoxic oestrogenism

Zearalenone is a potent non-steroidal oestrogen produced by certain *Fusarium* species, particularly *F. graminearum*, when growing on stored maize and other cereals. Pasture levels of zearalenone in some countries may be sufficient to cause reproductive problems in cattle and sheep. Pigs, particularly prepubertal gilts, may be affected within weeks of ingesting contaminated food. Vulval oedema and hypertrophy of the mammary glands and uterus are features of the disease in gilts. In multiparous sows, anoestrus, pseudopregnancy and infertility may suggest oestrogenism. The mycotoxin can be detected by chromatography. Oestrogen activity in feed can be assayed by injection of extracts into sexually immature mice. An ELISA technique has been developed for detecting zearalenone in pasture samples and urine.

Tremorgen intoxications

Tremorgens, a heterogeneous group of mycotoxins, produce neurological effects including muscular tremors, ataxia, incoordination and convulsive seizures following ingestion.

Perennial ryegrass staggers is one of the most common mycotoxicoses of ruminants and horses in New Zealand, Australia, Europe and the USA. *Acremonium lolii*, growing on perennial ryegrass, produces lolitrems which are responsible for the clinical signs. Although morbidity may be high in affected herds or flocks, deaths are rare and recovery is rapid if animals are moved from contaminated pasture.

Paspalum staggers is caused by the ingestion of tremorgens present in the sclerotia of *Claviceps paspali* which are found in the seed-heads of paspalum grasses. The mycotoxins paspaline and paspalitrems A and B produce typical tremorgen ataxia. Many *Penicillium* species and some *Aspergillus* species produce tremorgens when growing on pasture plants or stored feed. The clinical signs resemble those which occur with ryegrass staggers.

Table 47.1 Mycotoxicoses of domestic animals.

Disease / Mycotoxins	Fungus / Crop or substrate	Species affected / Geographical distribution	Functional or structural effects / Clinical findings
Aflatoxicosis / Aflatoxins B_1, B_2, G_1, G_2	*Aspergillus flavus, A. parasiticus* / Maize, stored grain groundnuts, soyabeans	Pigs, poultry, cattle, dogs, trout / Worldwide	Hepatotoxicity, immunosuppression, mutagenesis, teratogenesis, carcinogenesis / Ill-thrift, drop in milk yield, rarely death from acute toxicity
Citrinin toxicosis / Citrinin	*Penicillium citrinum, P. expansum, Aspergillus terreus* / Wheat, oats, maize, barley, rice	Pigs, cattle, poultry / Worldwide	Kidney lesions in pigs, haemorrhagic syndrome in cattle / Increased water consumption in pigs, dilute urine, haemorrhages in cattle
Cyclopiazonic acid toxicosis / Cyclopiazonic acid	*Aspergillus* species, some strains of *Penicillium camembertii* / Stored grain, meal	Pigs, poultry / Worldwide	Interference with ion transport across cell membranes / Weakness, food refusal
Diplodiosis / Unidentified neurotoxin	*Diplodia maydis* / Maize cobs	Sheep, cattle, goats, horses / South Africa, Argentina	Neurotoxicity / Ataxia, paresis and paralysis in adults, perinatal deaths in lambs and calves
Ergotism / Ergotamine, ergometrine, ergocristine	*Claviceps purpurea* / Seed-heads of ryegrass and other grasses, cereals	Cattle, sheep, deer, horses, pigs, poultry / Worldwide	Neurotoxicity and vasoconstriction / Convulsions, gangrene of extremities, agalactia, hyperthermia in hot climates
Facial eczema / Sporidesmin	*Pithomyces chartarum* / Pasture litter from ryegrass and white clover	Cattle, sheep, goats / New Zealand, Australia, South Africa, South America, occasionally USA and parts of Europe	Hepatotoxicity, biliary occlusion / Photosensitization, jaundice
Fescue toxicosis / Ergovaline	*Neotyphodium coenophialum* / Tall fescue grass	Cattle, sheep, horses / New Zealand, Australia, USA, Italy	Vasoconstriction / Dry gangrene in cold weather in cattle and sheep (fescue foot); hyperthermia and low milk yields (fescue summer toxicosis)
Fumonisin toxicosis / Fumonisins, especially B_1 and B_2	*Fusarium verticillioides*, other *Fusarium* species / Standing or stored maize	Horses, other *Equidae*, pigs / Egypt, South Africa, USA, Greece	Mycotoxic leukoencephalomalacia in horses, porcine pulmonary oedema / Neurological signs in horses include weakness, staggering, circling, depression
Mouldy sweet potato toxicosis / Derivative of 4-ipomeanol	*Fusarium solani, F. semitectum* / Sweet potatoes	Cattle / USA, Australia, New Zealand	Cytotoxicity producing interstitial pneumonia and pulmonary oedema / Respiratory distress, sudden death may occur
Mycotoxic lupinosis / Phomopsins A, B, C, D and E	*Diaporthe toxica* / Growing lupins with stem blight	Sheep, occasionally cattle, horses, pigs / Worldwide	Hepatotoxicity / Inappetence, stupor, jaundice, ruminal stasis, often fatal
Ochratoxicosis / Ochratoxins A, B, C and D	*Aspergillus alutaceus*, other *Aspergillus* species, *Penicillium verrucosum*, other *Penicillium* species / Stored barley, maize and wheat	Pigs, poultry / Worldwide	Degenerative renal changes / Polydipsia and polyuria in pigs, fall in egg production in birds

SECTION III

Table 47.1 *Continued*

Disease / Mycotoxins	Fungus / Crop or substrate	Species affected / Geographical distribution	Functional or structural effects / Clinical findings
Oestrogenism / Zearalenone	*Fusarium graminearum*, other *Fusarium* species / Stored maize and barley, pelleted cereal feeds, maize silage	Pigs, cattle, occasionally sheep / Worldwide	Oestrogenic activity / Hyperaemia and oedema of vulva and precocious mammary development in young gilts; anoestrus and reduced litter size in mature sows; reduced fertility in cattle and sheep
Patulin toxicosis / Patulin	*Penicillium expansum*, *Aspergillus* species / Rotting fruit, especially apples, apple juice, mouldy bread	Cattle, sheep, pigs / Worldwide	Antibiotic-like effect on ruminal flora, acidosis, vomiting and anorexia in pigs / Poor feed utilization in ruminants, weight loss in pigs
Slaframine toxicosis / Slaframine	*Rhizoctonia leguminicola* / Legumes, especially red clover, in pasture or hay	Sheep, cattle, horses / USA, Canada, Japan, France, the Netherlands	Cholinergic activity / Salivation, lacrimation, bloating, diarrhoea, sometimes death
Sterigmatocystin toxicosis / Sterigmatocystin	*Aspergillus versicolor*, *A. flavus*, other *Aspergillus* species / Stored wheat flour, cereals, peanuts, dried beans	Cattle, poultry / Many countries	Hepatotoxicity, enteric lesions / Drop in milk yield, dysentery
Tremorgen intoxications			
Perennial ryegrass staggers / Lolitrem B	*Neotyphodium lolii* / Perennial ryegrass	Cattle, pigs, poultry, sheep, horses, deer / USA, Australia, New Zealand, Europe	Neurotoxicity / Muscular tremors, incoordination, convulsive seizures, collapse
Paspalum staggers / Paspalinine, paspalitrems A, B, C	*Claviceps paspali* / Seed-heads of paspalum grasses	Cattle, sheep, horses / New Zealand, Australia, USA, South America	Neurotoxicity / Muscular tremors, incoordination, convulsive seizures, collapse
Penitrem staggers / Penitrem A, Verruculogen, other mycotoxins	*Penicillium crustosum*, some *Aspergillus* species / Stored feed and pasture	Ruminants, other domestic animals / Probably worldwide	Neurotoxicity / Muscular tremors, incoordination, convulsive seizures, collapse
Aspergillus clavatus-induced tremors / Unidentified neurotoxin	*Aspergillus clavatus* / Sprouted wheat, miller's malt culms	Cattle / China, South Africa, Europe	Neurotoxicity, degeneration of neurons / Frothing from mouth and knuckling of limbs when forced to move
Trichothecene toxicoses			
Deoxynivalenol toxicosis / deoxynivalenol	*Fusarium graminearum*, *Fusarium culmorum* / Cereal crops	Pigs, rarely other species / Countries with temperate or cold climates	Neurotoxicity / Contaminated feed refused, vomition, poor growth
T-2 toxicosis / T-2 toxin	*Fusarium sporotrichioides*, *F. poae*, other *Fusarium* species / Mouldy wheat, other cereals	Cattle, pigs, poultry / USA	Cytotoxicity, immunosuppression / feed refusal in pigs, rumenitis in cattle, beak lesions in chicken
Diacetoxyscirpenol toxicosis / Diacetoxyscirpenol	*Fusarium tricinctum*, other *Fusarium* species / Cereals	Cattle, pigs, poultry / North America, some other regions	Necrotic lesions, mucosal haemorrhages, vomition / Necrotic lesions in alimentary tract, haemorrhages in skin
Stachybotryotoxicosis / Satratoxin, roridin, verrucarin	*Stachybotrys chartarum* / Stored cereals, straw, hay	Horses, cattle, sheep, pigs / Former USSR, Europe, South Africa	Cytotoxicity, coagulopathy, immunosuppression / Stomatitis, necrotic lesions in alimentary tract, haemorrhages
Myrotheciotoxicosis / Roridin	*Myrothecium verrucaria*, *M. roridum* / Ryegrass, rye stubble, straw	Sheep, cattle, horses / Former USSR, New Zealand, south-eastern Europe	Inflammation of many tissues, pulmonary congestion / Unthriftiness, sudden death

Pathogenic algae and cyanobacteria

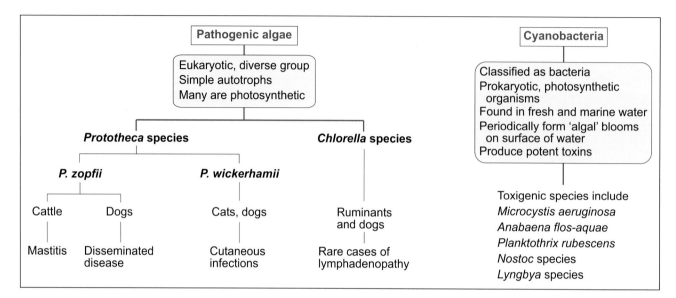

Algae are saprobic eukaryotic organisms which are widely distributed in the environment especially in water. Many contain chlorophyll. Infrequently, some species of algae have been implicated in disease of domestic animals. Colourless eukaryotic algae belonging to the genus *Prototheca* can invade tissues causing cutaneous and disseminated disease in a number of species and mastitis in cattle. Green algae belonging to *Chlorella* species have been associated with tissue invasion in ruminants on rare occasions. The prokaryotic cyanobacteria (formerly known as blue-green algae) produce potent toxins which can affect hepatic and neurological function.

Prototheca species

The saprobic colourless algae, *Prototheca* species, are widely distributed. It is thought that *Prototheca* species may be achlorophyllous descendents of *Chlorella* species. *Prototheca zopfii* has been associated with disseminated protothecosis in dogs and with mastitis in cows. Three biotypes of *P. zopfii* have been described. Subsequent studies based on sequence analysis of the 18S rRNA gene have led to the proposal that *P. zopfii* should be reclassified as genotypes 1 (biotype 1) and 2 (biotype 2), and a new species *P. blaschkeae* (biotype 3). The majority of bovine protothecal mastitis cases are caused by *P. zopfii* genotype 2. Cutaneous protothecosis in cats and dogs is caused by *P. wickerhamii*. *Prototheca* species grow aerobically forming yeast-like colonies on Sabouraud dextrose agar and on blood agar. During asexual reproduction two to sixteen sporangiospores develop within a sporangium.

Infections due to *Prototheca* species are opportunistic and infrequent. Organisms can enter tissues at sites of minor trauma in skin and mucous membranes or through the teat canal. Some outbreaks in cattle have been associated with the use of contaminated intramammary products. A cutaneous form of protothecosis, caused by *P. wickerhamii*, is the only manifestation of the disease reported in cats characterized by large, firm, discrete nodules on limbs and feet. Infection of dogs with *P. zopfii* probably occurs through the intestinal mucosa as dissemination is often preceded by haemorrhagic colitis. Affected dogs present with protracted bloody diarrhoea along with signs of neurological or ocular disturbance. There may be progressive weight loss and debility. *Prototheca zopfii* can cause chronic progressive pyogranulomatous lesions in bovine mammary glands and associated lymph nodes. Indurative mastitis may affect a number of quarters. *Prototheca zopfii* can persist in the tissues throughout a dry period and may be excreted during the next lactation. Treatment of protothecosis is difficult and may ultimately be unsuccessful.

Suitable specimens for laboratory examination include milk samples and biopsy or postmortem tissues. An indirect ELISA has been described for the detection of antibodies in serum and whey. Methenamine silver or PAS techniques can be used to demonstrate algal cells and sporangia in histological sections of granulomatous lesions. Immunofluorescent techniques are used to identify *P. zopfii* and *P. wickerhamii* in tissues. The organisms grow on blood agar and Sabouraud dextrose agar without cycloheximide. Culture plates are incubated aerobically at 35–37°C for two to five days.

Chlorella species

Green algae cause disease in ruminants on rare occasions. *Chlorella* species are morphologically similar to *Prototheca*

Concise Review of Veterinary Microbiology, Second Edition. P.J. Quinn, B.K. Markey, F.C. Leonard, E.S. FitzPatrick and S. Fanning.
© 2016 John Wiley & Sons, Ltd. Published 2016 by John Wiley & Sons, Ltd.
Companion website: www.wiley.com/go/quinn/concise-veterinary-microbiology

species. However, they are photosynthetic, possessing chloroplasts containing green pigment which imparts colour to infected tissues. In Australia, the organisms have been recovered from liver and associated lymph nodes of sheep and from cattle with lymphadenitis. Disseminated chlorellosis has been described in a dog.

The cyanobacteria

These prokaryotic photosynthetic organisms are found worldwide in fresh and marine water and in soil. Blue-green 'algal' blooms may form when conditions allow rapid replication of cyanobacteria. They occur in water, enriched with phosphates or nitrogen, when its temperature is between 15 and 30°C, its pH is neutral or alkaline, and wind disturbance is minimal. Domestic or wild animals drinking contaminated water are likely to be exposed to toxin released from the organisms. More than 40 species of cyanobacteria are known to produce potent hepatotoxins or neurotoxins. *Microcystis aeruginosa* is hepatotoxic and the species most often incriminated in episodes of poisoning. Some species such as *Anabaena flos-aquae* can generate both hepatotoxin and neurotoxin.

Toxins of the cyanobacteria, their modes of action and their clinical effects are presented in Table 48.1. Although death may occur within a short time after ingestion of a lethal dose of toxin, the dose–response curve is relatively steep and animals can ingest nearly 90% of a lethal dose without noticeable effects. Birds and ruminants are usually more susceptible to the toxins than monogastric animals.

Affected animals may have a history of access to contaminated water with an 'algal' bloom and their mouths or legs may be stained green. Samples of bloom should be examined microscopically for the presence of cyanobacteria. Toxin must be demonstrated in the bloom or in stomach contents by chemical, biological or immunoassay techniques in a reference laboratory.

Table 48.1 Toxins of cyanobacteria, their modes of action and clinical effects.

Toxins	Mode of action	Clinical effects
Microcystins and nodularins	Hepatotoxic; inhibition of protein phosphatases	Hepatomegaly and hepatoencephalopathy; photosensitization; raised serum liver enzyme levels; severe toxicity results in intrahepatic haemorrhage and death from hypovolaemic shock
Anatoxin-a	Neurotoxic; postsynaptic cholinergic agonist; mimics the activity of acetylcholine	Involuntary muscular contractions, convulsions; severe toxicity results in death
Anatoxin-a(s)	Neurotoxic; anti-acetylcholinesterase activity	Similar to the effects of anatoxin-a; hypersalivation
Saxitoxins and neosaxitoxins	Blockade of signal transmission in motor neurons	Flaccid paralysis; death from respiratory failure

Affected horses and ruminants should be removed from the source of toxin and housed out of direct sunlight. Emetics administered to recently exposed dogs may aid recovery. Activated charcoal slurry or ion-exchange resins may be used for adsorbing toxins from the gastrointestinal tract. Animal access to contaminated water must be restricted. The treatment of an 'algal' bloom with algicides results in the liberation of toxins from dead cells into the water.

49 Antifungal chemotherapy

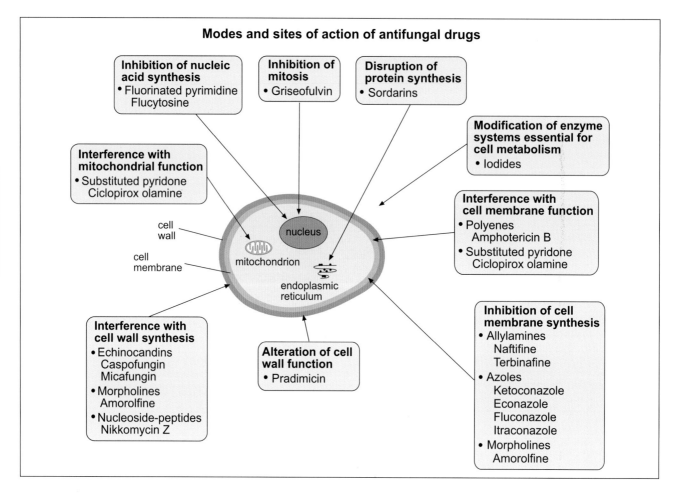

Modes and sites of action of antifungal drugs

Inhibition of nucleic acid synthesis
• Fluorinated pyrimidine Flucytosine

Inhibition of mitosis
• Griseofulvin

Disruption of protein synthesis
• Sordarins

Modification of enzyme systems essential for cell metabolism
• Iodides

Interference with mitochondrial function
• Substituted pyridone Ciclopirox olamine

Interference with cell membrane function
• Polyenes Amphotericin B
• Substituted pyridone Ciclopirox olamine

cell wall

cell membrane

nucleus

mitochondrion

endoplasmic reticulum

Interference with cell wall synthesis
• Echinocandins Caspofungin Micafungin
• Morpholines Amorolfine
• Nucleoside-peptides Nikkomycin Z

Alteration of cell wall function
• Pradimicin

Inhibition of cell membrane synthesis
• Allylamines Naftifine Terbinafine
• Azoles Ketoconazole Econazole Fluconazole Itraconazole
• Morpholines Amorolfine

Based on the location of lesions, fungal infections can be classified into three broad categories: superficial mycoses, subcutaneous mycoses and systemic mycoses. Superficial mycoses are limited to the skin, other keratinized structures including hair and nails and also mucous membranes. Subcutaneous mycoses affect the dermis, subcutaneous tissues and occasionally adjacent structures. Systemic mycoses are infections that usually originate in the lungs and spread to many other organs. Factors that predispose to opportunistic fungal infections include alteration of the normal microbial flora as a consequence of prolonged antibacterial therapy, primary or secondary immunodeficiency, immunosuppression due to drug therapy, acute viral infections and exposure to high doses of infectious fungal spores. As most antifungal drugs have a fungistatic action, with clearance of infection dependent on the host's response, it is unrealistic to expect antifungal therapy to clear infections from the tissues of immunosuppressed animals or from animals with primary or secondary immunodeficiency diseases. Accordingly, the

host's immune response should be considered carefully when designing antifungal treatment regimes.

There are four major classes of antifungal drugs: allylamines, azoles, echinocandins and polyenes. Other antifungal compounds include griseofulvin, flucytosine, iodides and morpholines. The modes and sites of action of antifungal drugs range from compounds which interfere with fungal cell wall synthesis to drugs that inhibit mitosis of fungal cells (Table 49.1).

Allylamines

Two compounds in this category of synthetic drugs, naftifine and terbinafine, are used therapeutically. Allylamines inhibit the activity of squalene epoxidase, an enzyme required for the production of ergosterol, the principal sterol in the membrane of fungal cells. Decreased synthesis of ergosterol and accumulation of squalene produce a toxic effect on the fungal pathogen. Terbinafine, a lipophilic drug, becomes concentrated in the dermis, epidermis, adipose tissue and nails. It has a broad spectrum

Concise Review of Veterinary Microbiology, Second Edition. P.J. Quinn, B.K. Markey, F.C. Leonard, E.S. FitzPatrick and S. Fanning.
© 2016 John Wiley & Sons, Ltd. Published 2016 by John Wiley & Sons, Ltd.
Companion website: www.wiley.com/go/quinn/concise-veterinary-microbiology

SECTION III

Table 49.1 Antifungal drugs and their modes of action.

Antifungal drug / Example	Mode of action	Comments
Allylamines Naftifine Terbinafine	These drugs inhibit the activity of squalene epoxidase, an enzyme required for ergosterol synthesis, the principal sterol in the membrane of fungal cells	Allylamines are particularly effective against dermatophytes. Terbinafine can be used orally or topically and is well absorbed
Antimitotic antibiotic Griseofulvin	This fungistatic antibiotic binds to microtubular proteins and interferes with fungal cell mitosis	Although formerly popular for the treatment of dermatophytosis, it has largely been replaced by more effective antifungal drugs in small animals but may still be used in horses

Azoles
Imidazoles
  Clotrimazole
  Ketoconazole
  Miconazole
  Econazole
Triazoles
  Fluconazole
  Itraconazole
  Voriconazole
	Imidazoles and triazoles interfere with the biosynthesis of ergosterol for the cytoplasmic membrane and lead to accumulation of 14-α-methylsterols. These changes disrupt cell membrane activities and inhibit fungal growth	Fluconazole and itraconazole are widely used for treating systemic fungal infections. Itraconazole is active against *Aspergillus* species and dimorphic fungi

Echinocandins Caspofungin Micafungin Anidulafungin	Echinocandins are semisynthetic lipopeptides which interfere with 1,3-β-glucan synthase, which is required for synthesis of 1,3-β-glucan, a major component of fungal cell walls	Caspofungin is effective against *Aspergillus* species and most *Candida* species
Fluorinated pyrimidine Flucytosine	This fluorinated pyrimidine enters cells by the action of cytosine deaminase and is converted to 5-fluorouracil, which interferes with RNA and protein synthesis	Flucytosine is active against *Cryptococcus neoformans* and *Candida* species. Often used with amphotericin B to delay the emergence of fungal resistance to flucytosine
Iodides Potassium iodide Sodium iodide	Although used for many years, the antifungal activity of iodides is not well understood. Direct antifungal effect and enhancement of immune responses may contribute to their antifungal activity	Prolonged treatment is often required. Sodium iodide has been used to treat sporotrichosis and nasal aspergillosis in dogs. There is a risk of iodism if treatment is prolonged
Morpholines Amorolfine	This antifungal compound is an inhibitor of sterol biosynthesis	Amorolfine is considered to be a highly effective antifungal agent for treating onychomycosis in human patients
Polyenes Amphotericin B	The polyenes are macrolide antibiotics with broad-spectrum antifungal activity. They bind preferentially to sterols, especially ergosterol. Amphotericin B binds to ergosterol and disrupts the osmotic integrity of the fungal cell membrane	Because of the toxic effects of the micellar suspension, three lipid-based formulations which are less toxic than the micellar suspension are available
Sordarins	Sordarin derivatives selectively inhibit fungal growth by blocking elongation factor 2 and disrupting protein synthesis	Sordarins are reported to have a broad antifungal spectrum with activity against dermatophytes, *Aspergillus* species, dimorphic fungi and *Pneumocystis carinii*
Substituted pyridone Ciclopirox olamine	This substituted pyridone exerts its antifungal activity by altering active membrane transport, cell membrane integrity and respiratory processes	Ciclopirox olamine is a broad-spectrum, topical, antifungal compound. It is reported to be effective against dermatophytes, yeasts and saprobes

of activity which includes dermatophytes, *Aspergillus* species, some dimorphic fungi and yeasts.

Griseofulvin

Although griseofulvin was formerly used extensively for the treatment of dermatophyte infections, it has been largely superseded by safer and more effective antifungal drugs. This fungistatic drug interferes with microtubule formation and inhibits mitosis of susceptible fungal cells. Griseofulvin has been used for treating dermatophyte infections in large and small animals. Treatment for several weeks may be required. Because of its teratogenic effects, griseofulvin is contraindicated in pregnant animals, especially queens and mares.

Azoles

Two chemically different groups of azole compounds, imidazoles and triazoles, are used therapeutically for their fungistatic activity. The antifungal activity of these compounds derives from their inhibition of fungal cytochrome 14-α-demethylase, an enzyme involved in the conversion of lanosterol to ergosterol. Depletion of ergosterol and accumulation of 14-α-methylsterols in fungal cell membranes disrupts their function and fungal growth ceases. The fungistatic action of azole compounds is slow and prolonged treatment regimens are required to ensure clinical recovery. Itraconazole and fluconazole have wider spectra of activity than ketoconazole. Fluconazole is effective against dermatophytes, *Candida* species, *Cryptococcus neoformans*, *Histoplasma capsulatum*, *Coccidioides immitis* and *Sporothrix schenckii* but ineffective against *Aspergillus* species. Itraconazole has a broader antifungal spectrum than fluconazole and is also active against *Aspergillus* species. It is the drug of choice for treating invasive aspergillosis. Because of the risk of teratogenicity, azole drugs are contraindicated in pregnant animals.

Echinocandins

This group of semisynthetic glycopeptides inhibits the synthesis of 1,3-β-glucan, a major component of many fungal cell walls. By acting as non-competitive inhibitors of 1,3-β-glucan synthase, echinocandins interfere with fungal cell division and also with cell growth. Because mammalian cells do not contain 1,3-β-glucan, echinocandins are selectively toxic for fungi. Three echinocandins, caspofungin, micafungin and anidulafungin, appear to have similar antifungal spectra. Caspofungin is effective against *Candida species*, most *Aspergillus* species and *Pneumocystis carinii* but not against *Cryptococcus neoformans* or zygomycetes.

Flucytosine

This fluorinated pyrimidine gains entry into susceptible fungal cells aided by cytosine permease. Inside the cell, it is converted into 5-fluorouracil and later into 5-fluorouridylic acid, which competes with uracil in the synthesis of RNA. This results in RNA miscoding and inhibition of DNA and protein synthesis. Flucytosine has a narrow spectrum of activity, principally the yeasts, *Candida* species and *Cryptococcus neoformans*. As resistance to flucytosine can develop quickly during treatment, this drug is used in combination with amphotericin B or fluconazole. Combination therapy is used for the treatment of cryptococcosis, especially in cats.

Iodides

Sodium iodide and potassium iodide have been used for treating fungal infections for many years. Their modes of action may be related to interference with fungal cell metabolism. A high percentage of human patients with sporotrichosis recovered following oral administration of potassium iodide. Sodium iodide has been used successfully to treat sporotrichosis in animals. Prolonged treatment with iodine compounds may be required and may lead to the risk of iodism.

Polyenes

The polyenes are macrolide antibiotics which have a broad antifungal spectrum. Many of these compounds are too toxic for therapeutic use but amphotericin B is suitable for antifungal therapy. Amphotericin B binds preferentially to sterols, especially ergosterol in the fungal cell membrane, resulting in altered permeability and cell death. The spectrum of activity of this antifungal drug includes pathogenic yeasts, dimorphic fungi, *Aspergillus* species and zygomycetes. Due to problems associated with amphotericin B as formerly used, new formulations of this drug offer greater efficacy with reduced toxicity.

Resistance to antifungal drugs

Fungal pathogens may be inherently resistant or become resistant to drugs that interfere with their replication or alter their metabolism. Primary resistance denotes natural resistance of a particular fungal genus or species. Secondary resistance is the development of resistance following the pressure of antifungal therapy. Mutation and selection account for much of the secondary resistance observed in fungal pathogens.

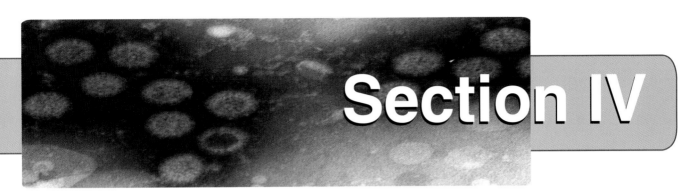

Section IV

Viruses and Prions

Nature, morphology and classification of viruses

- Small infectious agents ranging in size from 20 to 400 nm
- Composed of nucleic acid surrounded by a protein coat; in addition, some have envelopes
- Contain only one type of nucleic acid, either DNA or RNA

- Viable host cells are required for replication
- Some have an affininty for particular cell types
- A number are stable in the environment; many labile viruses are sensitive to heat, desiccation, detergents and disinfectants

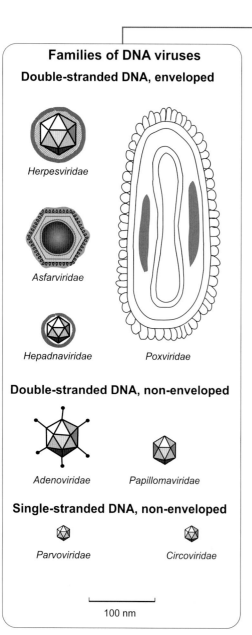

Families of DNA viruses

Double-stranded DNA, enveloped

Herpesviridae

Asfarviridae

Hepadnaviridae

Poxviridae

Double-stranded DNA, non-enveloped

Adenoviridae

Papillomaviridae

Single-stranded DNA, non-enveloped

Parvoviridae

Circoviridae

100 nm

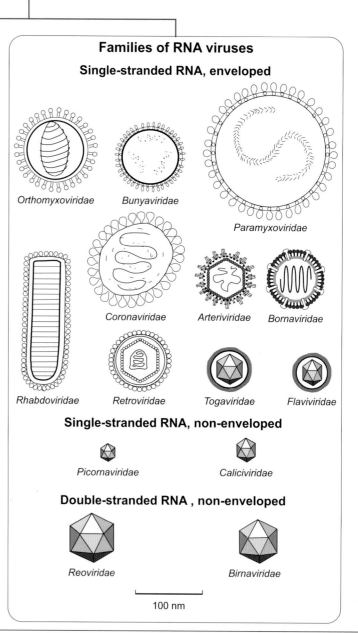

Families of RNA viruses

Single-stranded RNA, enveloped

Orthomyxoviridae

Bunyaviridae

Paramyxoviridae

Coronaviridae

Arteriviridae

Bornaviridae

Rhabdoviridae

Retroviridae

Togaviridae

Flaviviridae

Single-stranded RNA, non-enveloped

Picornaviridae

Caliciviridae

Double-stranded RNA , non-enveloped

Reoviridae

Birnaviridae

100 nm

Concise Review of Veterinary Microbiology, Second Edition. P.J. Quinn, B.K. Markey, F.C. Leonard, E.S. FitzPatrick and S. Fanning.
© 2016 John Wiley & Sons, Ltd. Published 2016 by John Wiley & Sons, Ltd.
Companion website: www.wiley.com/go/quinn/concise-veterinary-microbiology

SECTION IV

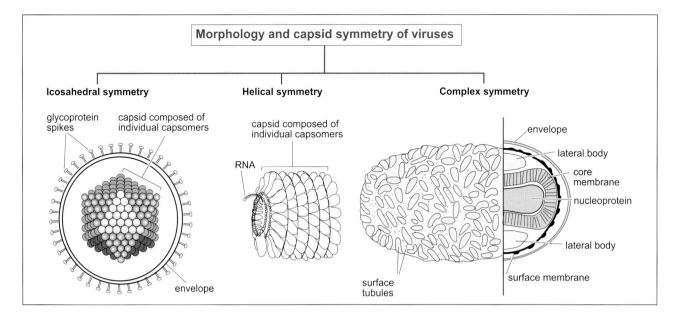

Morphology and capsid symmetry of viruses

Icosahedral symmetry

glycoprotein spikes

capsid composed of individual capsomers

envelope

Helical symmetry

capsid composed of individual capsomers

RNA

Complex symmetry

envelope

lateral body

core membrane

nucleoprotein

lateral body

surface membrane

surface tubules

The term 'virus' (Latin *virus*, poison) refers to members of a unique class of infectious agents which are extremely small, contain only one type of nucleic acid and are dependent on living cells for replication (Box 50.1). The genomes of the viruses which infect animals are smaller than those of prokaryotic cells, ranging from about 2 kbp to 800 kbp. In most viruses, the nucleic acid is present as a single molecule; in some RNA viruses the nucleic acid occurs in separate segments. Although the nucleic acid of viral genomes is usually linear, in some viruses it is circular. Genomes of DNA viruses can be single-stranded or double-stranded.

A fully assembled infective virus is termed a virion. The fundamental component of the virion is a nucleoprotein core with the ability to infect host cells and replicate in them, thus ensuring continued survival. The genome of vertebrate viruses is enclosed within a shell of proteins, called a capsid. Each subunit of the capsid is composed of a folded polypeptide chain. Collections of these subunits constitute structural units or protomers which, in turn, comprise assembly units. The term 'capsomer' or 'morphological unit' is used to describe features such as protrusions seen on the surface of virus particles in electron micrographs. These structures often correspond to groups of protein subunits arranged about a local axis of symmetry. Capsids are composed

of multiples of one or more types of protein subunits. The utilization by viruses of a small number of repeated protein subunits ensures minimal cost in coding space. The orderly arrangement of similar protein–protein interfaces results in a symmetrical structure. Icosahedral and helical symmetries are the types of capsid symmetry described in viruses.

Closed-shell, isometric viruses have a structure based on icosahedral symmetry. This structural form offers the maximum capacity and greatest strength for a given surface area. The protective, helical capsid of many RNA viruses is formed by the insertion of protein subunits between each turn of the nucleic acid helix.

In many types of viruses, the nucleocapsid is covered by an envelope composed of a lipid bilayer and associated glycoproteins. The envelope is acquired when the nucleocapsid buds through a membrane of the cell. Proteins, encoded by viral nucleic acid and integrated as glycoprotein into the appropriate membrane by the compartmentalization mechanisms of the host cell, are an integral part of the viral envelope. Peplomers or spikes are knob-like projections on the envelope of certain viruses. These structures are formed from oligomers of surface glycoproteins.

Taxonomically, viruses are assigned to five main hierarchical levels, namely order, family, subfamily, genus and species. The species taxon is regarded as the most important level of classification. A virus species is defined by a combination of multiple properties and characteristics; no single or unique property is essential for species definition. In the present scheme of virus taxonomy, the primary delineating criteria are the type and nature of the genome, the mode and site of viral replication and the structure of the virion. Currently, more than 1,900 virus species are recognized by the International Committee on Taxonomy of Viruses, with the periodic addition of new species. In addition, international specialist groups monitor large numbers of strains and subtypes. No universal agreement on terminology appropriate for description of strains and subtypes of virus species has been ratified internationally.

Box 50.1 Characteristics of viruses which are pathogenic for animals

- Small infectious agents, usually ranging in size from 20 to 400 nm
- Composed of nucleic acid surrounded by a protein coat; in addition, some have envelopes
- Contain only one type of nucleic acid, either DNA or RNA
- Unlike bacteria and fungi, viruses cannot replicate on inert media; viable host cells are required for replication
- Some viruses have an affinity for particular cell types

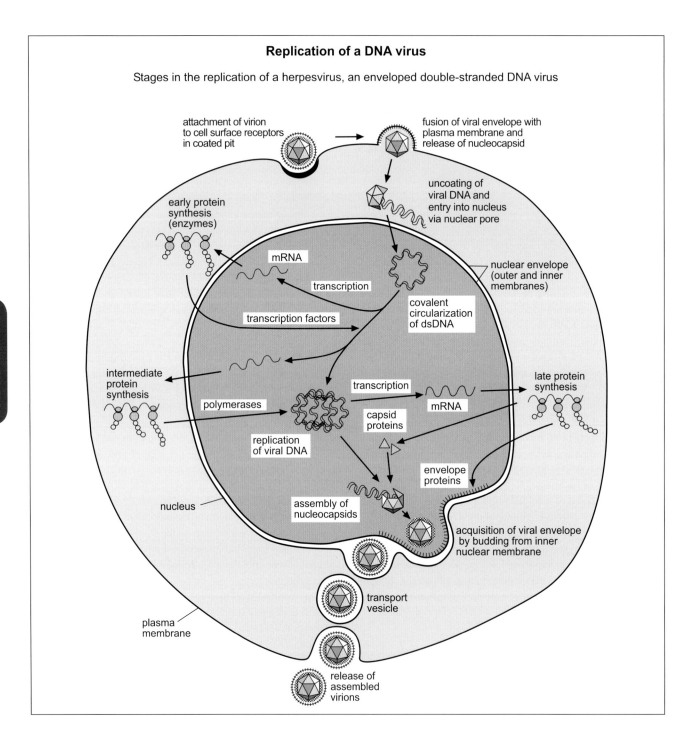

Replication of a DNA virus

Stages in the replication of a herpesvirus, an enveloped double-stranded DNA virus

attachment of virion to cell surface receptors in coated pit

fusion of viral envelope with plasma membrane and release of nucleocapsid

uncoating of viral DNA and entry into nucleus via nuclear pore

early protein synthesis (enzymes)

mRNA

transcription

transcription factors

nuclear envelope (outer and inner membranes)

covalent circularization of dsDNA

intermediate protein synthesis

polymerases

transcription

mRNA

late protein synthesis

capsid proteins

replication of viral DNA

envelope proteins

nucleus

assembly of nucleocapsids

acquisition of viral envelope by budding from inner nuclear membrane

plasma membrane

transport vesicle

release of assembled virions

Concise Review of Veterinary Microbiology, Second Edition. P.J. Quinn, B.K. Markey, F.C. Leonard, E.S. FitzPatrick and S. Fanning.
© 2016 John Wiley & Sons, Ltd. Published 2016 by John Wiley & Sons, Ltd.
Companion website: www.wiley.com/go/quinn/concise-veterinary-microbiology

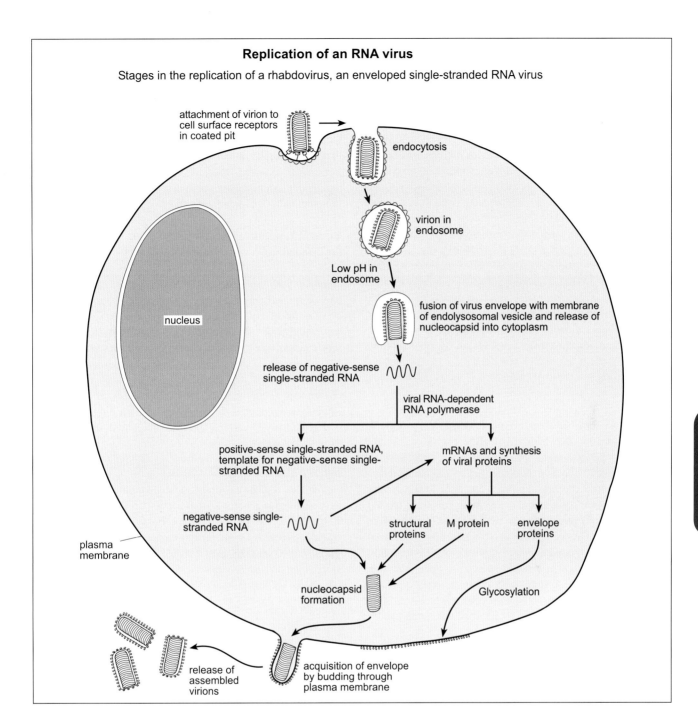

Replication of an RNA virus

Stages in the replication of a rhabdovirus, an enveloped single-stranded RNA virus

attachment of virion to cell surface receptors in coated pit

endocytosis

virion in endosome

Low pH in endosome

fusion of virus envelope with membrane of endolysosomal vesicle and release of nucleocapsid into cytoplasm

release of negative-sense single-stranded RNA

viral RNA-dependent RNA polymerase

nucleus

positive-sense single-stranded RNA, template for negative-sense single-stranded RNA

mRNAs and synthesis of viral proteins

negative-sense single-stranded RNA

structural proteins

M protein

envelope proteins

plasma membrane

Glycosylation

nucleocapsid formation

release of assembled virions

acquisition of envelope by budding through plasma membrane

Unlike bacteria, which can grow on inert media, viruses are obligate intracellular parasites and can multiply only in viable cells. This requirement arises from their limited genomic composition which obliges them to utilize host cell organelles, enzymes and other macromolecules for replication. The effects of viral multiplication on host cells range from minor changes in cellular metabolism to cytolysis.

The replicative cycle of a virus can be conveniently divided into a number of stages (Box 51.1). A virion must first attach to cell surface receptors in order to produce infection. Initial virus–cell interaction is a random event which relates to the number of virus particles present and the availability of appropriate receptor molecules. Virus–cell interaction determines both the host range and the tissue tropism of viral species. Viruses have evolved to the point where they can utilize a wide range of host cell

surface proteins as receptors. Many of these surface molecules are highly conserved and are essential for fundamental cellular functions. Some viruses have more than one type of ligand molecule and they may bind to several cell surface receptors

---

Box 51.1 Stages in replication of viruses

- Attachment to a surface receptor on a susceptible host cell
- Entry into the cell
- Uncoating of viral nucleic acid
- Replication of viral nucleic acid and synthesis of virus-encoded proteins
- Assembly of newly formed virus particles and release from host cell

in sequential order during attachment. Some viral species can detach and adsorb to another cell when infection of a particular host cell does not proceed. Detachment of orthomyxoviruses and paramyxoviruses from host cells is mediated by viral neuraminidase, a receptor-destroying enzyme.

Virus uptake or penetration of the cell's plasma membrane is an energy-dependent process that can occur in two main ways, endocytosis or direct entry. Several endocytic mechanisms are described including clathrin-mediated, caveolar/raft-mediated and macropinocytosis. Acidification within the endosome leads to structural changes in the internalized virus that facilitate its entry into the cytosol. The envelopes of some viruses, such as orthomyxoviruses, rhabdoviruses and flaviviruses, fuse with the membrane of endosomes, releasing nucleocapsids directly into the cytoplasm. An alternative strategy which is used by some enveloped viruses, including paramyxoviruses, retroviruses and herpesviruses, involves fusion of the viral envelope with the plasma membrane. This allows release of the nucleocapsid directly into the host cell cytoplasm. The entry of some non-enveloped viruses such as picornaviruses involves the direct passage or translocation of viral genomes into the cytoplasm through channels or pores in the plasma membrane.

Uncoating is the process whereby the viral genome is released in a form suitable for transcription. In the case of enveloped viruses, in which the nucleocapsid is discharged directly into the cytoplasm, transcription can usually proceed without complete uncoating. For other viruses, uncoating results from disruption of the capsid protein–nucleic acid relationship as a result of proteolytic enzyme activity or following binding to particular 'replication' sites. In reoviruses, the genome may express all functions without complete release from the capsid. For the majority of non-enveloped viruses complete uncoating occurs. Poxviruses are uncoated in two stages. The initial stage is mediated by host enzymes, with complete release of viral DNA from the core requiring virus-specified proteins. In some viruses which replicate in the cell nucleus, uncoating may be completed at the nuclear pore complex.

The synthesis of viral proteins by host cells, which is the central event in replication of viruses, requires the production of viral mRNA. While DNA viruses which replicate in the nucleus can employ host cell transcriptases to synthesize viral mRNA, other viruses use their own enzymes to generate mRNA. Viruses have evolved strategies which facilitate interference with the activity of cellular mRNA. Viruses direct the synthesis of either a separate mRNA for each gene or mRNA encompassing several genes. Eukaryotic cell protein-synthesizing mechanisms, however, translate only monocistronic messages. If a large precursor protein molecule is produced, cleavage into individual proteins is required and each family of viruses employs unique strategies for this purpose.

Based on the nature of the genome and the method of mRNA synthesis, viruses of veterinary importance can be grouped into seven classes, the Baltimore classification. Central to this scheme is the designation of the genome of single-stranded RNA viruses as positive-sense or negative-sense nucleic acid. In this context, the word 'sense' refers to nucleic acid polarity. The nucleic acid of positive-sense single-stranded RNA viruses is mRNA in sense and can be translated directly on host ribosomes, forming viral proteins.

Replication of DNA viruses

Double-stranded DNA viruses, such as herpesviruses, papovaviruses and adenoviruses that replicate in the nucleus of the cell, have a relatively direct replication strategy. The viral DNA is transcribed by cellular DNA-dependent RNA polymerase (transcriptase), forming mRNA. In contrast, the single-stranded DNA viruses, parvoviruses and circoviruses, which also replicate in cell nuclei, utilize cellular DNA polymerase to synthesize double-stranded DNA. This is then transcribed to mRNA by cellular transcriptases. Parvoviruses and circoviruses require dividing cells for their replication. The replication of large DNA viruses (poxviruses and African swine fever virus), which encode all enzymes required for replication, occurs primarily in the cytoplasm.

A defined temporal sequence of events occurs during transcription and replication of DNA viruses. Specified genes encode for early proteins, which include the enzymes and other proteins necessary for virus replication and for suppression of the synthesis of host cell proteins. Subsequently, replication of viral nucleic acid and transcription of the genes which encode the late proteins occur. These late proteins, which are also often transcribed from newly formed viral nucleic acid, are structural components synthesized late in the infection cycle. This temporal sequence is not clearly demonstrable in the replicative cycles of RNA viruses in which most of the genetic information is expressed contemporaneously.

Replication of RNA viruses

Reoviruses and birnaviruses, double-stranded RNA viruses, have segmented genomes. Transcription occurs in the cytoplasm under the direction of a viral transcriptase. The negative-sense strand of each segment is transcribed to produce individual mRNA molecules. In contrast, the genomes of positive-sense single-stranded RNA viruses can act directly as mRNA after infection. The enzymes necessary for genome replication in these viruses are produced after infection by direct translation of virion RNA. This RNA can bind directly to ribosomes and is translated to yield a single polyprotein which is then cleaved to yield both functional and structural proteins. Because direct translation can occur, naked RNA extracted from such viruses is infectious. The positive-sense single-stranded RNA viruses utilize a number of different synthetic pathways during replication. In togaviruses, only about two-thirds of the viral RNA is directly translated during the first round of protein synthesis. Subsequently, full-length negative-sense RNA is synthesized and, from this, a full-length positive-sense RNA destined for encapsidation and a one-third length positive-sense RNA strand are formed. The genomes of caliciviruses, coronaviruses and arteriviruses also encode for mRNA which can be partial or full length.

Negative-sense single-stranded RNA viruses possess an RNA-dependent RNA polymerase. The naked RNA of these viruses, unlike that of the positive-sense single-stranded RNA viruses, cannot initiate infection. After infection by the virion, the genomic RNA functions as a template for transcription of positive-sense mRNA and also for virus replication, utilizing the same polymerase. The positive-sense RNA subsequently serves as the template for synthesis of negative-sense genomic RNA. Most single-stranded negative-sense RNA viruses replicate in the cytoplasm of the cell. Notable exceptions are orthomyxoviruses and Borna disease virus, which replicate in the nucleus. Part of the segmented genome of some members of the *Bunyaviridae* is ambisense, utilizing a mixed replication strategy with features characteristic of both positive-sense and negative-sense single-stranded RNA viruses.

The genome of retroviruses consists of positive-sense single-stranded RNA which does not function as mRNA. Instead, a single-stranded DNA copy is produced by RNA-dependent DNA polymerase (reverse transcriptase) using the viral RNA as a template. As the second strand of DNA is formed, the parental RNA is removed from the RNA–DNA hybrid molecule. The double-stranded DNA is integrated into the host cell genome as a provirus and can subsequently be transcribed to new viral RNA.

Protein synthesis

Within the cell, the sites at which particular proteins are synthesized relate to the type and function of the protein. Membrane proteins and glycoproteins are synthesized on membrane-bound ribosomes, while soluble proteins including enzymes are synthesized on ribosomes free in the cytoplasm. Short specific amino acid sequences, known as sorting sequences, facilitate the incorporation of proteins at various cellular locations where they are required for metabolic activity. Most viral proteins undergo post-translational modification including proteolytic cleavage, phosphorylation and glycosylation. During glycosylation, sugar side-chains are added to viral proteins in a programmed manner as the proteins are being transferred from the rough endoplasmic reticulum to the Golgi apparatus. This event occurs in preparation for the final assembly of intact virions prior to their release from the cell.

Assembly and release of virions

The mechanisms required for the assembly and release of enveloped and non-enveloped viruses are distinct. Non-enveloped viruses of animals have an icosahedral structure. The structural proteins of these viruses associate spontaneously in a symmetrical and stepwise fashion, forming procapsids. Subsequently, viral nucleic acid is incorporated into the procapsid. Proteolytic cleavage of specific procapsid polypeptides may be required for the final formation of infectious particles. Non-enveloped viruses are usually released following cellular disintegration. The assembly of picornaviruses and reoviruses occurs in the cytoplasm of the cell, whereas parvoviruses, adenoviruses and papovaviruses are assembled in the nucleus.

The final step in the process of virion assembly for enveloped viruses involves acquisition of an envelope by budding from membranes of the cell. Prior to budding, cell membranes are modified by the insertion of virus-specified transmembrane glycoproteins which aggregate in patches in the plasma membrane. Their presence alters the antigenic composition of infected cells which become targets for cytotoxic T lymphocytes. In the case of icosahedral viruses, the proteins of their nucleocapsids bind to the hydrophilic domains of the virus-specified membrane glycoprotein spikes which project slightly into the cytoplasm. As a result, the nucleocapsid becomes surrounded by the altered portion of membrane during budding. The nucleocapsids of helical viruses bind to a virus-specified matrix (M) protein which in turn binds to the hydrophilic domains of the virus-specified glycoproteins that line the cytoplasmic side of membrane patches.

Budding of viruses through the plasma membrane usually does not breach the integrity of the membrane and, as a result, many enveloped viruses are non-cytopathic and may be associated with persistent infections. However, unlike most other enveloped viruses, togaviruses, paramyxoviruses and rhabdoviruses are cytolytic. Flaviviruses, coronaviruses, arteriviruses and bunyaviruses acquire their envelopes inside cells by budding through the membranes of the rough endoplasmic reticulum or the Golgi apparatus. These viruses are then transported in vesicles to the cell surface where the vesicle fuses with the plasma membrane releasing the virion by exocytosis. Herpesviruses, which replicate in the nucleus, are unique in that they bud through the inner lamella of the nuclear membrane and accumulate in the space between inner and outer lamellae, in the cisternae of the endoplasmic reticulum and in cytoplasmic vesicles.

Release from the cell occurs either by exocytosis or by cytolysis. Epithelial cells exhibit polarity and infecting viruses show a tendency to bud from either the apical surface which facilitates shedding from the host or from the basolateral surface which facilitates systemic spread. The assembly and release of poxviruses is a complex process taking several hours. Although replication occurs entirely in the cytoplasm of the host cell at discrete sites, termed viroplasms or 'viral factories', nuclear factors may be involved in transcription and assembly. Maturation leading to the formation of infectious intracellular mature virus follows. Virus particles then move out of the assembly area and become enveloped in a double membrane derived from the trans-Golgi network. At the periphery of the cell, fusion with the plasma membrane results in loss of the outer layer of the double membrane and release of extracellular enveloped virus.

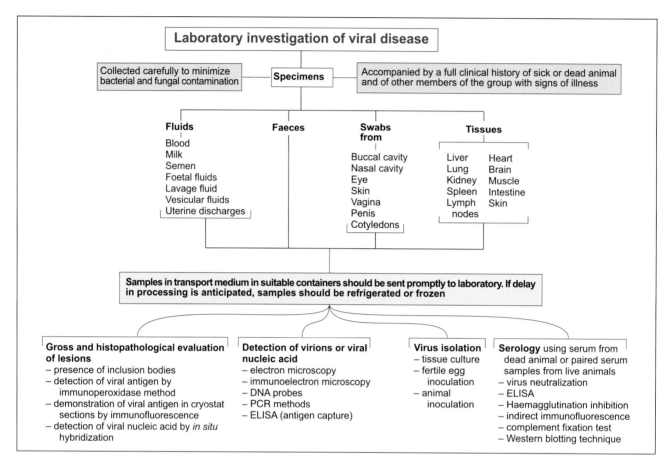

Laboratory investigation of viral disease

Collected carefully to minimize bacterial and fungal contamination — **Specimens** — Accompanied by a full clinical history of sick or dead animal and of other members of the group with signs of illness

Fluids
Blood
Milk
Semen
Foetal fluids
Lavage fluid
Vesicular fluids
Uterine discharges

Faeces

Swabs from
Buccal cavity
Nasal cavity
Eye
Skin
Vagina
Penis
Cotyledons

Tissues
Liver   Heart
Lung   Brain
Kidney   Muscle
Spleen   Intestine
Lymph   Skin
nodes

Samples in transport medium in suitable containers should be sent promptly to laboratory. If delay in processing is anticipated, samples should be refrigerated or frozen

Gross and histopathological evaluation of lesions
– presence of inclusion bodies
– detection of viral antigen by immunoperoxidase method
– demonstration of viral antigen in cryostat sections by immunofluorescence
– detection of viral nucleic acid by *in situ* hybridization

Detection of virions or viral nucleic acid
– electron microscopy
– immunoelectron microscopy
– DNA probes
– PCR methods
– ELISA (antigen capture)

Virus isolation
– tissue culture
– fertile egg inoculation
– animal inoculation

Serology using serum from dead animal or paired serum samples from live animals
– virus neutralization
– ELISA
– Haemagglutination inhibition
– indirect immunofluorescence
– complement fixation test
– Western blotting technique

Many viral diseases of animals can be diagnosed on the basis of clinical signs together with postmortem findings and histopathological findings. However, confirmation of the involvement of specific viral pathogens often requires special laboratory procedures. Surveillance for particular viruses is an important aspect of the management of valuable animals such as bulls used for artificial insemination and stallions which have the potential to spread infection to many other animals. As part of international trade regulations, certification of freedom from particular viral diseases must accompany animals exported to countries in which the diseases are exotic. Moreover, rapid and accurate laboratory confirmation of exotic viral diseases, including those with zoonotic potential, is essential for the successful implementation of eradication policies and for the protection of human health. Surveillance of animal populations for new or emerging viral diseases is an important responsibility of national veterinary services.

More than 200 major viral diseases of veterinary importance affect animal species. Because of the considerable resources required for the provision of comprehensive diagnostic services in virology, national diagnostic services usually concentrate on those diseases prevalent in a country. Moreover, laboratories often provide diagnostic services for particular animal species. Special laboratory containment facilities are mandatory for some viruses which cause highly contagious diseases such as foot-and-mouth disease. The Office International des Épizooties (OIE) in Paris, also known as the World Organization for Animal Health, monitors and publishes details of significant animal disease outbreaks worldwide. This surveillance work relies on international cooperation and a network of laboratories dealing with viral diseases of international importance.

Collection, preservation and transportation of samples

Failure to provide a suitably selected specimen for the diagnostic laboratory is the single most important cause of unreliable laboratory results. Ideally, specimens for laboratory examination should be collected as early as possible from affected animals before secondary bacterial infections become established. It is advisable to collect samples from apparently normal in-contact animals because some of these animals may be actively shedding

Concise Review of Veterinary Microbiology, Second Edition. P.J. Quinn, B.K. Markey, F.C. Leonard, E.S. FitzPatrick and S. Fanning.
© 2016 John Wiley & Sons, Ltd. Published 2016 by John Wiley & Sons, Ltd.
Companion website: www.wiley.com/go/quinn/concise-veterinary-microbiology

virus. The specimens selected for examination should relate to the clinical signs or to lesion distribution at postmortem.

Preservation of the infectivity or antigenicity of viruses may be required for particular tests. As many viruses are labile, specimens for virus isolation should be collected into transport medium, refrigerated and transmitted to the laboratory without delay. Samples should be frozen at –70°C if delay in delivery is anticipated. Freezing in a domestic freezer at –20°C significantly decreases the infectivity of most viruses. Transport medium consists of buffered isotonic saline containing a high concentration of protein, such as bovine albumin or foetal calf serum, which prolongs virus survival. Antibiotics and antifungal drugs are added in order to inhibit growth of contaminants. Samples for electron microscopy, in which the demonstration of virion morphology is the primary objective, require less exacting conditions for storage and transportation. Air-dried smears for fluorescent antibody (FA) staining should be fixed in either acetone or methyl alcohol for up to 10 minutes in order to preserve viral antigens. This fixation process allows penetration of FA conjugates into cells. A similar fixation procedure is required for cryostat sections of frozen tissues prior to FA staining. Formalin-fixed tissue samples embedded in paraffin wax can be stored for many years and used to demonstrate the presence of viral antigen by immunohistochemical techniques.

Guidance from clinicians regarding the possible aetiology of the disease under investigation is essential for deriving maximum benefit from laboratory tests. This requires an accurate assessment of the history and clinical signs, together with a tentative clinical diagnosis. In some instances, postmortem and histopathological examination of tissues may be sufficient for diagnostic purposes, particularly if characteristic inclusion bodies are found in infected tissues.

Detection of virus, viral antigens or nucleic acid

The presence of virus in tissues can be confirmed by isolation of live virus, by demonstration of virus particles or viral antigen and by detecting viral nucleic acid. Virus isolation using cell culture, fertile eggs or experimental animals is the standard against which other diagnostic methods are usually compared. Diagnostic laboratories usually have a limited range of cell lines, appropriate for the range of samples received. Embryonated eggs are widely used for the isolation of influenza A virus and avian viruses. Because of ethical considerations and cost, virus isolation in experimental animals is now employed infrequently.

Virus isolation is a sensitive procedure when cultural conditions are optimal for a particular virus and this method also generates a supply of virus for further studies. However, it is labour-intensive, slow and expensive. A number of blind passages may be required before a virus becomes adapted to a particular cell line and, as a consequence, a test result may not be available for some weeks. Because some viruses do not produce a cytopathic effect, additional detection procedures such as haemadsorption and FA staining may be needed to demonstrate their presence in cell cultures. Even when a virus produces a pronounced cytopathic effect, additional tests are often required for definitive identification.

The sensitivity and versatility of methods for the detection of viral nucleic acids have greatly improved in recent years and these procedures are now becoming the methods of choice for viral identification. These methods are particularly valuable when dealing with viruses which are either difficult to grow or cannot be grown *in vitro*. They are useful for detecting latent infections in which infectious virus is absent and also for specimens containing inactivated virus. Cloned viral DNA is available for the probing of samples and tissues by nucleic acid hybridization. This technique, however, has been largely replaced in recent years by PCR, which has the advantage of amplifying the target gene sequences. Application of this technique has been extended for detection of RNA viruses through the use of reverse transcriptase. Because of their exquisite sensitivity, PCR techniques require rigorous standardization to exclude cross-contamination and to ensure reproducibility and reliability.

Diagnostic serology

Serological procedures can be used for the retrospective diagnosis of viral diseases and for epidemiological surveys. These procedures can be automated and diagnostic reagents for many viral pathogens are available commercially. Single blood samples from animals in susceptible populations suffice for establishing the prevalence of a disease. When using serological procedures for the diagnosis of endemic disease in flocks or herds, paired serum samples taken at an interval of at least three weeks are required to demonstrate rising antibody titres. The first samples should be collected when clinical signs are first evident and the second samples during convalescence. A single blood sample may be adequate for diagnosis if reagents are available for demonstrating IgM antibodies, which are indicative of a primary immune response. Difficulties with the interpretation of serological tests may arise due to cross-reactions with antigenically related viruses. In young animals, passively acquired maternal antibodies, which may persist for several months, can lead to difficulty in interpreting results.

Interpretation of test results

Because false-positive and false-negative results can occur in many test procedures, inclusion of positive and negative controls is essential. The sensitivity and specificity of a particular diagnostic test should be established. The sensitivity of a diagnostic test, expressed as a percentage, is the number of animals identified as positive out of the total number of animals with the disease. The specificity of a test is the percentage of uninfected animals in which the result is negative. In order to detect all animals with an important viral infection, a test with high sensitivity is required. For laboratory confirmation of a viral infection in an individual animal, a test with high specificity is essential.

The isolation of virus or the demonstration of antibody to a specific virus does not necessarily confirm an aetiological link with a disease state. For the conclusive confirmation of test results, it may be necessary to demonstrate a correlation between the site of virus recovery and the nature and extent of lesions. Circumstantial evidence for the aetiological involvement of a virus in a clinically affected animal is supported by the recovery of the same virus from susceptible in-contact animals. Moreover, a rising antibody titre to the putative causal virus is of diagnostic importance. Published reports on the potential importance of a similar disease syndrome and its aetiology may point to the suitability of particular laboratory investigations for that particular viral infection.

53 Antiviral chemotherapy

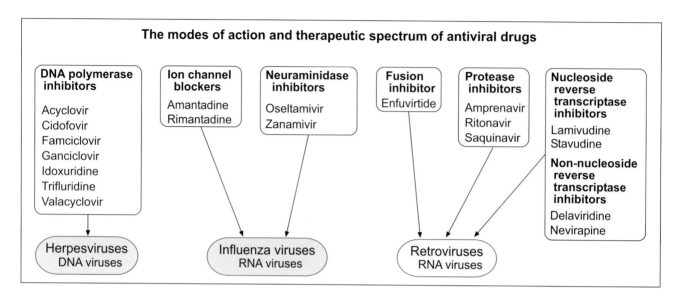

The modes of action and therapeutic spectrum of antiviral drugs

DNA polymerase inhibitors
Acyclovir
Cidofovir
Famciclovir
Ganciclovir
Idoxuridine
Trifluridine
Valacyclovir

Ion channel blockers
Amantadine
Rimantadine

Neuraminidase inhibitors
Oseltamivir
Zanamivir

Fusion inhibitor
Enfuvirtide

Protease inhibitors
Amprenavir
Ritonavir
Saquinavir

Nucleoside reverse transcriptase inhibitors
Lamivudine
Stavudine

Non-nucleoside reverse transcriptase inhibitors
Delaviridine
Nevirapine

Herpesviruses
DNA viruses

Influenza viruses
RNA viruses

Retroviruses
RNA viruses

Viral replication occurs in sequential steps. Attachment and penetration follow the binding of viral attachment protein to cell surface receptors. Once within the cell, uncoating with release of the viral genome follows. Expression of the viral genome, replication of the genome and translation of the viral proteins is followed by post-translational modifications of viral proteins, assembly of virion components and release by budding or cell lysis.

Antiviral drugs are employed to inhibit virus-specific events related to virus replication rather than host cell synthetic activities. Most antiviral drugs interfere with viral-encoded enzymes or viral structures essential for replication. Many antiviral drugs are nucleic acid analogues which interfere with DNA and RNA synthesis. Other mechanisms of action include interference with virus–cell binding, interruption of virus uncoating and interference with virus progeny release from infected host cells. Some antiviral substances such as interferons possess immunomodulatory activity. Stages of viral replication and possible points at which antiviral drugs or components of the immune system can interrupt replicative events are presented in Table 53.1. A major obstacle to the development of antiviral drugs is the inherent toxicity of inhibitory compounds for host cells. The other limiting factor in antiviral chemotherapy is the development of resistance.

Interferons

A number of immunomodulatory drugs induce interferon production and promote immune responses to viral pathogens. Interferons are proteins produced by virus-infected cells or by sentinel immune cells which act on adjacent cells, inhibiting virus replication. These protective molecules bind to specific cell

Table 53.1 Categories of antiviral drugs and immune components indicating the stages at which they act during virus replication.

Categories of drugs or immune components with antiviral activity	Stage of replication where antiviral drugs or immune components act
Peptide analogues of attachment proteins; fusion protein inhibitors; neutralizing antibodies	Attachment to host cell
Ion channel blockers	Uncoating
Inhibitors of viral DNA polymerase, RNA polymerase, reverse transcriptase	Transcription of viral genome
Nucleoside analogues	Replication of viral genome
Interferons, antisense oligonucleotides	Translation of viral proteins
Protease inhibitors	Post-translational changes in proteins
Interferons	Assembly of virion components
Neuraminidase inhibitors; specific antibodies plus complement; cytotoxic T cells and NK cells	Release of virions by budding or cell lysis

Concise Review of Veterinary Microbiology, Second Edition. P.J. Quinn, B.K. Markey, F.C. Leonard, E.S. FitzPatrick and S. Fanning.
© 2016 John Wiley & Sons, Ltd. Published 2016 by John Wiley & Sons, Ltd.
Companion website: www.wiley.com/go/quinn/concise-veterinary-microbiology

SECTION IV

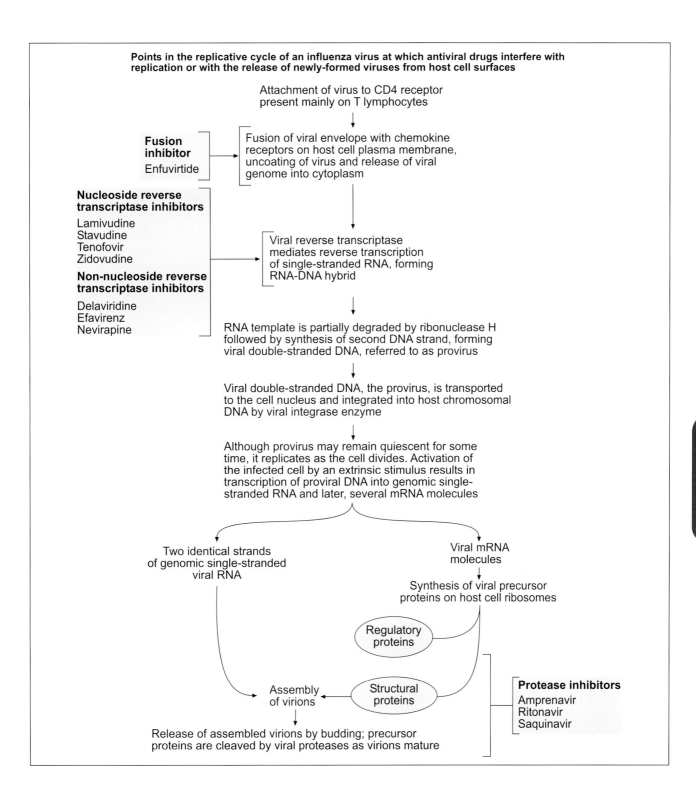

Points in the replicative cycle of an influenza virus at which antiviral drugs interfere with replication or with the release of newly-formed viruses from host cell surfaces

Attachment of virus to CD4 receptor present mainly on T lymphocytes

Fusion inhibitor

Enfuvirtide

Fusion of viral envelope with chemokine receptors on host cell plasma membrane, uncoating of virus and release of viral genome into cytoplasm

Nucleoside reverse transcriptase inhibitors

Lamivudine
Stavudine
Tenofovir
Zidovudine

Non-nucleoside reverse transcriptase inhibitors

Delaviridine
Efavirenz
Nevirapine

Viral reverse transcriptase mediates reverse transcription of single-stranded RNA, forming RNA-DNA hybrid

RNA template is partially degraded by ribonuclease H followed by synthesis of second DNA strand, forming viral double-stranded DNA, referred to as provirus

Viral double-stranded DNA, the provirus, is transported to the cell nucleus and integrated into host chromosomal DNA by viral integrase enzyme

Although provirus may remain quiescent for some time, it replicates as the cell divides. Activation of the infected cell by an extrinsic stimulus results in transcription of proviral DNA into genomic single-stranded RNA and later, several mRNA molecules

Two identical strands of genomic single-stranded viral RNA

Viral mRNA molecules

Synthesis of viral precursor proteins on host cell ribosomes

Regulatory proteins

Structural proteins

Assembly of virions

Protease inhibitors

Amprenavir
Ritonavir
Saquinavir

Release of assembled virions by budding; precursor proteins are cleaved by viral proteases as virions mature

surface receptors and initiate intracellular events, including the induction of particular enzymes, which render cells resistant to viral invasion. Interferons produced by recombinant technology and also by chemical synthesis are available for treating a number of viral infections in humans and also for use in animals. Recently, recombinant interferon-α2a, modified by attachment of polyethylene glycol, has become available. This modified interferon, referred to as pegylated interferon, is absorbed slowly from the injection site and has a much longer half-life than conventional interferon.

Antiviral drugs

Chemical compounds are selected for their ability to act at a particular point in the replicative cycle of a virus where they can exert inhibitory effects. The names applied to these chemical compounds reflect their modes of action or their chemical nature. Ion channel blockers, neuraminidase inhibitors, reverse transcriptase inhibitors, fusion inhibitor and inhibitors of genome replication are the titles applied to these antiviral drugs (Table 53.2).

Table 53.2 Chemical nature, mode of action and antiviral spectrum of selected antiviral drugs.

Antiviral drug	Chemical nature / Mode of action	Antiviral spectrum	Comments
Acyclovir	Acyclic guanine nucleoside / Inhibits viral DNA polymerase	Herpesviruses	Used for treating herpesvirus infections in avian species and cats; ineffective against latent viral infections
Amprenavir	Aminosulphonamide non-peptide protease inhibitor / Active site inhibitor of HIV protease	HIV	The therapeutic role of protease inhibitors in viral diseases of animals is not well defined
Cidofovir	Cytidine nucleotide analogue / Inhibits viral DNA synthesis	Herpesviruses, poxviruses, papillomaviruses, adenoviruses	Long tissue half-life allows infrequent dosing
Delaviridine	Bis-heteroarylpiperazine compound / Disrupts the catalytic activity of HIV-1 reverse transcriptase	HIV-1	Cross-resistance to other drugs in this class usually applies
Enfuvirtide	Synthetic peptide / Prevents fusion of HIV-1 with host cell membrane	HIV-1	Retains activity against viruses which have become resistant to other classes of antiviral drugs
Famciclovir and penciclovir	Nucleotide analogues / Inhibit viral DNA polymerase	Herpesviruses	Development of resistance during clinical use is reported to be low
Ganciclovir	Acyclic guanine nucleoside analogue / Inhibits viral DNA synthesis and preferentially inhibits viral rather than host cellular DNA polymerases	Herpesviruses	This drug is especially active against cytomegalovirus
Idoxuridine	Iodinated thymidine analogue / Incorporated into viral DNA with interference in nucleic acid synthesis and viral gene expression	Herpesviruses and poxviruses	Because of its toxic effects if given systemically, it is used for topical treatment only; ophthalmic solutions containing idoxuridine are used for treating herpesvirus keratitis in animals
Immunomodulators including interferons	Proteins, other novel compounds / Promote protective antiviral immune responses	Most RNA viruses are inhibited by interferons; many DNA viruses are insensitive to their antiviral effects	Interferons produced by recombinant technology and also by chemical synthesis are available for treating viral infections in humans and animals
Lamivudine	Cytosine analogue / Inhibits reverse transcriptase activity of retroviruses and also inhibits the DNA polymerase of hepatitis B virus	Retroviruses and hepatitis B virus	Resistance to lamivudine develops rapidly in patients with HIV; when combined with zidovudine, a marked synergistic effect results
Oseltamivir	Analogue of sialic acid / Potent selective inhibitor of neuraminidase	Influenza A virus and influenza B virus	Can be used prophylactically and therapeutically
Rimantadine	Tricyclic amine / Ion channel blocker which interferes with virus uncoating	Influenza A virus	Primary drug resistance is uncommon but has been reported in some avian and swine influenza viruses
Trifluridine	Fluorinated analogue of thymidine / Competitive inhibitor of the incorporation of thymidine into DNA	Used topically for keratoconjunctivitis in humans and ocular herpesvirus infections in animals	Because of its toxicity, unsuitable for systemic use
Valacyclovir	L-Valyl ester of acyclovir, a nucleoside analogue / Inhibits viral DNA synthesis	Herpesviruses	Enhanced oral bioavailability offers many advantages over acyclovir

Ion channel blocking compounds inhibit acid-mediated dissociation of the ribonucleoprotein complex early in the replication of influenza viruses, a process essential for uncoating of the single-stranded RNA genome. When influenza viruses complete their replicative cycle, they bud from the cell's membrane. Release of newly formed virions from infected cells requires neuraminidase for cleavage of sialic acid residues from the cell membrane envelope present on the budding virions. If this does not take place, the binding of haemagglutinin protruding from the virion surface with persisting sialic acid residues on newly released adjacent virions causes agglutination of the virions on the cell surface. Neuraminidase inhibitors are sialic acid analogues which specifically inhibit influenza A virus and influenza B virus neuraminidase activity. Points in the replicative cycle of an influenza virus at which antiviral drugs interfere with replication or with the release of newly-formed viruses from host cell surfaces are illustrated.

Many antiviral drugs which inhibit viral genome replication are nucleoside analogues. These compounds inhibit viral polymerases, especially DNA polymerases. Before these drugs can exert their antiviral effect, they must undergo intracellular phosphorylation to the active triphosphate form. Phosphorylated nucleoside analogues inhibit polymerases by competing with natural substrates and they are usually incorporated into the growing DNA chain where they often terminate elongation. Nucleoside analogues are widely used for treating infections caused by herpesviruses in humans and also in animals.

The activity of antiretroviral drugs includes prevention of fusion of the virus envelope with receptors on the host cell plasma membrane, interference with the activity of reverse transcriptase and inhibition of viral protease activity. Antiretroviral fusion inhibitors are drugs which interfere with virus attachment and entry into host cells, thereby preventing the subsequent stages of virus infection from proceeding. Such drugs also provide an opportunity for components of the immune system to clear viruses from body fluids and host tissues.

Non-nucleoside reverse transcriptase inhibitors induce conformational changes in reverse transcriptase which disrupt its catalytic activity. Nucleoside reverse transcriptase inhibitors are activated intracellularly by phosphorylation with cellular kinases and their triphosphate forms competitively inhibit reverse transcriptase. The triphosphate form of these antiviral agents terminates elongation of the proviral DNA chain. Together with genome replication, production of viral proteins is an essential part of the replicative cycle of all viruses. For a number of viruses, including human immunodeficiency virus (HIV)-1, assembly of proteins and nucleic acid into viral particles does not produce an infectious virion. An additional step, referred to as maturation, is required. New virus proteins require cleavage by virus-specific proteases to become fully functional. When introduced into an infected cell before virion budding commences, protease inhibitors prevent polyprotein cleavage and result in the production of non-infectious particles.

Resistance to antiviral drugs

All forms of microorganisms, including viruses, are capable of becoming resistant to inhibitory drugs and the development of resistance to antiviral compounds is an inevitable consequence of antiviral chemotherapy. As current antiviral drugs inhibit active replication, viral replication is likely to resume when treatment concludes. Effective antiviral host immune responses are essential, therefore, for clinical recovery from infection. Failure of antiviral therapy may relate to the host's immunological competence or to the emergence of drug-resistant variants. Of the many strategies that can be applied to the control of viral diseases in humans and animals, vaccination is the preferred option. In the absence of effective vaccination, antiviral chemotherapy offers the possibility of prophylactic and therapeutic treatment for a defined number of viral pathogens.

54 Herpesviridae

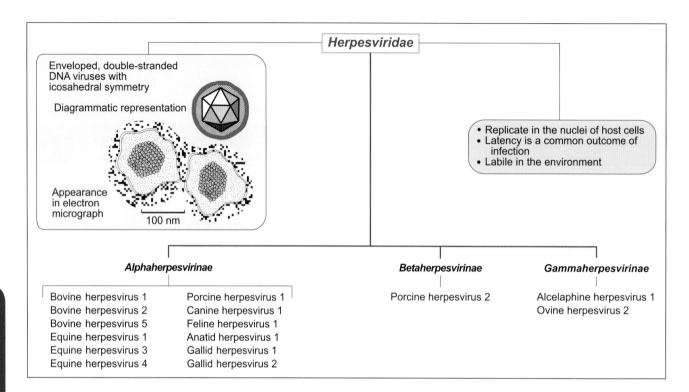

Herpesviridae

Enveloped, double-stranded DNA viruses with icosahedral symmetry

Diagrammatic representation

Appearance in electron micrograph

100 nm

- Replicate in the nuclei of host cells
- Latency is a common outcome of infection
- Labile in the environment

Alphaherpesvirinae

Bovine herpesvirus 1	Porcine herpesvirus 1
Bovine herpesvirus 2	Canine herpesvirus 1
Bovine herpesvirus 5	Feline herpesvirus 1
Equine herpesvirus 1	Anatid herpesvirus 1
Equine herpesvirus 3	Gallid herpesvirus 1
Equine herpesvirus 4	Gallid herpesvirus 2

Betaherpesvirinae

Porcine herpesvirus 2

Gammaherpesvirinae

Alcelaphine herpesvirus 1
Ovine herpesvirus 2

The family *Herpesviridae* contains more than 100 viruses. Fish, amphibians, reptiles, birds and mammals including humans are susceptible to herpesvirus infection. These viruses are of special importance because of their widespread occurrence, their evolutionary diversity and their involvement in many important diseases of domestic animals and humans. The name, herpesvirus (Greek *herpein*, to creep), refers to the sequential appearance and local extension of lesions in human infection. Herpesviruses are enveloped and range from 200 to 250 nm in diameter. They contain double-stranded DNA within an icosahedral capsid. Herpesviruses enter cells by fusing with the plasma membrane. Replication occurs in the cell nucleus. The envelope is probably derived from the nuclear membrane of the host cell, incorporating at least 10 viral-encoded glycoproteins. Release from the cell is by exocytosis. Active infection results in cell death. Intranuclear inclusions are characteristic of herpesvirus infections. Extension of viral infection occurs through points of cell contact without exposure of virus to neutralizing antibodies in blood or interstitial fluids. Protective antibody responses are usually directed against the envelope glycoproteins. Herpesvirus virions, which are fragile and sensitive to detergents and lipid solvents, are unstable in the environment.

The family is divided into three subfamilies comprising 13 genera. Alphaherpesviruses replicate and spread rapidly, destroying host cells and often establishing latent infections in sensory ganglia. Betaherpesviruses, which replicate and spread slowly, cause infected cells to enlarge, hence their common name, cytomegaloviruses. They may become latent in cells of the monocyte series. Gammaherpesviruses, which infect lymphocytes, can produce latent infections in these cells. When lymphocytes become infected, there is minimal expression of viral antigen. Some gammaherpesvirus species also replicate in epithelial and fibroblastic cells, causing cytolysis. A number of herpesviruses are implicated in neoplastic transformation of lymphocytes.

Clinical infections

Herpesviruses establish lifelong infections with periodic reactivation resulting in bouts of clinical disease. Shedding of virus may be periodic or continuous. During latency, the episomal viral genome becomes circular and gene expression is limited. Reactivation of infection is associated with various stress factors including transportation, adverse weather conditions, overcrowding and intercurrent infection. Natural infections with particular herpesviruses are usually restricted to defined host species. Because these viruses are highly adapted to their natural hosts, infections may be inapparent or mild. However, in very young or immunosuppressed animals, infection can be life-threatening.

Concise Review of Veterinary Microbiology, Second Edition. P.J. Quinn, B.K. Markey, F.C. Leonard, E.S. FitzPatrick and S. Fanning.
© 2016 John Wiley & Sons, Ltd. Published 2016 by John Wiley & Sons, Ltd.
Companion website: www.wiley.com/go/quinn/concise-veterinary-microbiology

Table 54.1 Herpesvirus infections of ruminants.

Virus	Genus	Comments
Bovine herpesvirus 1	*Varicellovirus*	Causes respiratory (infectious bovine rhinotracheitis) and genital (infectious pustular vulvovaginitis, balanoposthitis) infections. Occurs worldwide
Bovine herpesvirus 2	*Simplexvirus*	Causes ulcerative mammillitis in temperate regions and pseudo-lumpy-skin disease in tropical and subtropical regions
Bovine herpesvirus 5	*Varicellovirus*	Causes encephalitis in calves; described in several countries
Ovine herpesvirus 2	*Macavirus*	Causes subclinical infection in sheep and goats worldwide. Causes malignant catarrhal fever in cattle and in some wild ruminants
Alcelaphine herpesvirus 1	*Macavirus*	Causes subclinical infection in wildebeest in Africa and in zoos. Causes malignant catarrhal fever in cattle, deer and in other susceptible ruminants

Table 54.3 Herpesvirus infections of horses.

Virus	Genus	Comments
Equine herpesvirus 1	*Varicellovirus*	Causes abortion, respiratory disease, neonatal infection and neurological disease. Occurs worldwide
Equine herpesvirus 3	*Varicellovirus*	Causes mild venereal infection (equine coital exanthema) in both mares and stallions
Equine herpesvirus 4	*Varicellovirus*	Causes rhinopneumonitis in young horses. Occurs worldwide

Table 54.4 Herpesvirus infections of domestic carnivores.

Virus	Genus	Comments
Canine herpesvirus 1	*Varicellovirus*	Causes a fatal generalized infection in neonatal pups
Feline herpesvirus 1	*Varicellovirus*	Causes feline viral rhinotracheitis in young cats

Herpesviruses can cause respiratory, genital, mammary and CNS diseases in cattle (Table 54.1). Aujeszky's disease, which affects pigs and other domestic species, is the major porcine herpesvirus infection (Table 54.2). Equine herpesvirus infections are presented in Table 54.3; those of domestic carnivores are listed in Table 54.4 and those of birds in Table 54.5.

Infectious bovine rhinotracheitis and pustular vulvovaginitis

Infection with bovine herpesvirus 1 (BoHV-1) is an important cause of losses in cattle worldwide. It is associated with several clinical conditions including infectious bovine rhinotracheitis (IBR), infectious pustular vulvovaginitis (IPV), balanoposthitis, conjunctivitis and generalized disease in newborn calves. Iso-

lates of BoHV-1 can be divided into subtypes 1.1 (IBR-like) and 1.2 (IPV-like) using restriction endonuclease analysis of the genome.

The virus is usually acquired through aerosols (subtype 1.1) or genital secretions (subtypes 1.2a and 1.2b). Aerosol transmission is most efficient over short distances and is facilitated by the close proximity of animals. Replication occurs in the mucous membranes of the upper respiratory tract and large amounts of virus are shed in nasal secretions. Virus also enters local nerve cell endings and is transported intra-axonally to the trigeminal ganglion, where it remains latent. In most instances, infection is contained within two weeks by a strong immune response. However, tissue necrosis may facilitate secondary bacterial infection, with severe systemic effects and, possibly, death. Rarely, viraemia in pregnant cows may produce foetal

Table 54.2 Herpesvirus infections of pigs.

Virus	Genus	Comments
Porcine herpesvirus 1 (Aujeszky's disease virus)	*Varicellovirus*	Causes Aujeszky's disease in pigs. Encephalitis, pneumonia and abortion are features of the disease. In many species other than pigs, pseudorabies manifests as a neurological disease with marked pruritis. Occurs worldwide but USA (occurs in feral pigs), Canada, New Zeland and several EU states have eradicated this disease
Porcine herpesvirus 2	Unassigned	Causes disease of the upper respiratory tract in young pigs (inclusion body rhinitis)

Table 54.5 Herpesvirus infections of birds.

Virus	Genus	Comments
Gallid herpesvirus 1	*Iltovirus*	Causes infectious laryngotracheitis. Present in many countries
Gallid herpesvirus 2 (Marek's disease virus)	*Mardivirus*	Causes Marek's disease, a lymphoproliferative condition in 12- to 24-week-old chickens. Occurs worldwide
Anatid herpesvirus 1	*Mardivirus*	Causes acute disease in ducks (duck plague), geese and swans characterized by oculonasal discharge, diarrhoea and high mortality. Occurs worldwide

infection and abortion. Following genital infection, virus replicates in the mucosa of the vagina or prepuce, and latent infection may become established in the sacral ganglia. Focal necrotic lesions on genital mucosae may eventually coalesce, forming large ulcers.

In outbreaks of disease, either the respiratory or the genital form usually predominates. Swabs collected from the nares and genitalia of several affected animals during the early acute phase of the disease are suitable for virus isolation, viral DNA detection or the preparation of smears for the rapid demonstration of viral antigen using immunofluorescence. Inactivated, subunit, modified live and marker vaccines are available for control. Vaccination reduces the severity of clinical signs but may not prevent infection or alter the carrier state.

Aujeszky's disease

This disease is caused by porcine herpesvirus 1, also referred to as Aujeszky's disease virus (ADV). The pig is the natural host of the virus and infection is endemic in the pig population in many countries. The virus is shed in oronasal secretions, milk and semen. Transmission usually occurs by nose-to-nose contact or by aerosols. Following infection, the virus replicates in the epithelium of the nasopharynx and tonsils. Virus spreads to regional lymph nodes and to the CNS along axons of the cranial nerves. Virulent strains produce a brief viraemia and become widely distributed around the body, particularly in the respiratory tract. Transplacental transfer results in generalized infection of foetuses. Latency occurs in a high percentage of infected animals, with virus localized in the trigeminal ganglia and tonsils.

The age and susceptibility of infected pigs and the virulence of the infecting strain influence the severity of the clinical signs. Young pigs are most severely affected; mortality may approach 100% in suckling piglets. Neurological signs predominate in young pigs. Mortality is much lower in weaned pigs, although neurological and respiratory signs are often present. Infection in sows may result in resorption of foetuses, abortion or stillbirths. In herds with endemic ADV infection, neonatal animals are protected by maternally-derived antibody.

Specimens of brain, spleen and lung from acutely affected animals are suitable for virus isolation and viral nucleic acid detection, while cryostat sections of tonsil or brain are suitable for detection of viral antigen by immunofluorescence. If used strategically, vaccination can prevent the development of clinical disease. Modified live, inactivated and gene-deleted marker vaccines are available.

Disease in other domestic animals occurs sporadically and is characterized by neurological signs resembling those of rabies, hence the name pseudorabies. Marked pruritis is a feature of the disease. The clinical course is short, with most affected animals dying within a few days.

Equine rhinopneumonitis and equine herpesvirus abortion

Infection with equine herpesvirus 1 (EHV-1) is associated with respiratory disease, abortion, fatal generalized disease in neonatal foals and encephalomyelitis. Close contact facilitates transmission of these fragile viruses. Transmission usually occurs by the respiratory route following contact with infected nasal secretions, aborted foetuses, placentae or uterine fluids. The viruses

replicate initially in the upper respiratory tract and regional lymph nodes with spread, in some cases, to the lower respiratory tract and lungs.

Abortion caused by EHV-1 occurs several weeks or months after exposure, usually during the last four months of gestation. Equine herpesvirus 1 has a predilection for vascular endothelium. Vasculitis and thrombosis in the placenta, along with transplacental infection of the foetus, results in abortion. Infected mares rarely abort during subsequent pregnancies and their fertility is unaffected. Infection close to term may result in the birth of an infected foal which usually dies due to interstitial pneumonia and viral damage in other tissues, sometimes complicated by secondary bacterial infection. Vasculitis and thrombosis in EHV-1 infection may affect the CNS, especially the spinal cord. Neurological changes appear to be related to infection with particular strains of EHV-1. Although neurological signs associated with EHV-1 infection are relatively uncommon, they may present in several horses during an outbreak of abortion or respiratory disease on a farm. The signs range from slight incoordination to paralysis, recumbency and death.

Respiratory disease caused by equine herpesvirus 4 (EHV-4) occurs in foals over two months of age, in weanlings and in yearlings. Following an incubation period of two to ten days, there are signs of fever, pharyngitis and serous nasal discharge. Secondary bacterial infection is common, giving rise to mucopurulent nasal discharge, coughing and, in some cases, bronchopneumonia. Outbreaks of respiratory disease caused by EHV-1 are clinically indistinguishable from respiratory infections caused by EHV-4 but occur less frequently.

Virus isolation and viral nucleic acid detection are used routinely for the laboratory confirmation of herpesvirus infection in horses. Viral antigen may be demonstrated in cryostat sections of lung, liver and spleen from aborted foetuses using immunofluorescence.

Effective management practices and vaccination are essential for control. Animals returning from sales, races or other events should be segregated for up to four weeks. On large stud farms, horses should be kept in small, physically separated groups. Modified live and inactivated virus vaccines are commercially available. As vaccination is not considered to be fully protective, frequent boosters are recommended. Vaccination appears to reduce the severity of clinical signs and to decrease the likelihood of abortion.

Canine herpesvirus infection

Infection in domestic and wild *Canidae* caused by canine herpesvirus 1 (CHV-1) is common worldwide. Clinical disease occurs in neonatal pups and is characterized by generalized infection and high mortality.

Infection usually occurs by the oronasal route following direct contact between infected and susceptible animals. During periods of stress, latent infections may be reactivated, with shedding of virus. The sites of latency include sensory ganglia. Virus is shed in oronasal and vaginal secretions. Newborn pups, which can acquire infection either during parturition or *in utero*, may transmit infection to littermates.

Following infection, CHV-1 replicates in the nasal mucosa, pharynx and tonsils. The virus replicates most effectively at temperatures below normal adult body temperature. Because the hypothalamic regulatory centre is not fully operational in pups under four weeks of age, they are particularly dependent on ambient temperature and maternal contact for maintenance of normal body temperature. A cell-associated viraemia and widespread viral replication in visceral organs can occur in infected neonatal animals with subnormal body temperatures. Affected pups stop sucking, show signs of abdominal pain, whine incessantly and die within days. Morbidity and mortality rates in affected litters are high. Bitches whose pups are affected tend to produce healthy litters subsequently.

Diagnostically significant postmortem findings include focal areas of necrosis and haemorrhage, particularly in the kidneys. Intranuclear inclusions are usually present. Specimens from liver, kidney, lung and spleen are suitable for virus isolation or detection of viral nucleic acid. A commercial vaccine is available. Affected bitches and their litters should be isolated to prevent infection of other whelping bitches.

Feline viral rhinotracheitis

This acute upper respiratory tract infection of young cats is caused by feline herpesvirus 1 (FHV-1). The virus, which occurs worldwide, accounts for about 40% of respiratory infections in cats.

Close contact is required for transmission. Most recovered cats are latently infected. Reactivation with virus replication and shedding is particularly associated with periods of stress such as parturition, lactation or change of housing. Initially, FHV-1 replicates in oronasal or conjunctival tissues before infecting the epithelium of the upper respiratory tract. Secondary bacterial infections, which commonly occur, exacerbate the clinical signs. Young cats display signs of acute upper respiratory tract infection including fever, sneezing, inappetence, hypersalivation, conjunctivitis and oculonasal discharge. In more severe disease, pneumonia or ulcerative keratitis may be evident. The mortality rate is low except in young or immunosuppressed animals.

Clinical differentiation of feline viral rhinotracheitis from feline calicivirus infection is difficult. Virus can be isolated from suitable tissue specimens or viral DNA can be detected in oropharyngeal or conjunctival swabs. Specific viral antigen can be demonstrated in acetone-fixed nasal and conjunctival smears using immunofluorescence. Good husbandry practices and disease control procedures should be implemented in catteries together with regular vaccination to minimize the impact of clinical disease. Commercial vaccines also contain feline calicivirus. The protection provided by vaccination against these two viruses is incomplete as vaccinated cats can become infected but clinical signs tend to be much reduced.

Marek's disease

This contagious lymphoproliferative disease of chickens is caused by gallid herpesvirus 2 (Marek's disease virus), which is cell-associated and oncogenic. The disease, which is of major economic significance in the poultry industry, occurs worldwide. Productive replication with release of infective virus occurs only in the epithelium of the feather follicle. Cell-free virus is released from the follicles along with desquamated cells. This dander can remain infective for several months in dust and litter in poultry houses. Infected birds remain carriers for life and their chicks, which are protected initially by maternally-derived antibody, acquire infection within a few weeks, usually by the respiratory route. In addition to the virulence of the infecting strain of herpesvirus, host factors which contribute to the severity of the disease include the sex, age at the time of infection and genotype. Female birds are more susceptible than male birds, while resistance to the development of disease increases with age. The bird's genotype influences the susceptibility of T lymphocytes to transformation and development of lymphoid tumours. Birds between 12 and 24 weeks of age are most commonly affected when clinically affected birds present with partial or complete paralysis of the legs and wings.

The diagnosis of Marek's disease is based on clinical signs and pathological findings. Differentiation from lymphoid leukosis is based on the age of affected birds, the incidence of clinical cases and the histopathological findings. The use of appropriate management strategies, genetically resistant stock and vaccination have reduced losses from Marek's disease. Disinfection, all-in/all-out policies, and rearing young chicks away from older birds for the first two or three months of life reduce exposure to infection, decreasing the likelihood of serious disease. A range of modified live vaccines are commercially available. Although a single dose of virus injected into day-old chicks provides good lifelong protection, it does not prevent superinfection with virulent field viruses. Automated *in ovo* vaccination is used in large commercial units.

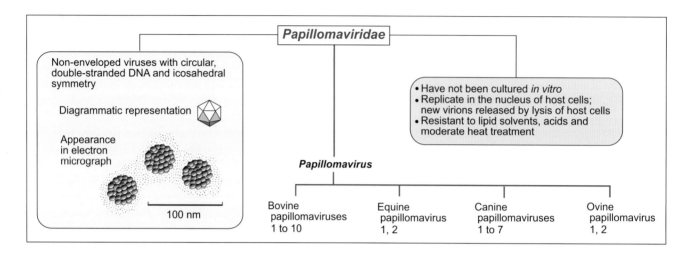

Papillomaviridae

Non-enveloped viruses with circular, double-stranded DNA and icosahedral symmetry

Diagrammatic representation

Appearance in electron micrograph

100 nm

- Have not been cultured *in vitro*
- Replicate in the nucleus of host cells; new virions released by lysis of host cells
- Resistant to lipid solvents, acids and moderate heat treatment

Papillomavirus

Bovine papillomaviruses 1 to 10

Equine papillomavirus 1, 2

Canine papillomaviruses 1 to 7

Ovine papillomavirus 1, 2

Formerly, papillomaviruses were grouped with polyomaviruses in the family *Papovaviridae*. Infections with polyomaviruses are of minor veterinary significance, sometimes causing disease in psittacine birds and laboratory animals. Some 30 genera are recognized in the family *Papillomaviridae* (Latin *papilla*, nipple, combined with Greek suffix *-oma* used to denote tumours). The taxonomy of papillomaviruses is confusing, particularly at the level of species and below. Further refinements by the International Committee on Taxonomy of Viruses (ICTV) including the creation of new genera, the reconciliation of genotype and species names, and the renaming of species are ongoing. Papillomaviruses typically infect the basal cells of squamous epithelium as a result of minute abrasions. Infected cells proliferate and differentiation is delayed. Viral gene expression is restricted during this proliferative phase. Full gene expression results in the production of viral capsids only after cellular differentiation begins in the upper layers of the epithelium. The release of virus occurs during desquamation of infected cells from the epithelial surface of lesions.

Clinical infections

The epitheliotropic, host-specific papillomaviruses cause proliferative lesions (warts) in many mammalian and avian species. Although they have not been grown in conventional cell culture, the DNA sequences of several papillomaviruses have been elucidated, allowing specific detection in lesions. In infected cells, the viral DNA is usually episomal. Papillomaviruses may be used experimentally for inserting foreign DNA into cultured cells.

Each papillomavirus tends to be host-specific and to produce proliferative lesions in specific anatomical sites. Although infections with papillomaviruses occur in many animal species, those which affect humans, cattle, horses and dogs are of most clinical

significance. Infections, which are often persistent, are usually established early in life. Lesions are most commonly observed in young animals and usually regress spontaneously after weeks or months. Regression is attributed to the development of cell-mediated immunity. Typical papillomas are composed of finger-like projections of proliferating epithelium supported by a thin core of mature fibrous tissue. In fibropapillomas, the fibrous tissue component predominates. More than 100 genotypes have been identified in humans, while in cattle at least 10 types are recognized. Several new papillomavirus types have been described in recent years in a range of species including horses and dogs. Individual types of virus share less than 50% sequence homology and exhibit differences in reciprocal immunological assays. Progression of papillomas to malignant tumours has been documented in humans, cattle and rabbits.

Bovine cutaneous papillomatosis

Fibropapillomas arising from infection with bovine papillomavirus (BPV) types 1 or 2 are often found on the head and neck of cattle under two years of age. Spontaneous regression of the lesions generally occurs within one year. Cutaneous papillomas caused by BPV-3 tend to persist. Because infection with BPV is usually self-limiting, treatment is seldom required. Teat fibropapillomas, associated with BPV-5 infection, have smooth surfaces and are described as 'rice grain' type. In contrast, 'frond' type teat papillomas arise from infection with BPV-6. Recently described genotypes, BPV 7–10, are associated with papillomas on the teats of cows. If interference with milking occurs, surgical removal of large lesions on teats may be required.

Bovine alimentary papilloma–carcinoma complex

Papillomas of the oesophagus, rumen and reticulum are associated with BPV-4 infection. The lesions, which are often solitary

Concise Review of Veterinary Microbiology, Second Edition. P.J. Quinn, B.K. Markey, F.C. Leonard, E.S. FitzPatrick and S. Fanning.
© 2016 John Wiley & Sons, Ltd. Published 2016 by John Wiley & Sons, Ltd.
Companion website: www.wiley.com/go/quinn/concise-veterinary-microbiology

and relatively small, are found incidentally at postmortem examination. Epidemiological and experimental studies have demonstrated that there is an increased frequency in the occurrence of malignant transformation of virus-induced alimentary papillomas to squamous cell carcinomas when animals are ingesting bracken fern. Such malignant lesions may cause difficulty in swallowing, ruminal tympany and loss of condition. Nodular fibropapillomas caused by BPV-2, which are occasionally found in similar upper alimentary tract locations to BPV-4 induced lesions, do not appear to become malignant.

Enzootic haematuria

Enzootic haematuria is encountered worldwide in cattle on poor pastures with abundant bracken fern growth. The haemorrhage originates from tumours in the bladder wall. Individual neoplastic lesions derive from either epithelial or mesenchymal tissues. Experimental studies suggest that BPV-2 and toxic compounds from bracken contribute to oncogenesis. It is probable that immunosuppression following ingestion of bracken may allow activation of latent BPV-2 in bladder tissues and this effect, together with the action of carcinogens also present in bracken, are responsible for the induction and progression of neoplastic lesions.

Equine papillomatosis

Papillomas are commonly encountered in horses between one and three years of age. Based on DNA studies, two types of equine papillomavirus have been identified. Type 1 is associated with papillomas on the muzzle and legs while type 2 is associated with papillomas of the genital tract. Spread may occur by direct or indirect contact. The lesions usually regress spontaneously after several months and recovered animals are immune to reinfection.

Equine sarcoid

Equine sarcoid is a locally invasive fibroblastic skin tumour and the most common neoplasm of horses, donkeys and mules. Viral DNA with a high degree of homology to BPV has been identified in tissue from sarcoids using both *in situ* hybridization and PCR. Experimental inoculation with BPV types 1 and 2 results in fibromatous lesions which resemble sarcoids but which regress spontaneously.

Lesions usually develop in horses between three and six years of age. Multiple cases can occur in families or groups of horses in close proximity. However, the incidence of equine sarcoid (estimated at 0.5–2%) is comparatively low for a viral disease, indicating that the horse may be a non-permissive host. Sarcoids can occur on any part of the body, either singly or in clusters. The most commonly affected sites are the head, ventral abdomen and limbs. They are highly variable in appearance but can be arbitrarily categorized as verrucous or fibroblastic. Clinical diagnosis should be confirmed histologically. Surgical removal is the usual form of treatment. Recurrence is common following conventional surgery and cryosurgery is more successful. Radiation therapy, CO_2 laser surgery and chemotherapy have also been used with varying degrees of success. Immunotherapy, aimed at stimulating cell-mediated immunity, may be effective in some cases. This involves intralesional injection of BCG or cell wall extract of *Mycobacterium bovis* into horses previously sensitized to tuberculoprotein.

Canine oral papillomatosis

Multiple transmissible papillomas in the oropharyngeal region of dogs are often encountered. The disease, which is caused by canine papillomavirus 1 (canine oral papillomavirus), is common in young dogs. The virus is readily transmitted by direct and indirect contact. The incubation period is up to eight weeks. Lesions are usually multiple and although generally confined to the oral mucosa are sometimes found on the conjunctiva, eyelids and muzzle. The papillomas initially appear as smooth, white, raised lesions but later become rough and cauliflower-like. Spread may occur inside the oral cavity. There is spontaneous regression within months. Surgical removal is generally unnecessary unless the papillomas persist or cause physical discomfort. Inactivated vaccines have been used but do not appear to be effective. Live, unattenuated vaccines, which are effective, may produce neoplastic lesions at the injection site.

Diagnosis

The clinical appearance of papillomas (warts) is distinctive. Laboratory confirmation is not usually required for typical papillomatous lesions. Histopathological examination may be required to determine the nature of some lesions, especially equine sarcoids. Electron microscopic examination of specimens from the epidermis may reveal characteristic virus particles. Hybridization assays and PCR methods are available for the detection of papillomavirus DNA, but are not used routinely. Isolates can be typed by extraction of DNA and restriction endonuclease analysis or by Southern blotting.

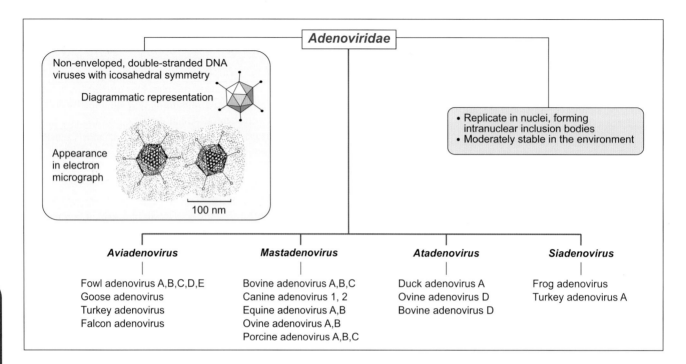

Non-enveloped, double-stranded DNA viruses with icosahedral symmetry

Diagrammatic representation

Appearance in electron micrograph

100 nm

Adenoviridae

- Replicate in nuclei, forming intranuclear inclusion bodies
- Moderately stable in the environment

Aviadenovirus

Fowl adenovirus A,B,C,D,E
Goose adenovirus
Turkey adenovirus
Falcon adenovirus

Mastadenovirus

Bovine adenovirus A,B,C
Canine adenovirus 1, 2
Equine adenovirus A,B
Ovine adenovirus A,B
Porcine adenovirus A,B,C

Atadenovirus

Duck adenovirus A
Ovine adenovirus D
Bovine adenovirus D

Siadenovirus

Frog adenovirus
Turkey adenovirus A

Adenoviruses (Greek *adenos*, gland) were first isolated from explant cultures of human adenoids. These non-enveloped, double-stranded DNA viruses comprise five genera: *Mastadenovirus* (mammalian adenoviruses), *Aviadenovirus* (avian adenoviruses), *Atadenovirus* (viruses of vertebrates), *Siadenovirus* (amphibian and avian viruses) and *Ichtadenovirus* (fish adenoviruses). Serogroups and serotypes are based on neutralization assays.

Clinical infections

Adenoviruses have a natural host range generally confined to a single species or to closely related species. Infection is common in animals and humans. Adenoviruses of veterinary importance are presented in Table 56.1. Adenovirus infections can be particularly severe in dogs and domestic fowl. In most domestic mammals, adenovirus infections are associated occasionally with enteric or respiratory problems. Avian adenoviruses occur worldwide in a wide range of species. Infection is extremely common in poultry flocks. Most of these infections are either subclinical or associated with relatively mild disease. However, severe disease may follow infection with duck adenovirus A (egg-drop syndrome) and turkey adenovirus A (haemorrhagic enteritis).

Infectious canine hepatitis

This worldwide, generalized viral disease of dogs principally affects the liver and vascular endothelium. Infectious canine

hepatitis has become relatively uncommon because of the widespread use of effective vaccines. Although dogs are the most commonly affected species, foxes, wolves, coyotes, skunks and bears are also susceptible. Transmission can occur following ingestion of urine, faeces or saliva from infected animals. The immune response usually eliminates virus from host tissues by 14 days after initial infection. However, virus may persist in the kidneys and may be excreted in urine for more than six months.

Following ingestion, canine adenovirus 1 (CAV-1) localizes in the tonsils and Peyer's patches. As viraemia develops, replication in vascular endothelium results in rapid distribution of virus throughout the body. Virus replication also occurs in the parenchymal cells of the liver and kidneys. Clinical recovery in most dogs coincides with the production of neutralizing antibodies about 10 days after infection. Glomerulonephritis, corneal oedema and anterior uveitis, attributed to immune complex deposition, may develop in some infected animals.

The incubation period is up to seven days. Dogs of all ages are susceptible and subclinical infection is common. Clinical disease is most frequently encountered in young dogs. The mortality rate ranges from 10 to 30% in mature dogs and up to 100% in young pups. In peracute disease, death occurs so rapidly that poisoning may be suspected. In acute disease, affected dogs present with fever, depression, anorexia, increased thirst, vomiting and diarrhoea. Abdominal palpation may elicit pain and,

Concise Review of Veterinary Microbiology, Second Edition. P.J. Quinn, B.K. Markey, F.C. Leonard, E.S. FitzPatrick and S. Fanning.
© 2016 John Wiley & Sons, Ltd. Published 2016 by John Wiley & Sons, Ltd.
Companion website: www.wiley.com/go/quinn/concise-veterinary-microbiology

SECTION IV

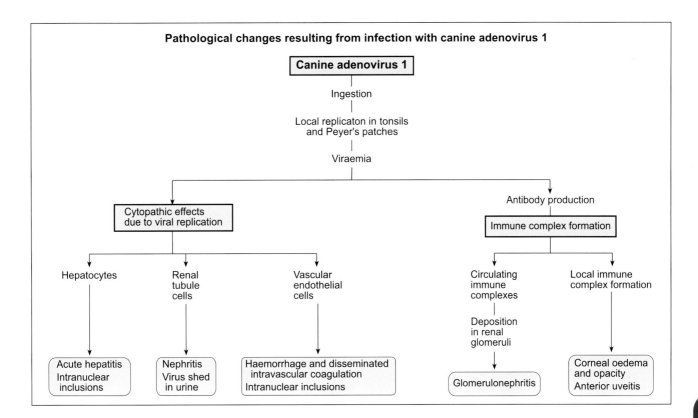

Pathological changes resulting from infection with canine adenovirus 1

```
                        Canine adenovirus 1
                                |
                            Ingestion
                                |
                    Local replicaton in tonsils
                       and Peyer's patches
                                |
                            Viraemia
                                |
        ┌───────────────────────┴───────────────────────┐
        |                                        Antibody production
Cytopathic effects                                       |
due to viral replication                      Immune complex formation
        |                                                |
  ┌─────┼─────────────┐                      ┌───────────┴───────────┐
Hepatocytes  Renal    Vascular          Circulating          Local immune
             tubule   endothelial       immune               complex formation
             cells    cells             complexes
                                             |
                                        Deposition
                                        in renal
                                        glomeruli
        |        |           |                |                       |
  Acute hepatitis  Nephritis   Haemorrhage and disseminated   Glomerulonephritis   Corneal oedema
  Intranuclear     Virus shed  intravascular coagulation                           and opacity
  inclusions       in urine    Intranuclear inclusions                             Anterior uveitis
```

Table 56.1 Adenoviruses of veterinary importance.

Virus	Comments
Canine adenovirus	Two strains are recognized, canine adenovirus (CAV)-1 and CAV-2. CAV-1 causes infectious canine hepatitis, with lesions arising from direct cytopathic effects and immune complex formation. CAV-2 is involved in infectious tracheobronchitis (kennel cough), a highly contagious respiratory disease
Equine adenovirus A	Usually a subclinical or mild respiratory infection in the horse population. In Arabian foals with severe combined immunodeficiency disease, associated with pneumonia, which is invariably fatal
Bovine adenoviruses	Associated with occasional outbreaks of respiratory and enteric disease
Ovine adenoviruses	Associated with occasional outbreaks of respiratory and enteric disease
Porcine adenoviruses	Usually subclinical infections; occasionally cause diarrhoea
Fowl adenoviruses	Frequently isolated from healthy birds or following respiratory disease. Associated with quail bronchitis, inclusion body hepatitis and hepatitis–hydropericardium syndrome
Duck adenovirus A	Causes egg drop syndrome in laying hens
Turkey adenovirus A	Causes turkey haemorrhagic enteritis (dysentery in 4 to 12-week-old poults with mortality rate of up to 60%) and marble spleen disease in pheasants (characterized by sudden death, pulmonary oedema and splenic necrosis in 2 to 8-month-old birds)

although hepatomegaly may be detected, jaundice is uncommon. Corneal opacity, either unilateral or bilateral, which may occur within weeks of clinical recovery in about 20% of affected animals, usually resolves spontaneously. Recovered animals have lifelong immunity.

A history of fever, sudden collapse and abdominal pain in young, unvaccinated dogs may suggest infectious canine hepatitis. In dogs that have died, the demonstration of basophilic intranuclear inclusion bodies in hepatocytes, Kupffer cells and endothelial cells is confirmatory. Viral antigen can be demonstrated by immunofluorescence in cryostat sections of liver. A PCR method for detecting viral DNA in clinical specimens has been described.

Vaccination with modified live CAV-1 vaccines occasionally results in mild nephropathy with shedding of virus in urine and, in some instances, corneal opacity. These side effects do not occur with modified live CAV-2 vaccines which stimulate effective long-lasting immunity to CAV-1.

Infection with canine adenovirus type 2

Canine adenovirus type 2, which is readily transmitted by aerosols, replicates in both the upper and lower respiratory tract. Clinical signs are generally mild or inapparent. Affected dogs may present with clinical signs similar to those of canine infectious tracheobronchitis (kennel cough). Most dogs recover and are immune to subsequent challenge. Occasional cases of bronchopneumonia may develop due to secondary bacterial infection. Virus shedding continues for about nine days after infection.

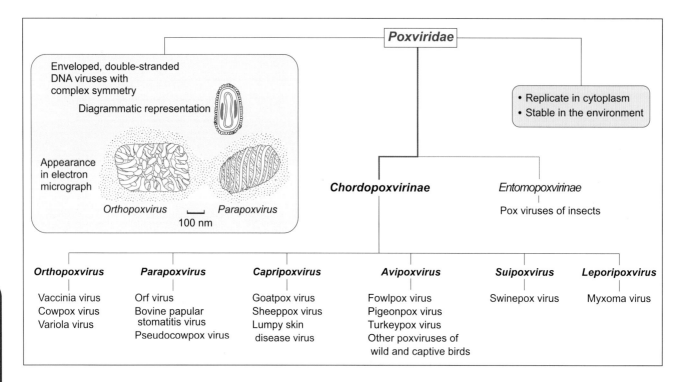

The family *Poxviridae* contains the largest viruses which cause disease in domestic animals. The family is divided into two subfamilies, *Chordopoxvirinae*, the poxviruses of vertebrates, and *Entomopoxvirinae*, the poxviruses of insects. Genetic recombination within genera results in extensive serological cross-reactions and cross-protection. These double-stranded DNA viruses replicate in the cytoplasm and are stable in the environment under dry conditions.

Infections with poxviruses usually result in vesicular skin lesions (Table 57.1). Smallpox, caused by variola virus, was formerly a human disease of major international significance. The use of vaccinia virus for the prevention of smallpox, first introduced by Jenner in the late eighteenth century, eventually led to the global eradication of this highly contagious disease at the close of the twentieth century.

Clinical infections

Transmission of poxviruses can occur by aerosols, by direct contact, by mechanical transmission through arthropods and through fomites. Skin lesions are the principal feature of these infections. Several virus-encoded proteins are released from infected cells, including a homologue of epidermal growth factor which stimulates cell proliferation. Typically, pox lesions begin as macules and progress through papules, vesicles and pustules to scabs which detach, leaving a scar. In generalized infections there is a cell-associated viraemia and recovered animals have solid immunity. Some localized pox infections may induce transient immunity and reinfection can occur.

Three closely related parapoxviruses, namely pseudocowpox virus, bovine papular stomatitis virus and orf virus, infect ruminants. These viruses are transmissible to humans, producing lesions which are clinically similar. Moreover, the three viruses are morphologically indistinguishable and identification of the causal agent relies on nucleic acid analysis.

Capripoxviruses are economically important viruses producing generalized infections with significant mortality in domestic ruminants. Sheeppox virus, goatpox virus and lumpy skin disease virus are closely related and share a group-specific structural protein (p32), which allows the same vaccine to be used against each virus.

Many avian species are susceptible to infection with members of the genus *Avipoxvirus*. Although antigenic relationships exist among avian poxviruses, this relatedness is variable. Virus species within the genus, named in accordance with their affinity for particular host species, include fowlpox virus, canarypox virus, pigeonpox virus and turkeypox virus. The type species of the genus is fowlpox virus.

Diagnosis

Diagnosis can often be made solely on clinical grounds. Skin biopsies or postmortem specimens may be used for laboratory confirmation. Eosinophilic intracytoplasmic inclusions may

Concise Review of Veterinary Microbiology, Second Edition. P.J. Quinn, B.K. Markey, F.C. Leonard, E.S. FitzPatrick and S. Fanning.
© 2016 John Wiley & Sons, Ltd. Published 2016 by John Wiley & Sons, Ltd.
Companion website: www.wiley.com/go/quinn/concise-veterinary-microbiology

Table 57.1 Members of the *Poxviridae* of veterinary significance.

Virus	Genus	Host species	Significance of infection
Vaccinia virus	*Orthopoxvirus*	Wide host range	Infections in sheep, water buffaloes, rabbits, cattle, horses and humans. Used as a recombinant virus vector for rabies vaccine
Cowpox virus	*Orthopoxvirus*	Rodents, cats, cattle	Species of small rodents are the likely reservoir hosts. Cats are the principal incidental hosts; infection results in skin lesions. Rare cause of teat lesions in cattle. Transmissible to humans
Uasin gishu virus	*Orthopoxvirus*	Unknown wildlife reservoir, horses	Rare disease, reported in Kenya and neighbouring African countries. Causes papilloma-like skin lesions in horses
Camelpox virus	*Orthopoxvirus*	Camel	Widely distributed in Asia and Africa. Causes systemic infection with typical pox lesions; severe infection in young camels
Pseudocowpox virus	*Parapoxvirus*	Cattle	Common cause of teat lesions in milking cows; causes milker's nodule in humans
Bovine papular stomatitis virus	*Parapoxvirus*	Cattle	Produces papular lesions on the muzzle and in the oral cavity of young cattle. Transmissible to humans
Orf virus	*Parapoxvirus*	Sheep, goats	Primarily affects young lambs; causes proliferative lesions on the muzzle and lips. Transmissible to humans
Sheeppox/goatpox virus	*Capripoxvirus*	Sheep, goats	Endemic in Africa, Middle East and India. Causes generalized infection with characteristic skin lesions and variable mortality
Lumpy skin disease virus	*Capripoxvirus*	Cattle	Endemic in Africa. Causes generalized infection with severe lesions and variable mortality
Swinepox virus	*Suipoxvirus*	Pigs	Causes mild skin disease. Occurs worldwide. Transmitted by the pig louse (*Haematopinus suis*)
Fowlpox virus	*Avipoxvirus*	Chickens, turkeys	Causes lesions on the head and on the oral mucous membrane. Occurs worldwide. Transmitted by biting arthropods
Myxoma virus	*Leporipoxvirus*	Rabbits	Causes mild disease in cottontail rabbits, the natural host, and severe disease in European rabbits (myxomatosis). Introduced into Europe, Australia and Chile as a biological control measure
Squirrelpox virus	Unassigned	Red and grey squirrels	Important factor in decline of native red squirrels (*Sciurus vulgaris*) in Great Britain; carried by grey squirrel (*Sciurus carolinensis*) introduced from North America
Nile crocodilepox virus	*Crocodylidpoxvirus*	Nile crocodile	Cause of skin lesions in wild and farmed crocodiles

be demonstrable histologically in epidermal cells. Electron microscopy can be used for the rapid identification of poxvirus particles in material from lesions. Parapoxviruses can be readily distinguished from members of the other genera. For some species, virus may be isolated in testis or kidney cell monolayers. An antigen-trapping ELISA has been developed for the detection of capripoxvirus antigen. Protocols for PCR assays for the detection of viral DNA are also available.

Control

Vaccines are available for a number of poxviruses and control is based on annual vaccination. Inactivated vaccines are less effective than modified live vaccines because cell-mediated immunity is the predominant protective response. A recombinant vaccine providing protection against lumpy skin disease and peste des petits ruminants has been developed. In flocks endemically infected with orf virus, control is based on the use of a fully virulent live vaccine derived from scab material or cell culture. Ewes should be vaccinated by scarification in the axilla at least eight weeks before lambing. Close to lambing, ewes must be moved to a new grazing area in order to minimize exposure of lambs to infectious vaccinal scab material.

58 *Asfarviridae*

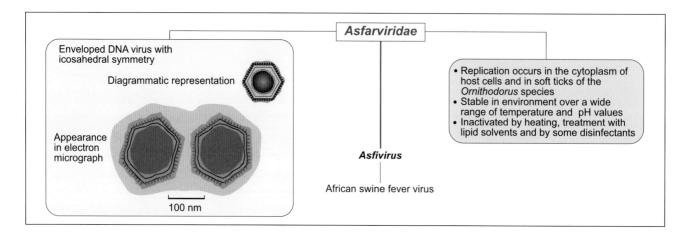

Asfarviridae

Enveloped DNA virus with icosahedral symmetry

Diagrammatic representation

Appearance in electron micrograph

100 nm

- Replication occurs in the cytoplasm of host cells and in soft ticks of the *Ornithodorus* species
- Stable in environment over a wide range of temperature and pH values
- Inactivated by heating, treatment with lipid solvents and by some disinfectants

Asfivirus

African swine fever virus

African swine fever virus (ASFV) is the sole member of the genus *Asfivirus* in the family *Asfarviridae*. Virions are 175 to 215 nm in diameter and consist of a membrane-bound nucleoprotein core inside an icosahedral capsid, surrounded by an outer lipid-containing envelope. The genome consists of a single molecule of linear double-stranded DNA. Following replication in the cytoplasm of host cells, virus is released either by budding through the plasma membrane or following cellular disintegration. African swine fever virus is stable in the environment over a wide range of temperature (4 to 20°C) and pH values. The virus may persist for months in meat.

African swine fever

African swine fever (ASF) is an economically important viral disease of pigs, characterized by fever, haemorrhages in many tissues and a high mortality rate. It is endemic in sub-Saharan Africa, Madagascar and Sardinia. A large outbreak beginning in Georgia in 2007 has spread across Russia, Belarus and Ukraine. Domestic and wild pigs are the only species susceptible to infection. In Africa, ASFV is maintained in a sylvatic cycle involving soft ticks of the genus *Ornithodorus* and inapparent infection of warthogs and bushpigs. Replication of virus occurs in the ticks and both transovarial and trans-stadial transmission have been described. Soft ticks feed for short periods on hosts before dropping off and sheltering in crevices in walls or cracks in the ground. The presence of infected ticks in a particular region makes the eradication of ASF difficult. Virulent strains of ASFV, producing high mortality in infected animals, are widely distributed in Africa. Many isolates from other parts of the world are less virulent and mortality rates are usually below 50%.

Feeding uncooked swill is an important mechanism of spread of ASF internationally, with outbreaks often starting in herds close to airports and harbours. Pigs which have recovered from clinical disease may remain infected for long periods. Carrier pigs are considered to be important sources of virus dissemination.

Infection in domestic pigs is usually acquired via the oronasal route. The virus replicates primarily in cells of the lymphoreticular system. Lesions include splenic enlargement, swollen haemorrhagic gastrohepatic and renal lymph nodes, subcapsular petechiation in the kidneys, petechial and ecchymotic haemorrhages on serosal surfaces, oedema of the lungs and hydrothorax. The widespread haemorrhages result from disseminated intravascular coagulation, endothelial damage and destruction of megakaryocytes. The clinical signs of ASF, which range from inapparent to peracute, relate to the challenge dose and virulence of the virus and to the route of infection. The incubation period is typically five to seven days in acute cases. Mortality rates, which are variable, depend on the age and general health of infected pigs. Animals may recover and appear clinically normal or may develop a chronic form of the disease, which usually occurs in regions where ASFV is endemic.

Laboratory confirmation of ASF is based on detection of ASFV using tests such as PCR, direct immunofluorescence and haemadsorption. Suitable samples include blood, serum, tonsil, spleen and lymph nodes. Antibodies persist for long periods in recovered animals and serological testing may be the only means of detecting animals infected with strains of low virulence.

Restriction of pig movement, serological monitoring of carrier pigs, and prevention of contact between domestic pigs and warthogs or ticks are important control measures in countries where the disease is endemic. Eradication of tick species which act as vectors of ASFV is an essential part of a control programme. An effective vaccine is not yet available. The occurrence of strains of low virulence renders eradication difficult.

SECTION IV

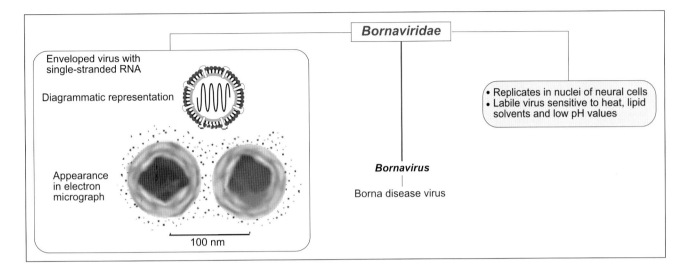

The family *Bornaviridae* contains a single genus, *Bornavirus*. The sole member of the genus is Borna disease virus (BDV). This enveloped virus, which has only recently been demonstrated by electron microscopy, is spherical, with a diameter of about 90 nm. The envelope surrounds an inner core, 50–60 nm in diameter. The genome consists of a single molecule of negative-sense, single-stranded RNA. Replication occurs in the nucleus of host cells with budding at the cell surface. This labile virus is sensitive to heat, lipid solvents and low pH values.

Borna disease

This fatal neurological disease of horses is named after Borna, the town in Saxony where a large outbreak occurred in 1895. The disease occurs sporadically in Germany, Switzerland and other parts of Europe. Sero-epidemiological studies, however, indicate a wide geographical distribution. Neurological disease attributed to BDV has been described in horses, sheep and cats. Serological evidence of infection has been recorded in other species including rabbits, cattle and ostriches. It is thought that virus may be transmitted through ingestion or inhalation. Most cases of Borna disease occur in spring and early summer; prevalence varies from year to year. There is evidence that rodents such as shrews may act as reservoir hosts. Persistent infections can be established experimentally in rats. It has been suggested that proventricular dilatation disease, a fatal disorder of parrots, is caused by an avian bornavirus. 'Staggering disease' in cats has been associated with BDV infection.

Following oronasal infection, the virus gains entry to the CNS by intra-axonal spread, either through the olfactory nerve or through nerves supplying the oropharyngeal and intestinal regions. Spread within the CNS and into the peripheral nerves also occurs within axons. A non-suppurative encephalitis with lymphocytic perivascular cuffing is largely confined to grey matter and neuronal degeneration is prominent. Borna disease has been described mainly in young horses. The incubation period, which is highly variable, ranges from weeks to several months. Factors which may influence the severity of clinical signs include the age and immunological status of the infected animal and the strain of infecting virus. On farms where infection in horses is present, clinical disease is usually confined to individual animals. Clinical signs include fever, somnolence and evidence of neurological disturbance. Ataxia, pharyngeal paralysis and hyperaesthesia may be present. The course of the disease is up to three weeks and mortality rates may reach 100%. Surviving horses have permanent CNS damage and may exhibit recurrent episodes of neurological disturbance.

Borna disease may vaguely resemble other neurological conditions in the horse. However, the distribution of lesions in the CNS differs from that in other equine encephalomyelitides and if eosinophilic intranuclear inclusions (Joest–Degen bodies) are present, they may be confirmatory. Viral antigen can be demonstrated in the brain by immunohistochemical methods. Demonstration of antibodies in serum or in cerebrospinal fluid by immunofluorescence, immunoblotting or ELISA may aid diagnosis. Reverse transcriptase-PCR for the demonstration of BDV-RNA is a valuable diagnostic tool. Control is difficult due to the sporadic nature of the disease. Although BDV does not appear to be readily transmitted by infected horses, seropositive animals should be isolated. Standard hygienic measures should be applied to suspect animals.

Concise Review of Veterinary Microbiology, Second Edition. P.J. Quinn, B.K. Markey, F.C. Leonard, E.S. FitzPatrick and S. Fanning.
© 2016 John Wiley & Sons, Ltd. Published 2016 by John Wiley & Sons, Ltd.
Companion website: www.wiley.com/go/quinn/concise-veterinary-microbiology

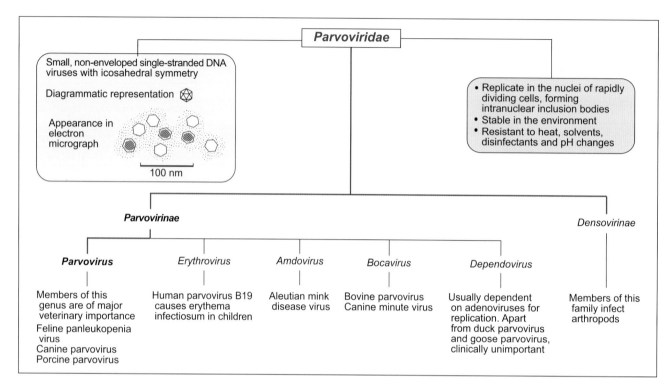

Viruses belonging to the family *Parvoviridae* (Latin *parvus*, small) range in size from 18 to 26 nm in diameter and possess a linear genome of single-stranded DNA. Parvoviruses replicate only in the nuclei of dividing host cells, a feature which determines the tissues targeted. After entering a cell, the virion is uncoated and its single-stranded DNA genome is converted to double-stranded DNA by DNA polymerases in the nucleus. Following viral replication, cell lysis occurs as virions are released. Many parvoviruses of vertebrates agglutinate erythrocytes and haemagglutination inhibition by specific antisera is widely used for their identification. Parvoviruses are very stable in the environment.

Clinical infections

Parvoviruses can infect many domestic and wild animals (Table 60.1). Mink enteritis virus, canine parvovirus and racoon parvovirus are considered to be host-range mutants of feline panleukopenia virus. Although most members of the group produce acute systemic diseases, some such as canine minute virus and bovine parvovirus, are of uncertain pathogenic significance. The most important parvoviral diseases of domestic animals are feline panleukopenia, canine parvovirus infection and porcine parvovirus infection.

Feline panleukopenia

Feline panleukopenia, also known as feline infectious enteritis or feline distemper, is a highly contagious generalized disease of domestic and wild cats. The disease, which is worldwide in distribution, is one of the most common feline viral infections.

Infection is generally endemic in unvaccinated cat populations with disease occurring predominantly in young recently weaned kittens as maternally-derived antibody levels wane. The disease may have a cyclical or seasonal pattern which is related to the births of kittens. Transplacental infection occurs in fully susceptible queens with effects on the foetus ranging from cerebellar hypoplasia to foetal death. High rates of virus excretion occur during the acute stage of the disease, mainly in faeces. In cool, moist, dark environments, infectivity may last for more than a year.

The incubation period is typically five days. Subclinical infections are common, particularly in older cats and kittens partially protected by maternally-derived immunity. Following ingestion or inhalation, replication occurs in the oropharynx and associated lymph nodes. Viraemia develops within 24 hours, producing infection of mitotically active cells in other tissues, particularly the cells of the intestinal crypts and also in bone marrow, thymic, lymph node and splenic cells. Destruction of these target tissues results in panleukopenia and villous atrophy. Disease is characterized by sudden onset of pronounced depression, anorexia and fever. Vomiting, sometimes accompanied by diarrhoea or dysentery, follows. The mortality rate ranges from 25 to 90%.

Concise Review of Veterinary Microbiology, Second Edition. P.J. Quinn, B.K. Markey, F.C. Leonard, E.S. FitzPatrick and S. Fanning.
© 2016 John Wiley & Sons, Ltd. Published 2016 by John Wiley & Sons, Ltd.
Companion website: www.wiley.com/go/quinn/concise-veterinary-microbiology

Table 60.1 Parvoviruses of veterinary significance.

Virus	Hosts	Consequences of infection
Feline panleukopenia virus	Domestic and wild cats	Highly contagious systemic and enteric disease most common in weaned kittens, manifested as depression, vomiting, diarrhoea. Intrauterine infection: abortion or cerebellar ataxia in neonatal kittens
Canine parvovirus (Canine parvovirus 2)	Dogs	Highly contagious enteric disease with depression, vomiting, dysentery and immunosuppression. Intrauterine or perinatal infection: myocarditis in pups (now rare)
Porcine parvovirus	Pigs	Major cause of stillbirths, mummified foetuses, embryonic deaths and infertility (SMEDI syndrome)
Mink enteritis virus	Mink	Generalized disease of mink kits, analagous to feline panleukopenia
Aleutian mink disease virus	Mink, ferrets	Chronic, progressive disease of mink homozygous for pale coat colour. Persistent viraemia, plasmacytosis, hypergammaglobulinaemia and immune complex-related lesions
Goose parvovirus (goose plague virus)	Geese	Highly contagious, fatal disease of 8 to 30-day-old goslings (Derzsy's disease): hepatitis, myositis, including myocarditis
Canine minute virus (Canine parvovirus 1)	Dogs	Serological surveys suggest the virus is widespread; ability of virus to produce disease is uncertain
Bovine parvovirus	Cattle	Associated with sporadic outbreaks of diarrhoea in calves

Diagnosis is usually based on demonstration of virus particles by electron microscopy or detection of virus by ELISA, PCR or haemagglutination using faecal samples from cats with acute disease. Typical histopathological changes may be present in sections of the ileum and jejunum.

Vaccination is the principal control measure. There is only one serotype of feline panleukopenia virus and immunity following natural infection is strong and long-lasting. As clinical infections cause heavy environmental contamination, premises should be thoroughly cleaned and disinfected with effective preparations such as 1% sodium hypochlorite or 2% formalin.

Canine parvovirus infection

Infection with canine parvovirus (CPV) emerged in the late 1970s as a worldwide disease in dogs, with high morbidity and mortality. Acute or subacute heart failure in pups infected *in utero* or during the perinatal period was a common manifestation of the disease. With the gradual development of immunity in the adult dog population, the clinical pattern of the disease changed. The most common clinical presentation now encoun-

tered is acute enteric disease in young dogs between weaning and six months of age. Many canine species are susceptible to infection and transmission is predominantly by the faecal–oral route. Since its emergence, CPV has continued to evolve through mutation and three subtypes or variants are recognized (2a, 2b and 2c). Infection or vaccination with one subtype generally confers immunity against the other subtypes.

The virus replicates initially in pharyngeal lymphoid tissues and Peyer's patches. Viraemia develops and the main target tissues are those with rapidly multiplying cell populations. During the first two weeks of life, there is active cardiac myocyte division allowing viral replication, with resultant necrosis and myocarditis. In older pups, the virus invades the actively dividing epithelial cells of the crypts in the small intestine. There may be extensive haemorrhage into the intestinal lumen in severely affected pups. Destruction of lymphoid tissues contributes to immunosuppression which facilitates the proliferation of Gram-negative bacteria and may result in endotoxaemia.

After an incubation period of four to seven days, animals with enteric disease show sudden onset of vomiting and anorexia. Diarrhoea, often blood-stained, develops within 48 hours. Affected dogs deteriorate rapidly due to dehydration and weight loss. Definitive diagnosis early in the course of the disease relies on the demonstration of virus or viral antigen in faeces using electron microscopy, ELISA, PCR or haemagglutination. In fatal cases, the nature and distribution of the gross and microscopic enteric lesions may point to a parvoviral infection.

Vaccination is the principal control measure. However, as vaccination alone usually cannot be relied on to control the cycle of endemic parvovirus infection in kennels, thorough cleaning and disinfection of premises must be carried out following a disease outbreak.

Porcine parvovirus infection

Porcine parvovirus is an important cause of reproductive failure in pigs worldwide. On farms where the disease is endemic, many sows are immune. Maternally-derived immunity usually persists for about four months, but it can persist in some pigs until they are six to nine months of age. During this period, the maternally derived antibodies may interfere with the development of active immunity following vaccination or natural infection. As a result, some gilts can be seronegative and susceptible to infection at mating and during pregnancy. The virus has a predilection for the mitotically active cells in foetal tissues. Transplacental infection in pregnant sows occurs 10–14 days after exposure to the virus. The major damage to foetuses arises before onset of immunocompetence, at about 60–70 days of gestation. Infection of embryos in the first weeks of life results in death and resorption. When infection occurs later in gestation, but before day 70, foetuses die and become mummified. Infection after 70 days of gestation usually results in the birth of healthy seropositive piglets. Demonstration of viral antigen in cryostat sections of foetal tissues such as lung, by immunofluorescence, is reliable and sensitive. Control is based on exposure of gilts and susceptible sows to porcine parvovirus prior to mating. This can be achieved by vaccination or by exposing animals to contaminated faeces or to placental or foetal tissue from infected sows.

61 *Circoviridae*

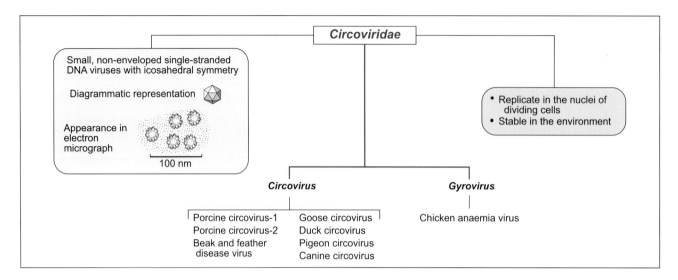

Circoviruses (20 to 25 nm in diameter) are non-enveloped with icosahedral symmetry. The genome consists of a molecule of circular single-stranded DNA. Replication occurs in the nuclei of dividing cells and these viruses are stable in the environment. Circoviruses are host-specific, have a worldwide distribution and infect cells of the haemolymphatic system. The majority of circoviruses identified have been isolated from avian species. Infections with chicken anaemia virus and with porcine circovirus are of particular veterinary interest. Beak and feather disease virus is associated with a debilitating, immunosuppressive disease of young psittacine birds, particularly cockatoos. Canine circovirus has been identified in dogs suffering form severe haemorrhagic gastroenteritis, vasculitis and granulomatous lymphadenitis.

Chicken anaemia virus infection

Young birds infected with chicken anaemia virus (CAV) develop aplastic anaemia and generalized lymphoid atrophy. This virus is present in poultry flocks worldwide. Both horizontal and vertical transmission occur. Infection is by the faecal–oral route. Once infection is established in a breeder flock, most birds develop antibodies before laying begins. Maternally-derived antibodies do not prevent chicks from becoming infected and shedding the virus. However, they prevent the development of clinical disease. An age-related resistance to disease but not to infection develops in chicks at about two weeks of age. However, age-related resistance and the protective effect of maternally-derived antibodies do not prevent clinical disease if immunosuppressive viruses such as infectious bursal disease virus or gallid herpesvirus 2 are present in the flock. The principal target cells are in the thymus and in the bone marrow. Chickens develop clinical signs at about two weeks of age. The mortality rate is usually about 10%. Subclinical infection in broilers from breeder flocks can adversely affect weight gains.

A presumptive diagnosis is based on the clinical signs and gross lesions at postmortem. Laboratory confirmation relies on detection of viral antigen by immunocytochemical techniques. Viral DNA can be demonstrated in bone marrow and thymus by *in situ* hybridization, by dot-blot hybridization or by PCR. Serum antibodies can be detected using virus neutralization, indirect immunofluorescence and ELISA. Commercial live vaccines are available and are designed to prevent vertical transmission of the virus from breeder hens. Vaccination does not prevent economic losses in broilers due to subclinical infection.

Pig circovirus infection

Porcine circovirus 2 (PCV-2) is consistently isolated from piglets with post-weaning multi-systemic wasting syndrome (PMWS). Sero-epidemiological studies indicate that infection is widespread in pig populations worldwide. The virus has also been linked to porcine dermatitis and nephropathy syndrome and to reproductive problems.

Co-factors appear to be necessary for the development of the full clinical disease. It is thought that immune stimulation may be an important trigger. A generalized depletion of lymphocyctes resulting in immunosuppression is a consistent feature of the disease.

Diagnosis of PMWS is based on clinical signs and pathological findings. A definitive diagnosis requires demonstration of PCV-2 antigen or viral nucleic acid in association with lesions. Due to the widespread nature of the virus, control is largely directed towards eliminating the co-factors and triggers of the disease that may be present on individual farms: good husbandry, rapid removal of affected animals and the elimination of other infectious agents. Commercial inactivated and subunit vaccines are available.

Concise Review of Veterinary Microbiology, Second Edition. P.J. Quinn, B.K. Markey, F.C. Leonard, E.S. FitzPatrick and S. Fanning.
© 2016 John Wiley & Sons, Ltd. Published 2016 by John Wiley & Sons, Ltd.
Companion website: www.wiley.com/go/quinn/concise-veterinary-microbiology

146

62 *Astroviridae*

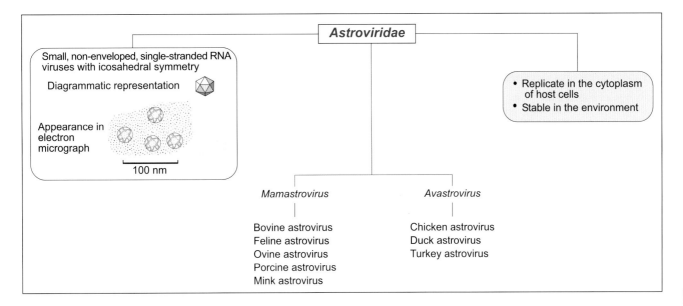

The family *Astroviridae* (Greek *aster*, star) contains viruses with a surface structure which imparts a star-like appearance. Astroviruses, 28 to 30 nm in diameter, are non-enveloped with icosahedral symmetry. The genome consists of a single molecule of positive-sense, linear, single-stranded RNA. These viruses are resistant to low pH values, various detergents and heating at 60°C for five minutes. Replication occurs in the cytoplasm of host cells and virions are released by cell lysis. Trypsin is required for cultivation of these viruses.

The family contains two genera: *Avastrovirus*, whose members infect avian species, and *Mamastrovirus*, whose members infect mammalian species. Viral species are designated according to the host of origin, while serotypes are specified by cross-neutralization tests.

Clinical infections

Astroviruses, which are distributed worldwide, have been detected in the faeces of humans, cattle, pigs, sheep, dogs, cats, deer, chickens, ducks and turkeys. Transmission occurs by the faecal–oral route. Infections are mild in most species. In general, isolates from different host species are antigenically distinct and host species-specific. However, new findings indicate that classification based on the host of origin is not always reliable, particularly in relation to astroviruses of birds and bats. The International Committee on Taxonomy of Viruses (ICTV) has approved a new classification system based on genetic criteria: mamastroviruses 1 to 19, avastroviruses 1 to 3.

Mamastroviruses are associated with self-limiting gastroenteritis in animals and humans. Following an incubation period of up to four days, diarrhoea may develop. Infections, particularly with avastroviruses, may be more severe involving a number of organs. Infection of ducklings with duck astrovirus, now referred to as astrovirus 3, may cause severe hepatitis. A runting and stunting syndrome accompanied by lesions of interstitial nephritis are associated with chicken astrovirus infection of birds. Turkey astroviruses are associated with poult enteritis mortality syndrome.

Diagnosis is based on the detection of astroviruses in faeces using electron microscopy or ELISA. Detection of viral RNA using reverse transcriptase PCR and virus isolation in primary cell lines or embryonated eggs are also possible. Because astrovirus infections are generally mild, vaccines have not been developed except for duck astrovirus. Control is based on husbandry practices appropriate for the prevention of enteritis in young animals including thorough cleaning, all-in/all-out policies and effective disinfection and implementation of strict biosecurity measures.

Concise Review of Veterinary Microbiology, Second Edition. P.J. Quinn, B.K. Markey, F.C. Leonard, E.S. FitzPatrick and S. Fanning.
© 2016 John Wiley & Sons, Ltd. Published 2016 by John Wiley & Sons, Ltd.
Companion website: www.wiley.com/go/quinn/concise-veterinary-microbiology

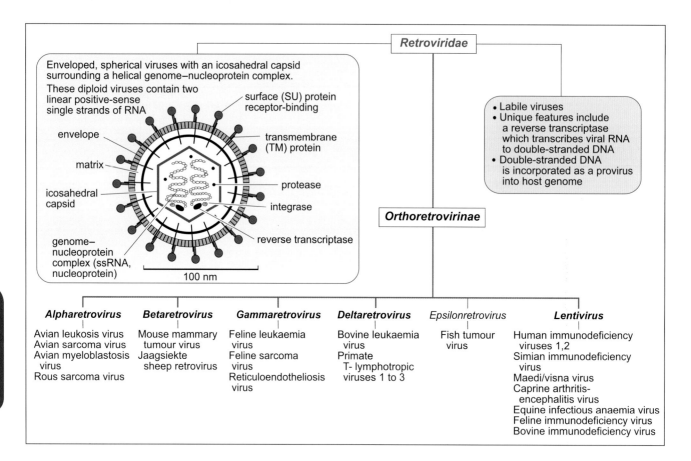

Enveloped, spherical viruses with an icosahedral capsid surrounding a helical genome–nucleoprotein complex.

These diploid viruses contain two linear positive-sense single strands of RNA

- envelope
- matrix
- icosahedral capsid
- genome–nucleoprotein complex (ssRNA, nucleoprotein)

100 nm

- surface (SU) protein receptor-binding
- transmembrane (TM) protein
- protease
- integrase
- reverse transcriptase

Retroviridae

- Labile viruses
- Unique features include a reverse transcriptase which transcribes viral RNA to double-stranded DNA
- Double-stranded DNA is incorporated as a provirus into host genome

Orthoretrovirinae

Alpharetrovirus
Avian leukosis virus
Avian sarcoma virus
Avian myeloblastosis virus
Rous sarcoma virus

Betaretrovirus
Mouse mammary tumour virus
Jaagsiekte sheep retrovirus

Gammaretrovirus
Feline leukaemia virus
Feline sarcoma virus
Reticuloendotheliosis virus

Deltaretrovirus
Bovine leukaemia virus
Primate T- lymphotropic viruses 1 to 3

Epsilonretrovirus
Fish tumour virus

Lentivirus
Human immunodeficiency viruses 1,2
Simian immunodeficiency virus
Maedi/visna virus
Caprine arthritis-encephalitis virus
Equine infectious anaemia virus
Feline immunodeficiency virus
Bovine immunodeficiency virus

Retroviruses (Latin *retro*, backwards) are labile enveloped RNA viruses, 80 to 100 nm in diameter. The family name refers to the presence in the virion of a reverse transcriptase which is encoded in the viral genome. Reverse transcriptase acts as an RNA-dependent DNA polymerase, which transcribes RNA to DNA. Under the influence of the reverse transcriptase, double-stranded DNA copies of the viral genome are synthesized in the cytoplasm of the host cell. During this process, repeat base sequences called long terminal repeats (LTR), containing several hundred base pairs, are added to the ends of the DNA transcripts. Transcripts are integrated into the chromosomal DNA as provirus, through the action of viral integrase. Integration occurs at random sites in the DNA and the sites of proviral integration determine the extent and nature of cellular changes. The LTR contain important promoter and enhancer sequences. Infectious viruses have four main genes: 5'-*gag-pro-pol-env*-3' as illustrated.

Because errors are relatively frequent during reverse transcription, a high mutation rate is a feature of retroviral replication. Recombination between retroviral genomes in doubly-infected cells can occur due to transfer of reverse transcriptase from one RNA template to another. Consequently,

quasispecies frequently form and definitive classification at the level of species or below often proves difficult.

Retroviruses can be categorized as exogenous or endogenous. Exogenous retroviruses are capable of horizontal transmission between members of the host species. Endogenous retroviruses occur widely among vertebrates, constituting up to 10% of the genomic DNA of the host. They are consistently present in germline cells and are transmitted (inherited in Mendelian fashion) only as provirus in germ-cell DNA from parent to offspring. They are regulated by cellular genes and are usually silent but may recombine with exogenous retroviruses.

Retroviruses in the genera *Alpharetrovirus*, *Betaretrovirus*, *Gammaretrovirus* and *Deltaretrovirus* are frequently referred to as oncogenic retroviruses because they can induce neoplastic transformation in cells which they infect (Table 63.1). On the basis of the interval between exposure to the virus and tumour development, exogenous oncogenic retroviruses are designated either as slowly transforming (*cis*-activating) viruses or as rapidly transforming (transducing) viruses. Slowly transforming retroviruses induce B-cell, T-cell or myeloid tumours after long incubation periods. For malignant transformation to occur,

Concise Review of Veterinary Microbiology, Second Edition. P.J. Quinn, B.K. Markey, F.C. Leonard, E.S. FitzPatrick and S. Fanning.
© 2016 John Wiley & Sons, Ltd. Published 2016 by John Wiley & Sons, Ltd.
Companion website: www.wiley.com/go/quinn/concise-veterinary-microbiology

Table 63.1 Oncogenic retroviruses of veterinary importance.

Genus	Virus	Hosts	Comments
Alpharetrovirus	Avian leukosis virus	Chickens, pheasants, partridge, quail	Endemic in commercial flocks. Exogenous and endogenous transmission of virus can occur. Causes lymphoid leukosis in birds between 5 and 9 months of age
Betaretrovirus	Jaagsiekte sheep retrovirus	Sheep	Causes jaagsiekte, a slowly progressive neoplastic lung disease of adult sheep which is invariably fatal. Occurs worldwide except in Australasia
	Enzootic nasal tumour virus	Sheep, goats	Closely related to jaagsiekte sheep retrovirus. Causes adenocarcinoma of low-grade malignancy, which affects the nares
Gammaretrovirus	Feline leukaemia virus	Cats	Important cause of chronic illness and death in young adult cats. Causes immunosuppression, enteritis, reproductive failure, anaemia and neoplasia. Worldwide distribution
	Reticuloendotheliosis virus	Turkeys, ducks, chickens, quail, pheasants	Infection usually subclinical. Sporadic disease may present with anaemia, feathering defects, impaired growth or neoplasia. Disease outbreaks have occurred following use of vaccine contaminated with reticuloendotheliosis virus
Deltaretrovirus	Bovine leukaemia virus	Cattle	Causes enzootic bovine leukosis in adult cattle. A small percentage of infected cattle develop lymphosarcoma

the provirus must be integrated into the host cell DNA close to a cellular oncogene (c-*onc*, protooncogene), resulting in interference with the regulation of cell division (insertional mutagenesis). Multiple insertions of the provirus into the host cell genome results in exaggerated gene expression and over-production of a transformation-associated protein. Rapidly transforming retroviruses, which can induce tumour formation after short incubation periods, contain viral oncogenes (v-*onc*). More than a dozen different oncogenes have been identified in transforming avian retroviruses. Viral oncogenes are considered to be cellular oncogenes acquired by recombination during virus evolution. If the oncogene is integrated into the viral genome without loss of replicative virus genes, as in Rous sarcoma virus, the retrovirus is described as replication-competent. Frequently, as a consequence of cellular oncogene integration, existing viral sequences necessary for replication are deleted. Such replication-defective retroviruses, which cannot multiply without helper viruses, are rarely transmitted under normal field conditions. The protein products of oncogenes may act as hormone or growth factor receptors, transcription control factors and kinases in signal transduction pathways. A third method of tumour induction is exemplified by bovine leukaemia virus, which depends on the *tax* gene encoding a protein capable of up-regulating both viral LTR and cellular promoter sequences, even when the provirus is integrated into a different chromosome (*trans*-activation).

Feline leukaemia and associated clinical conditions

Infection with feline leukaemia virus (FeLV) not only results in feline leukaemia but is also associated with a variety of other clinical conditions. Isolates of FeLV are assigned to four subgroups (A, B, C and T) on the basis of differences in the gp70 envelope glycoprotein. FeLV-A, the predominant subgroup, is isolated from all FeLV-infected cats. Viruses of subgroup B, which arise through recombination between the *env*

genes of FeLV-A and endogenous FeLV-related proviral DNA, are present in about 50% of isolates. Cats that are infected with both FeLV-A and FeLV-B have a higher risk of developing tumours than those infected with FeLV-A alone. Each FeLV-C isolate is unique, arising *de novo* in a FeLV-A infected cat through mutations in the receptor-binding region of the FeLV-A *env* gene. Once generated, FeLV-C viruses rapidly cause a fatal anaemia and consequently are not transmitted to other cats. Conversion of FeLV-A to FeLV-T requires a combination of an insertion and single amino acid changes to the envelope protein, giving rise to a T-cell tropic, cytopathic virus capable of inducing immunodeficiency.

Close contact is required for transmission of this labile virus and the incidence of infection is related to population density. Highest infection rates are found in catteries and multi-cat households. Large amounts of virus are shed in saliva. Infection is usually acquired by licking, grooming and through bite wounds. Young kittens are more susceptible to infection than adults and a significant proportion of those exposed before 14 weeks of age become persistently infected. Such animals constitute the main reservoir of FeLV and are prone to develop an FeLV-related disease. Because the production of virus particles requires cellular DNA synthesis, tissues with high mitotic activity, such as bone marrow and epithelia, are targeted. The virus causes tumours, particularly lymphosarcoma, by several means, including insertional mutagenesis and recombination with a variety of cellular protooncogenes, producing rapidly transforming, replication-defective viruses. Examples of the latter are FeLVs isolated from thymic lymphomas and also feline sarcoma viruses (FeSV) that are isolated from rare multicentric fibrosarcomas in young cats. These viruses are not transmitted under natural conditions. The majority of persistently infected cats die within three years of infection. About 80% of these cats die from non-neoplastic FeLV-associated disease.

Representation of important genes of oncogenic retroviruses and their encoded proteins

Oncogenic retroviruses   **Genomic composition**

Avian leukaemia virus
Feline leukaemia virus
5' | LTR | gag | pro | pol | env | LTR | 3'

Replication-defective, rapidly transforming retroviruses
5' | LTR | gag | pro | pol | env | V-onc | LTR | 3'

Rous sarcoma virus
5' | LTR | gag | pro | pol | env | V-src | LTR | 3'

Bovine leukaemia virus
5' | LTR | gag | pro | pol | env | tax | rex | LTR | 3'

Gene	Encoded protein
gag	Nucleocapsid
pro	Protease
pol	Enzymes: reverse transcriptase, integrase
env	Envelope glycoproteins
v-onc	Oncoprotein
v-src	Oncoprotein (tyrosine phosphokinase)
tax	Transcriptional activator
rex	Post-transcriptional activator

LTR: Long terminal repeats

Anaemia, reduction in reproductive performance, enteritis and a variety of secondary infections are important features of the disease.

Detection of viral antigen in blood or saliva is the method commonly used for the laboratory diagnosis of feline leukaemia. Commercial ELISA and rapid immunomigration tests are available. A test and removal policy has been shown to be effective in eradicating infection from catteries. Several commercial vaccines are available. Vaccination does not provide complete protection and does not alter the course of infection in persistently infected cats.

Enzootic bovine leukosis

This retroviral disease of adult cattle is characterized by persistent lymphocytosis and the development of B-cell lymphosarcoma in a number of infected animals. The labile virus is intimately cell-associated and transmission usually takes place through transfer of blood or secretions such as milk containing infected lymphocytes. Less than 10% of calves born to infected dams are infected at birth. Animals are usually infected between six months and three years of age. Iatrogenic transmission is important and has been linked to reuse of needles, multi-dose injectors, contaminated surgical instruments and rectal examination procedures. The primary target cell is the B lymphocyte. Although infections are lifelong, most animals remain subclinically infected. About 30% of infected animals develop persistent lymphocytosis without clinical signs of disease. From 1 to 5% of infected animals eventually develop lymphosarcoma as adults. The presenting signs relate to the sites of tumour formation.

Several serological tests including agar gel immunodiffusion (AGID) and ELISA are suitable for the detection of antibodies to bovine leukaemia virus. Vaccination is not used for control. Test and removal strategies are used in eradication programmes.

Jaagsiekte

This disease, also called ovine pulmonary adenomatosis, is a slowly progressing neoplastic disease of adult sheep caused by jaagsiekte sheep retrovirus (JSRV). Respiratory exudates from affected sheep are infectious and transmission occurs by the respiratory route. Close contact facilitates spread of infection with the incidence of disease highest in housed animals. Within an infected flock, disease incidence may be up to 20%. Multiple copies of endogenous retroviruses related to JSRV (enJSRV) have been found in the genomes of both sheep and goats.

The virus replicates in two types of pulmonary cells, type II alveolar cells and non-ciliated bronchial cells. Tumours arising from these cell types progressively replace normal lung tissue leading to death from asphyxia. The incubation period may range from several months up to two years. Affected animals are usually three to four years of age, in poor bodily condition, and display respiratory embarrassment. Secondary pasteurellosis is a frequent complication. A clinical diagnosis is usually confirmed by histopathological examination. The incidence of disease in a flock can be reduced by strict isolation, particularly during the rearing of lambs, and by elimination of suspect animals immediately after clinical or laboratory confirmation of the disease.

Lentiviruses

Lentiviruses (Latin *lentus*, slow) cause lifelong infections and are associated with diseases that have a long incubation period and an insidious protracted course. Lentiviruses of domestic animals are presented in Table 63.2.

Feline immunodeficiency virus infection

Feline immunodeficiency virus (FIV) infection of domestic cats was first reported in 1987 and is now recognized worldwide as an important cause of disease in cats. Five subtypes of FIV

Table 63.2 Lentiviruses of domestic animals.

Virus	Hosts	Comments
Feline immunodeficiency virus	Cats	Causes lifelong infection with persistent viraemia and immunosuppression in cats over 5 years of age. Worldwide distribution
Equine infectious anaemia virus	Horses, mules, donkeys	Causes lifelong infection with recurring febrile episodes. Anaemia is a prominent clinical sign
Maedi/visna virus	Sheep	Causes lifelong infection with progressive respiratory disease (maedi) and indurative mastitis in older sheep. Clinical signs develop in a small percentage of infected animals. Some infected sheep develop progressive neurological disease (visna)
Caprine arthritis-encephalitis virus	Goats	Causes lifelong infection. Associated with polyarthritis and indurative mastitis in adults and progressive nervous disease in kids. Common in dairy goat herds. Worldwide distribution
Bovine immunodeficiency virus	Cattle	Widely distributed; pathogenicity not determined

(A to E) have been identified. Virus is shed mainly in the saliva and transmission usually occurs through bites. Accordingly, infection rates are highest in free-roaming adult male cats. Animals remain infected for life but not all infected cats develop disease.

The virus replicates principally in $CD4^+$ (helper) T lymphocytes, producing a progressive decline in cell-mediated immunity due to depletion of these lymphocytes. The prevalence of clinical disease is highest in cats over six years of age. The course of the disease may be divided into an acute phase, a prolonged asymptomatic phase, a phase characterized by vague clinical signs and a terminal phase with marked immunodeficiency. Clinical signs are highly variable and include recurrent fever, leukopenia, anaemia, weight loss, lymphadenitis, chronic gingivitis and behavioural changes. Opportunistic infections are frequent in the terminal phase of the disease. Chronic stomatitis and gingivitis are common findings. Other manifestations include chronic respiratory, enteric and skin infections. Neurological signs, usually due to direct viral damage, develop in a small number of infected cats.

Diagnosis is primarily based on serological testing for antibodies. Commercial ELISA and immunoconcentration kits are available. Treatment is primarily aimed at the control of secondary infections. Control is based on prevention of exposure by separating infected and non-infected cats in multi-cat households, by preventing cats from roaming freely, by using seronegative queens for breeding and by screening all cats before introduction into seronegative populations. Commercial vac-

cines are available but there are concerns regarding the level of protection induced against heterologous strains.

Equine infectious anaemia

This disease affects horses, mules and donkeys in many countries. The virus is transmitted mechanically by haematophagous insects, particularly *Tabanus* species and *Stomoxys* species. Transmission occurs most often in the summer, during periods of high insect activity, in low-lying swampy areas close to woodlands. Iatrogenic transmission can occur through contaminated needles or surgical instruments.

The virus replicates in macrophages, monocytes and Kupffer cells. Infected horses fail to eliminate the virus despite mounting a strong immune response. In the course of viral replication, mutations, which arise frequently, can result in the emergence of new virus strains exhibiting antigenic variation in envelope glycoproteins (antigenic drift). Febrile episodes and marked immune stimulation signal the emergence of these new strains. Non-neutralizing antibodies produced against virus early in the course of infection lead to the formation of immune complexes. Such immune complexes activate complement, contributing to fever, anaemia and thrombocytopenia and can initiate glomerulonephritis. Haemolysis, enhanced erythrophagocytosis and depressed erythropoiesis are responsible for the anaemia in chronically affected horses. In most animals, clinical episodes eventually cease, probably as a consequence of a broad-based neutralizing response against a wide range of viral epitopes.

Laboratory confirmation of infection is based on the demonstration of serum antibodies to the core virus protein p26. The serological test recognized for international trade is the AGID (Coggins) test. Restriction of animal movement accompanied by detection and removal of seropositive animals are used to minimize the risk of disease spread.

Small ruminant lentivirus group

Two distinct lentiviruses have been described in sheep and goats, maedi/visna virus (MVV) and caprine arthritis-encephalitis virus (CAEV). These viruses are closely related and cause persistent infections and comparable disease syndromes. Each virus can infect both sheep and goats. Genomic analyses of these ovine and caprine lentivirus isolates suggest that they evolved from a common ancestral genotype. The current view is that they comprise a heterogeneous group with a variable host range and different pathogenic capabilities.

Infection is frequently subclinical. The clinical severity of disease is influenced by viral virulence, the age of the host when exposed and other host factors. Virus production is triggered following conversion of monocytes into macrophages. The immune response is not fully effective and probably contributes to the pathogenesis of the disease.

Laboratory confirmation relies on detection of virus-specific antibodies. The most commonly used assays are AGID and ELISA. Control is based on test and segregation programmes. The milk from infected animals is an important source of infection and newborn animals should be isolated and reared separately from their infected dams.

64 *Reoviridae*

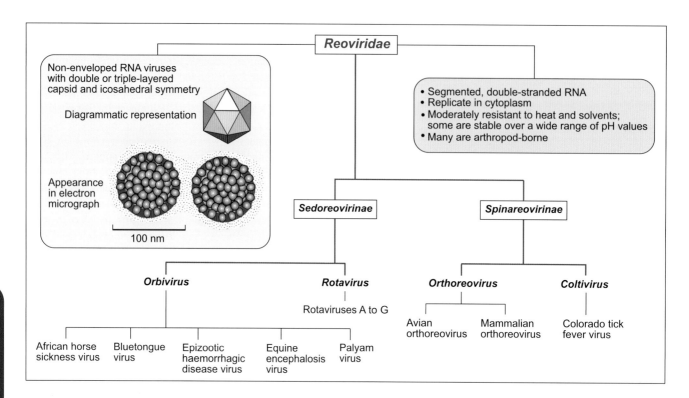

The family name *Reoviridae* is based on the acronym 'reo' because the initial isolates came from **r**espiratory and **e**nteric sources without any associated disease, so-called **o**rphan viruses. These icosahedral viruses, 60 to 80 nm in diameter, are non-enveloped and possess a layered capsid which is composed of up to three concentric protein shells. The genome of the virion is composed of nine to twelve segments of double-stranded RNA. Genetic reassortment readily takes place in cells co-infected with viruses of the same species (genetic shift). There is also a high rate of mutation (genetic drift). As a result, there are numerous serotypes and strains of each virus species. Replication occurs in the cytoplasm of host cells, often with the formation of intracytoplasmic inclusions. The family contains 15 genera in two subfamilies, *Sedoreovirinae* (six genera) and *Spinareovirinae* (nine genera). Members of the genera *Orthoreovirus*, *Rotavirus* and *Orbivirus* infect animals and humans. Members of the genera *Coltivirus* and *Seadornavirus* are arboviruses that may occasionally cause disease in humans. Other genera in the family contain viruses of plants, arthropods and fish. Viruses in the family are moderately resistant to heat, organic solvents and non-ionic detergents.

Clinical infections

Reoviruses, which are widespread in nature, have been isolated from many animal species (Table 64.1). Avian orthoreoviruses have been implicated in arthritis, tenosynovitis, chronic respiratory disease and enteritis. Rotaviruses cause acute diarrhoea in young intensively reared farm animals. Transmission of orthoreoviruses and rotaviruses occurs through contact with contaminated faeces.

African horse sickness and bluetongue are particularly important diseases caused by orbiviruses. Epizootic haemorrhagic disease of deer and Ibaraki disease in cattle, both caused by members of the epizootic haemorrhagic disease virus (EHDV) serogroup, have clinical effects in these species similar to those of bluetongue in sheep. The viruses of African horse sickness, bluetongue and epizootic haemorrhagic disease of deer are transmitted by blood-sucking arthropods, especially by *Culicoides* species.

Enteric disease caused by rotaviruses in young animals

Rotaviruses cause diarrhoea in intensively reared young farm animals worldwide. Isolates are divided into several antigenically distinct groups (A–G), also termed species, based on differences in the major capsid protein, VP6. Most isolates belong to group A. High titres of virus (10^9 virus particles per gram of faeces) are excreted by clinically affected animals. Because the virus is stable in the environment, premises may be heavily contaminated and, accordingly, intensively reared animals are those

Concise Review of Veterinary Microbiology, Second Edition. P.J. Quinn, B.K. Markey, F.C. Leonard, E.S. FitzPatrick and S. Fanning.
© 2016 John Wiley & Sons, Ltd. Published 2016 by John Wiley & Sons, Ltd.
Companion website: www.wiley.com/go/quinn/concise-veterinary-microbiology

Table 64.1 Viruses of veterinary importance in the family *Reoviridae*.

Genus	Virus	Comments
Orbivirus	African horse sickness virus	Arthropod-borne infection of *Equidae*, principal vector *Culicoides* species. Endemic in Africa. High mortality rate
	Bluetongue virus	Arthropod-borne infection of sheep, cattle, goats and wild ruminants. Principal vector *Culicoides* species. Severe disease in sheep. Clinical disease uncommon in cattle except for serotype 8. Teratogenic effects
	Epizootic haemorrhagic disease virus	Arthropod-borne infection of deer, cattle and buffalo. At least seven serotypes recognized. Principal vector *Culicoides* species. Clinically similar to bluetongue. Important disease of white-tailed deer in North America. Generally subclinical or mild infections in cattle except for Ibaraki virus (EHDV-2) in south-east Asia which causes an acute febrile disease
	Equine encephalosis virus	Reported in South Africa and Israel. Majority of infections subclinical. Sporadic cases of acute fatal disease. Cerebral oedema, fatty liver and enteritis are prominent features
	Palyam virus	Arthropod-borne disease of cattle. Causes abortion and teratogenic effects. Recorded in southern Africa, south-east Asia and Australia. Many viruses in the serogroup
	Peruvian horse sickness virus	Isolated from horses (neurological disease) in Peru and Northern Territories of Australia (Elsey virus). Mosquito vector
Rotavirus	Rotaviruses	Outbreaks occur in intensively reared neonatal animals. Mild to severe diarrhoea, severity influenced by virulence of viral strain, age, colostral intake and management factors
Orthoreovirus	Avian orthoreoviruses	Important cause of viral arthritis/tenosynovitis in chickens. Multiple serotypes described. Turkeys and other avian species susceptible
	Mammalian orthoreoviruses	Associated with mild enteric and respiratory disease in many species, severity dependent on secondary infections. Four serotypes recognized
Coltivirus	Colorado tick fever virus	Rodent species act as reservoirs. Arthropod-borne, mainly ticks and also mosquitoes. Primarily of significance in humans

most often affected. Diagnosis is based on electron microscopy or demonstration of viral antigen in faeces by ELISA or latex agglutination. Control involves measures aimed at reducing the levels of virus challenge in young animals while vaccination of pregnant dams can be used to raise antibody levels in mammary secretions.

African horse sickness

This is a non-contagious OIE-listed disease of *Equidae* caused by African horse sickness virus. Nine serotypes of this orbivirus constitute the African horse sickness serogroup. The disease is endemic in sub-Saharan Africa. The virus is transmitted by haematophagous insects, principally *Culicoides imicola*. Four forms of this febrile disease are recognized. A peracute pulmonary form is characterized by depression and nasal discharge, with rapid progression to severe respiratory distress. Mortality rates may approach 100%. A subacute cardiac form manifests as conjunctivitis, abdominal pain and progressive dyspnoea. Subcutaneous oedematous swellings of the head and neck are most obvious in the supraorbital fossae, palpebral conjunctiva and intermandibular space. In this form of the disease, the mortality rate is about 50%. A mixed form of intermediate severity (up to 70% mortality rate) presents with both cardiac and pulmonary features. A mild or subclinical form, termed horse sickness fever, may be observed in zebras and donkeys. Vector control, quaran-

tine of affected animals and vaccination are the main methods of preventing disease transmission.

Bluetongue

This non-contagious OIE-listed disease of sheep and other domestic and wild ruminants is transmitted by a range of *Culicoides* species. Twenty-six serotypes of bluetongue virus (BTV) have been described. Infection is of greatest significance in sheep and deer. In 2006, BTV-8 appeared in northern Europe and caused a severe epizootic. Clinical disease in cattle has been a feature of this epizootic with clinical signs similar but generally milder than those observed in sheep. The clinical presentation is highly variable, ranging from subclinical to severe disease with high mortality. Affected animals are febrile and depressed with vascular congestion of the lips and muzzle. Oedema of the lips, face, eyelids and ears develops. Lameness may result from coronitis and laminitis. Mortality rate may be up to 30%. A presumptive diagnosis may be based on clinical findings and postmortem lesions. Confirmation generally relies on detection of viral RNA by RT-PCR or demonstration of BTV-specific antibodies. Live attenuated vaccines have been used successfully for many years and provide protection against virulent viruses of homologous serotype. Polyvalent vaccines are essential in regions where a number of serotypes are present. Killed adjuvanted vaccines can induce protection but are more expensive to produce and require two inoculations.

65 *Orthomyxoviridae*

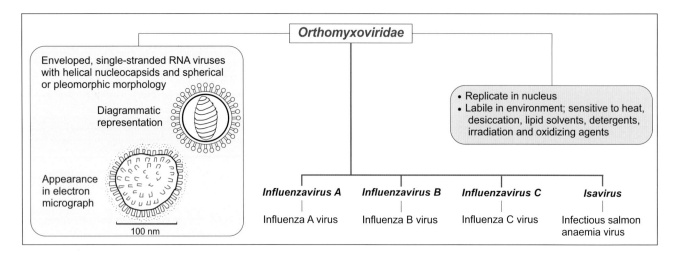

The family *Orthomyxoviridae* (Greek *orthos*, proper and *myxa*, mucus) contains those viruses which cause influenza in humans and animals. Orthomyxoviruses are spherical or pleomorphic, enveloped viruses, 80 to 120 nm in diameter. Long filamentous forms also occur. The envelope, which is derived from host cell membrane lipids, contains glycosylated and non-glycosylated viral proteins. Surface projections of glycoproteins form 'spikes' or peplomers which, in influenza A and B viruses, are of two types: a haemagglutinin (H) responsible for virus attachment and envelope fusion, and a neuraminidase (N) capable of cleaving viral receptors thus promoting both entry of virus into cells and release of virions from infected cells.

Influenza viruses haemagglutinate erythrocytes from a wide range of species. Antibodies to the H glycoprotein are mainly responsible for virus neutralization. The nucleocapsid has a helical symmetry. The genome, which is composed of six to eight segments, consists of linear, negative-sense, single-stranded RNA. Replication occurs in cell nuclei with release of virions by budding from plasma membranes. Virions are labile in the environment and are sensitive to heat, lipid solvents, detergents, irradiation and oxidizing agents.

The family contains six genera, namely *Influenzavirus A*, *Influenzavirus B*, *Influenzavirus C*, *Thogotovirus*, *Quaranjavirus* and *Isavirus*. Influenza B and C viruses are pathogens of humans; Thogoto virus and Dhori virus are tick-borne arboviruses isolated from camels, cattle and humans in parts of Africa, Europe and Asia; infectious salmon anaemia virus affects farmed salmon. Influenza A virus, the most important member of the family, is a significant pathogen of animals and humans.

Isolates of influenza A virus are grouped into subtypes on the basis of their H and N antigens. Currently, 18 H antigens and 11 N antigens are recognized and new subtypes of influenza A virus emerge periodically. A number of mechanisms – point mutation and recombination (genetic reassortment) – are responsible for the emergence of new strains and new subtypes respectively. Point mutations give rise to antigenic drift, in which variation occurs within a subtype. Genetic reassortment, a more complex process in which the genome segments of two or more related viruses infecting the same cell are exchanged, results in the development of new subtypes (antigenic shift). To assess the risk posed by the emergence of new variant viruses, a precise classification of isolates has been adopted by the World Health Organization. This system is based on the influenza virus type, host, geographical origin, strain number, year of isolation and subtype. An example of this classification system, influenza virus A/equine/Prague/1/56 (H7N7), indicates that this virus was isolated from a horse in Prague during 1956. Antigenic subtypes of influenza A virus which cause disease in humans and farm animals are presented in Table 65.1.

Clinical infections

Influenza A viruses cause significant infections in humans, pigs, horses and birds. All known subtypes (except H17N10 and H18N11, which have been found only in bats) can infect birds. Aquatic birds, particularly ducks which are reservoirs of influenza A virus, provide a genetic pool for the generation of the new subtypes capable of infecting mammals. Migratory waterfowl and trade in poultry and poultry products may disseminate avian viruses across international borders. Although isolates of influenza A virus are usually species specific, there are well-documented instances of transfer between species. The viruses replicate in the intestinal tract of birds and transmission of low pathogenic influenza viruses is mainly by the faecal–oral route. Human infection with avian influenza viruses has been attributed to the combined effects of poor hygiene and the close association of concentrated human populations with domestic

Concise Review of Veterinary Microbiology, Second Edition. P.J. Quinn, B.K. Markey, F.C. Leonard, E.S. FitzPatrick and S. Fanning.
© 2016 John Wiley & Sons, Ltd. Published 2016 by John Wiley & Sons, Ltd.
Companion website: www.wiley.com/go/quinn/concise-veterinary-microbiology

Table 65.1 Antigenic subtypes of influenza A virus isolated from humans and animals.

Hosts	Antigenic subtypes	Comments
Humans	H1N1 (1918, 1977, 2009)[a] H2N2 (1957) H3N2 (1968)	Subtypes which have been found in pigs such as H1N1 have been implicated in human pandemics. Sporadic or limited transmission of infections reported with H5N1, H7N2, H7N3, H7N7, H7N9, H9N2 and H10N8 in recent years
Birds	Many antigenic subtypes represented by different combinations of haemagglutinin (H) and neuraminidase (N) peplomers have been recognized	Disease is usually associated with subtypes expressing H5 or H7. Wild birds, especially migrating ducks, act as carriers
Pigs	Predominantly H1N1, H1N2 and H3N2	Severity of disease is determined by the antigenic subtype
Horses	Usually H7N7 or H3N8 (H7N7 has not been detected in horses for more than 20 years. H3N8 has replaced H7N7 as the predominant subtype)	Subtypes associated with disease, which are widely distributed geographically, are absent from Australia, New Zealand and Iceland
Dogs	H3N8 (originated from an equine H3N8 lineage), H3N2	H3N8 first reported in Florida in 2004. Large outbreak of influenza (H3N2) in dogs in USA in 2014

[a] Year of recognition.

fowl and pigs. Genetic reassortment in these animal populations can lead to the emergence of novel virulent influenza virus subtypes which are capable of infecting humans, thereby initiating pandemics. Avian influenza viruses usually replicate poorly in humans. However, both human and avian influenza subtypes replicate in pigs, a species in which genetic reassortment readily occurs with the emergence of new subtypes. Such novel subtypes may be implicated in major pandemics which occur at intervals of about 20 years. As there is limited immunity in the human population to new subtypes, spread from country to country tends to occur rapidly.

Subtypes of influenza A virus, which are well established as pathogens in particular animal populations, have also been implicated in crossing species barriers without genetic reassortment. An H1N1 avian subtype appeared in pigs in Europe in 1979. In 1997, following a large epidemic of avian influenza in chickens, a highly pathogenic avian influenza (HPAI) H5N1 subtype (first isolated from a goose in southern China in 1996) was isolated from a fatal case in a young child in Hong Kong. This subtype had not previously been described outside of avian species. Human health fears prompted the destruction of 1.2 million birds in Hong Kong. The virus reappeared in members of a Hong Kong family in 2003 and was subsequently found to be circulating across south-east Asia resulting in spread to the Middle East, Africa and Europe. Fortunately human-to-human transmission has not been demonstrated to any significant extent to date, although human cases (mortality rate approximately 60%) have continued to occur as a result of contact with infected poultry. Other subtypes of avian origin have caused human infections (Table 65.1), particularly in China where factors such as live bird markets appear to be important in disease transmission.

Avian influenza (fowl plague)

Influenza A subtypes occur worldwide. Outbreaks of severe clinical disease, usually caused by subtypes expressing H5 and H7 determinants, occur periodically in chickens and turkeys. In these species, acute infection is often referred to as fowl plague or HPAI and is categorized as a listed disease by the OIE. It is likely that the HPAI viruses in these acute outbreaks arise by mutation from low pathogenic avian influenza viruses. Spread of influenza virus in tissues is dependent on the type of proteases present in a given tissue and the structure of the viral haemagglutinin molecule. The production of infectious virions requires cleavage of the viral haemagglutinin. In the majority of influenza A virus subtypes, haemagglutinin cleavage takes place only in the epithelial cells of the respiratory and digestive tracts. Because of the amino acid composition at their cleavage sites, haemagglutinins of virulent subtypes are susceptible to cleavage in many tissues, facilitating the development of generalized infection. Highly virulent subtypes cause explosive outbreaks of disease with high mortality. Clinical signs are more apparent in birds which survive for a few days. Respiratory distress, diarrhoea, oedema in the cranial region, cyanosis, sinusitis and lacrimation are features of the clinical presentation. In countries free of the disease, test and slaughter policies are implemented. Vaccination is permitted in those countries with recurring outbreaks of disease but is prohibited in countries implementing a slaughter policy.

Equine influenza

Equine influenza is an economically important respiratory disease of horses. Outbreaks of disease are associated with the assembly of horses at shows, sales, racing or training. Affected animals develop a high temperature with nasal discharge and a dry cough. A number of inactivated vaccines are commercially available, but as immunity is short-lived, regular booster injections are required. Vaccinated horses, exposed to field virus, exhibit milder clinical signs than unvaccinated animals.

SECTION IV

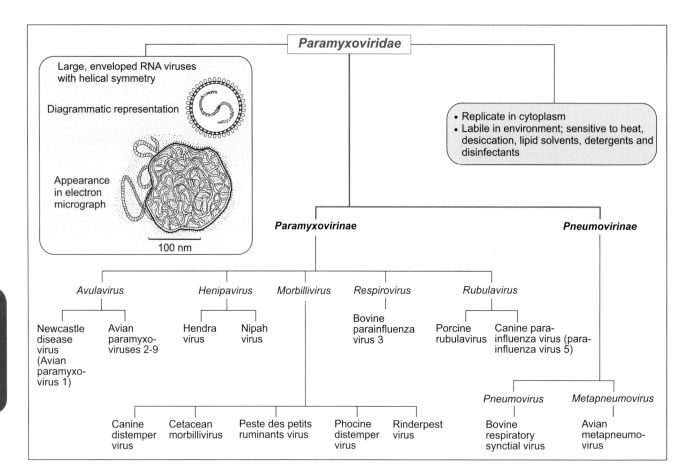

Paramyxoviruses and orthomyxoviruses were formerly grouped together as the 'myxoviruses' (Greek *myxa*, mucus), a name which describes their affinity for mucous membranes. Paramyxoviruses are pleomorphic, 150 nm or more in diameter and enveloped. They contain a single molecule of negative-sense, single-stranded RNA. Two types of glycoprotein 'spikes' or peplomers are present in the envelope, an attachment protein and a fusion protein (F). The attachment protein may be either a haemagglutinin–neuraminidase protein (HN) or a protein without neuraminidase activity (G or H). The attachment proteins allow the virus to bind to cell surface receptors and the fusion protein causes the virus envelope to fuse with the host cell membrane. However, there is significant variation between different paramyxoviruses in the mechanism of viral attachment, stimulation of the fusion protein and the process of viral entry into the cell. Both types of peplomers can induce production of virus neutralizing antibodies. Paramyxoviruses may exhibit haemagglutinating, haemolytic and neuraminidase activities. The nucleocapsid, which has helical symmetry, is 13 to 18 nm in diameter and has a characteristic herring-bone appearance. Replication

occurs in the cell cytoplasm and acidophilic inclusions are a feature of paramyxovirus infections. Virions are released by budding from the plasma membrane at sites containing virus envelope proteins. The labile virions are sensitive to heat, desiccation, lipid solvents, non-ionic detergents and disinfectants.

The family is divided into two subfamilies, *Paramyxovirinae* and *Pneumovirinae*, containing seven and two genera respectively. The genera *Aquaparamyxovirus* (viruses of fish) and *Ferlavirus* (viruses of reptiles) are the most recent members of the family to be designated as genera in a family that continues to expand as new virus species in wild animals are discovered. Although paramyxoviruses are genetically relatively stable and do not appear to undergo recombination, some antigenic variation occurs through mutational changes and selection.

Clinical infections

Paramyxoviruses, which typically have a narrow host range, infect mainly mammals and birds (Table 66.1). Following transmission through close contact or by aerosols, replication occurs

---

Concise Review of Veterinary Microbiology, Second Edition. P.J. Quinn, B.K. Markey, F.C. Leonard, E.S. FitzPatrick and S. Fanning.
© 2016 John Wiley & Sons, Ltd. Published 2016 by John Wiley & Sons, Ltd.
Companion website: www.wiley.com/go/quinn/concise-veterinary-microbiology

Table 66.1 Paramyxoviruses of veterinary importance.

Genus	Virus	Comments
Morbillivirus	Rinderpest virus	Cause of cattle plague, a highly contagious disease in domestic and wild ruminants, characterized by high morbidity and high mortality. Worldwide eradication announced by FAO in 2011
	Peste des petits ruminants virus	Produces severe disease, resembling rinderpest, in small ruminants, particularly sheep and goats, with high morbidity and high mortality rates
	Canine distemper virus	Acute disease in dogs and wild carnivores, characterized by multi-systemic involvement, including CNS signs, and variable mortality
Avulavirus	Newcastle disease virus (Avian paramyxovirus 1)	Generalized infection characterized by respiratory, intestinal and nervous signs in domestic and wild birds. Isolates vary widely in virulence; velogenic, mesogenic and lentogenic strains are recognized
	Avian paramyxovirus 2–9	Reported worldwide from a range of domestic and wild birds. Although infections with most avian paramyxoviruses are associated with mild or inapparent disease, infections with APMV-2 and APMV-3 have been associated with respiratory disease in turkeys
Rubulavirus	Porcine rubulavirus	Known as blue eye disease, characterized by mortality in young pigs, corneal opacity and reproductive failure; described only in Mexico
	Canine parainfluenza virus	Causes inapparent or mild respiratory disease in dogs; sometimes associated with kennel cough; also known as parainfluenza virus 5 (formerly simian virus 5)
Respirovirus	Bovine parainfluenza virus 3	Cause of subclinical or mild respiratory disease in cattle and sheep. Sometimes associated with shipping fever in cattle. Predisposes to secondary bacterial infection, particularly with *Mannheimia haemolytica*
Pneumovirus	Bovine respiratory syncytial virus	Common subclinical infection in adult cattle. Associated with respiratory disease outbreaks of varying severity in young cattle. Sheep and goats are also susceptible
Metapneumovirus	Avian metapneumovirus	Causes severe upper respiratory tract infection in turkeys, with coryza and swollen sinuses. In chickens, the disease is referred to as 'swollen head syndrome'

primarily in the respiratory tract. Disease outbreaks of viral infections in marine mammals has led to the recognition of new morbilliviruses, phocine distemper virus and cetacean morbillivirus. Fruit bats are the reservoir hosts of the zoonotic henipaviruses. Hendra virus was isolated during an outbreak of severe respiratory disease in horses in Australia during 1994. Two humans in contact with infected horses were also affected; 14 horses and their trainer died. A related virus, Nipah virus, was isolated in Malaysia during 1999 following outbreaks of disease in pigs and humans working in affected pig units. The disease, which caused a febrile encephalitis, resulted in more than 100 human deaths. New paramyxoviruses continue to be identified in bats, particularly fruit bats, including Menangle virus, Tioman virus, Mapuera virus and bat parainfluenza virus. Menangle virus and Tioman viruses can produce disease in pigs, while Mapuera virus is closely related to porcine rubulavirus.

Rinderpest

This acute OIE-listed disease, which occurred primarily in ruminants and is also referred to as cattle plague, has been recognized for centuries as a major cause of mortality in cattle and domestic buffalo. Originally an Asian disease, devastating outbreaks in Europe resulted in the foundation of the first veterinary school in Lyon in 1761. Following its introduction into the Horn of Africa a devastating outbreak followed throughout sub-Saharan Africa during the last decade of the nineteenth century. Due to the labile

nature of the virus, transmission, which occurs through aerosols, usually requires close contact. Epidemics usually occur following movement of susceptible animals into an endemic area or the introduction of infected animals into susceptible populations. Infected animals develop fever and become anorexic and depressed. Mucosal erosions in the mouth and nasal passages become evident within five days. Profuse salivation is accompanied by an oculonasal discharge. About three days after the appearance of the mucosal ulcers, fever regresses and a profuse diarrhoea develops. The dark fluid faeces often contain mucus, necrotic debris and blood. Morbidity may reach 90% and mortality can approach 100%. Following various regional initiatives, the Food and Agriculture Organization (FAO) launched a global eradication scheme in 1994 that involved movement restrictions, vaccination, active surveillance and culling. By the end of the twentieth century rinderpest was considered endemic only in the Somali pastoral ecosystem which straddles the borders of Kenya, Ethiopia and Somalia. However, the virus had not been confirmed in this area since 2001. The FAO announced the worldwide eradication of rinderpest in 2011, making it the first animal virus and, after smallpox virus, only the second virus to be eradicated.

Peste des petits ruminants

This condition, also referred to as goat plague, is an acute contagious disease of small ruminants, particularly goats. It is an

OIE-listed disease and occurs in sub-Saharan Africa north of the equator, the Middle East, India and Pakistan. Close contact is required for transmission of this labile virus which occurs through aerosols. The introduction of infection into a flock is invariably associated with movement of animals. Infection rates are similar in sheep and goats but the disease is generally more severe in goats. The disease is particularly severe in young animals with affected animals exhibiting fever, dry muzzle and a serous nasal discharge which becomes mucopurulent. Erosions in the buccal cavity are accompanied by marked salivation. Ulcers develop in the mucosae of the alimentary, respiratory and urinary tracts. Conjunctivitis with ocular discharge is a feature of the disease. A profuse diarrhoea, which results in dehydration, develops within days of infection. Signs of tracheitis and pneumonia are common. Pulmonary infections caused by *Pasteurella* species are common in the later stages of the disease. Pregnant animals may abort. Mortality rates in severe outbreaks often exceed 70%.

Laboratory confirmation is based primarily on RT-PCR. Antibodies can be detected by virus neutralization or by competitive ELISA. In regions where the disease is endemic, quarantine and vaccination are used for control.

Canine distemper

This highly contagious disease of dogs and other carnivores has a worldwide distribution. Outbreaks of disease have been documented in several wildlife species including lions. Canine distemper virus (CDV), a pantropic morbillivirus, produces a generalized infection involving many organ systems including the skin, respiratory, gastrointestinal, urinary and central nervous systems. The virus is relatively labile, requiring transmission by direct contact or by aerosols. Infection spreads rapidly among young dogs, usually between three and six months of age, when maternally derived immunity declines. The severity and duration of illness are variable and are influenced by the virulence of the infecting virus, the age and immune status of the infected animal and the rapidity of the immune response to infection. Acute disease, which may last for a few weeks, is followed either by recovery and lifelong immunity or by the development of neurological signs and, eventually, death. Modified live vaccines provide good protection when administered to pups after maternally derived antibody has declined to low levels, usually after 12 weeks of age. Clinical cases are comparatively rare in countries where vaccination is widely practised.

Old dog encephalitis, characterized by motor and behavioural deterioration many years after recovery from CDV infection, is invariably fatal. It is probably associated with non-cytolytic spread of virus from cell to cell, thereby evading immune detection.

Newcastle disease

Virulent strains of Newcastle disease virus (NDV), also known as avian paramyxovirus serotype 1 (APMV-1), cause disease in poultry worldwide. A wide range of avian species including chickens, turkeys, pigeons, pheasants, ducks and geese are susceptible. A reservoir of NDV exists in wild birds, especially pigeons and waterfowl.

Strains of NDV differ in their virulence and isolates are categorized into five pathotypes on the basis of virulence and tissue tropism in poultry:

- viscerotropic velogenic isolates causing severe fatal disease characterized by haemorrhagic intestinal lesions (Doyle's form);
- neurotropic velogenic isolates causing acute disease characterized by nervous and respiratory signs with high mortality (Beach's form);
- mesogenic isolates causing mild disease with mortality confined to young birds (Beaudette's form);
- lentogenic isolates causing mild or inapparent respiratory infection (Hitchner's form);
- asymptomatic enteric isolates associated with subclinical intestinal infection.

The extent of spread within the body relates to strain virulence which is determined by the amino acid sequence of the F glycoprotein. The fusion (F) glycoprotein of NDV is synthesized in an infected cell as a precursor molecule (F_0) which is cleaved by host cell proteases to F_1 and F_2 subunits. If cleavage fails to occur, non-infectious particles are produced. The F_0 molecules of virulent strains of NDV possess multiple basic amino acids at critical positions which facilitate intracellular cleavage by proteases such as furin, present in a wide range of host tissues. In contrast, the replication of lentogenic strains is confined to the respiratory and intestinal epithelia where suitable trypsin-like proteases are produced.

Virus is shed in all excretions and secretions. Transmission usually occurs by aerosols or by ingestion of contaminated feed or water. Respiratory, gastrointestinal and nervous signs occur in chickens. The mortality rate in fully susceptible flocks may be close to 100%. A presumptive clinical diagnosis may be made when the characteristic signs and lesions associated with virulent strains are present. Laboratory confirmation by isolation and identification of the virus is necessary. Molecular techniques are increasingly being used for the detection of NDV in clinical specimens. Primers are usually selected to cover the cleavage site of the F_0 protein gene, thus providing information on the virulence of the virus detected. The current OIE definition for reporting an outbreak of Newcastle disease is infection of birds by avian paramyxovirus serotype 1 with either an intracerebral pathogenicity index (ICPI) ≥ 0.7 in day-old chicks or with multiple (at least three) basic amino acids at the C-terminus of the F_2 protein and phenylalanine at residue 117 (N-terminus of the F_1 protein). A combination of vaccination and slaughter is frequently employed to control disease outbreaks. Vaccination is particularly important for birds in breeder flocks. Lentogenic or mesogenic strains of NDV propagated in eggs or tissue culture are used in live vaccines.

Pigeons are susceptible to all strains of NDV and may play a role in the transmission of Newcastle disease. Isolates from pigeons, often referred to as 'pigeon' paramyxovirus 1 (PPMV-1), are associated with clinical disease in racing pigeons resembling the neurotropic form of Newcastle disease. Many PPMV-1 viruses are also pathogenic for commercial poultry.

Bovine parainfluenza virus 3

Infection with bovine parainfluenza virus 3 (BPIV-3), which occurs worldwide, is often subclinical. Clinical disease is most common in calves with low levels of maternal antibodies. Transmission, which occurs by aerosols and direct contact, is facilitated by overcrowding in poorly ventilated conditions. Although uncomplicated infections are frequently subclinical, mild respiratory disease may be seen. The virus is commonly isolated from animals during outbreaks of serious respiratory disease such as enzootic calf pneumonia and shipping fever, conditions in which other respiratory viruses and bacteria are often involved. Various stress factors such as transportation or adverse environmental conditions may contribute to the severity of the disease.

Both inactivated and modified live BPIV-3 vaccines are available, often combined with other respiratory viruses. Modified live vaccines are designed either for intranasal administration or for intramuscular injection. Immunity tends to be short-lived and reinfection may occur after some months.

Bovine respiratory syncytial virus

Pulmonary disease, caused by bovine respiratory syncytial virus (BRSV), occurs in beef and dairy calves worldwide. The virus replicates mainly in ciliated epithelial cells of the upper respiratory tract. The virus derives its name from the characteristic syncytia which it induces in infected cells. Infection with BRSV stimulates production of proinflammatory cytokines and an excessive inflammatory reaction that results in respiratory disease. In adult animals, infection is usually mild or subclinical with persistent infection considered to be responsible for the maintenance of infection in herds. Moderate to severe respiratory signs typically develop in animals between three and nine months of age. Clinical signs, which range from mild to severe, include fever, nasal and lacrimal discharge, coughing and polypnoea. A biphasic pattern is commonly observed in outbreaks among beef calves. Mild respiratory disease is followed by apparent recovery and, within a few days, dyspnoea and pulmonary emphysema develop. Mortality in these outbreaks may reach 20%.

Clinical signs and pathological findings may permit a presumptive diagnosis. Laboratory confirmation by viral antigen detection, RT-PCR or serological testing is necessary for a definitive diagnosis. Suitable control measures include reducing stress factors, maintaining good hygiene in calf pens, rearing calves away from older age groups and implementing a closed herd policy. Modified live vaccines may be administered parenterally or intranasally. Although vaccination tends to reduce the likelihood of clinical disease in exposed animals, the duration of protection is short and frequent boosters may be required.

67 *Rhabdoviridae*

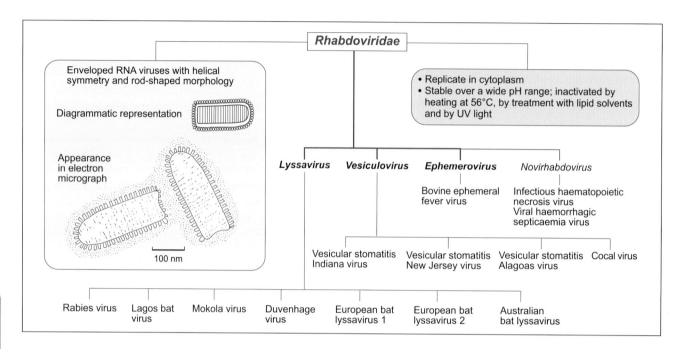

Rhabdoviridae

Enveloped RNA viruses with helical symmetry and rod-shaped morphology

Diagrammatic representation

Appearance in electron micrograph

100 nm

- Replicate in cytoplasm
- Stable over a wide pH range; inactivated by heating at 56°C, by treatment with lipid solvents and by UV light

Lyssavirus   *Vesiculovirus*   *Ephemerovirus*   *Novirhabdovirus*

Bovine ephemeral fever virus

Infectious haematopoietic necrosis virus
Viral haemorrhagic septicaemia virus

Vesicular stomatitis Indiana virus   Vesicular stomatitis New Jersey virus   Vesicular stomatitis Alagoas virus   Cocal virus

Rabies virus   Lagos bat virus   Mokola virus   Duvenhage virus   European bat lyssavirus 1   European bat lyssavirus 2   Australian bat lyssavirus

Members of the family *Rhabdoviridae* (Greek *rhabdos*, rod) have characteristic rod shapes. Rhabdoviruses possess a linear, non-segmented RNA genome of negative polarity encased in a ribonucleoprotein complex. This large family contains viruses of vertebrates, invertebrates and plants. Rhabdoviruses of vertebrates appear bullet- or cone-shaped. The family *Rhabdoviridae* comprises 11 genera. The genera *Vesiculovirus*, *Lyssavirus* and *Ephemerovirus* contain viruses of veterinary significance. Rhabdoviruses of importance in fish belong to the genera *Novirhabdovirus*, *Vesiculovirus* and *Perhabdovirus*. Replication occurs in the cytoplasm (with the exception of nucleorhabdoviruses of plants). Newly synthesized nucleocapsids acquire envelopes from the plasma membrane as virions bud from the cell. Virions (100 to 430 nm × 45 to 100 nm) are stable in the pH range 5 to 10. They are rapidly inactivated by heating at 56°C, by treatment with lipid solvents and by exposure to UV light.

Clinical infections

Rhabdoviruses of veterinary importance are presented in Tables 67.1 and 67.2. They can be transmitted by bites of mammals, arthropod vectors or direct contact. Infection may also be acquired through environmental contamination. The best-known and most important member of the *Rhabdoviridae* is rabies virus, a *Lyssavirus* (Greek *lyssa*, rage or fury). A number of distinct lyssaviruses, many isolated from bats, produce clinical signs indistinguishable from rabies. Novel lyssaviruses continue to be isolated from wildlife sources. The most important vesiculoviruses which infect domestic animals are the vesicular stomatitis Indiana virus and the vesicular stomatitis New Jersey virus. Bovine ephemeral fever virus, of significance in the tropics and subtropics of Africa, Asia and Australia, is the type species of the genus *Ephemerovirus*.

Rabies

This viral infection, which affects the central nervous system of most mammals including humans, is invariably fatal. However, mammalian species vary widely in their susceptibility. Most clinical cases are due to infection with rabies virus (genotype 1). A number of other neurotropic lyssaviruses, closely related to the rabies virus, produce clinical signs indistinguishable from rabies. Classical rabies caused by rabies virus is endemic on continental land masses, with the exception of Australia and Antarctica. Many island countries are also free of the disease.

Several species-adapted genotypes or strains of rabies virus have been described. Strains affecting a particular species are transmitted more readily to members of that species than to other animal species. In a given geographical region, rabies is usually maintained and transmitted by particular mammalian reservoir hosts. Two epidemiologically important infectious cycles are recognized, urban rabies in dogs and sylvatic rabies in wildlife. More than 95% of human cases in developing countries are as a result of bites from rabid dogs. Racoons, skunks, foxes and bats are important reservoirs of rabies virus in North America. In continental Europe, the principal reservoir is the red fox. The vampire bat is an important reservoir of the virus in Central and South America and in the Caribbean islands. Although virus may be transmitted through scratching and licking, transmission

Concise Review of Veterinary Microbiology, Second Edition. P.J. Quinn, B.K. Markey, F.C. Leonard, E.S. FitzPatrick and S. Fanning.
© 2016 John Wiley & Sons, Ltd. Published 2016 by John Wiley & Sons, Ltd.
Companion website: www.wiley.com/go/quinn/concise-veterinary-microbiology

SECTION IV

Table 67.1 Lyssaviruses which cause rabies and rabies-like diseases.

Virus	Phylogroup	Genotype	Serotype	Geographical distribution	Comments
Rabies virus	1	1	1	Apart from Australia and Antarctica, rabies virus (genotype 1) occurs on all continents. Many island countries are free of the disease	Causes fatal encephalitis in many mammalian species. Transmitted by wildlife species, including foxes, racoons and bats; domestic carnivores also involved in transmission. Rabies is a major zoonotic disease with more than 50,000 human fatalities worldwide each year
Lagos bat virus	2	2	2	Africa	Isolated initially from fruit bats; also isolated from domestic animals with encephalitis
Mokola virus	2	3	3	Africa	Isolated initially from shrews; also isolated from domestic animals. Human infection reported
Duvenhage virus	1	4	4	Africa	Originally isolated from a human bitten by an insectivorous bat; additional cases reported in humans. Not reported in domestic animals
European bat lyssavirus 1	1	5	—	Europe	Identified with increasing frequency in insectivorous bats. Human infection reported
European bat lyssavirus 2	1	6	—	Europe	Present in insectivorous bats. Initially isolated from a human with symptoms of rabies and subsequently from other human cases; not reported in domestic animals
Australian bat lyssavirus	1	7	—	Australia	Identified in fruit bats and in insectivorous bats; human infection reported

usually occurs through bites. The saliva of infected animals may contain rabies virus for some time before the onset of clinical signs.

The incubation period, which is highly variable and can be as long as six months or more, is influenced by various factors including host species, virus strain, the amount of inoculum and the site of introduction of the virus. The clinical course in domestic carnivores, which usually lasts for days or for a few weeks, may encompass prodromal, furious (excitative) and dumb (paralytic) phases. Antemortem diagnostic tests for rabies are not generally used. The brains of animals which develop clinical signs should be examined for the presence of virus using the direct fluorescent antibody test. Other methods include demonstration of intracytoplasmic inclusions (Negri bodies) histologically, virus isolation or RT-PCR. Rapid laboratory confirmation

is essential for the implementation of appropriate treatment of human patients.

Most countries which are free of rabies rely on rigorous quarantine measures to prevent the introduction of disease. In countries where rabies is endemic, control methods are aimed mainly at reservoir species. Urban rabies can be effectively controlled by vaccination and restriction of movement of dogs and cats and by the elimination of stray animals. Control of sylvatic rabies requires special measures. Vaccination of red foxes with live oral vaccines delivered in baits has eliminated sylvatic rabies from several regions of western Europe. Although attenuated virus vaccines were used initially, there was uncertainty about their ultimate safety. A vaccinia–rabies virus glycoprotein (VRG) vaccine was developed and has proved effective for vaccinating foxes, coyotes and racoons.

Table 67.2 Viruses of veterinary significance in the genera *Vesiculovirus* and *Ephemerovirus*.

Genus/Virus	Hosts	Comments
Vesiculovirus		
Vesicular stomatitis Indiana virus	Cattle, horses, pigs, humans	Causes febrile disease with vesicular lesions; resembles foot-and-mouth disease clinically. Occurs in North and South America
Vesicular stomatitis New Jersey virus	Cattle, horses, pigs, humans	Causes febrile disease with vesicular lesions; infection more severe than that caused by the Indiana virus. Occurs in North and South America
Vesicular stomatitis Alagoas virus (Brazil virus)	Horses, mules, cattle, humans	Originally isolated from mules in Brazil
Cocal virus (Argentina virus)	Horses	Isolated initially from mites in Trinidad; occurs in South America
Ephemerovirus		
Bovine ephemeral fever virus	Cattle	Arbovirus that causes febrile illness of short duration; occurs in Africa, Asia and Australia

68 *Bunyaviridae*

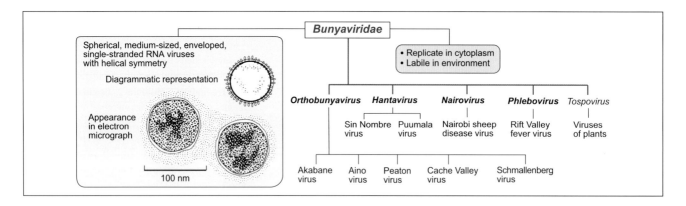

The family *Bunyaviridae* contains more than 300 viruses. The name of this family is derived from Bunyamwera, the place in Uganda where the type species Bunyamwera virus was first isolated. Virions (80 to 120 nm in diameter) are spherical and enveloped. Glycoprotein peplomers project from the surface of the envelope which encloses three circular, helical nucleocapsid segments. The genome consists of three single-stranded RNA segments designated small, medium and large. Genetic reassortment occurs between closely related viruses. Based on antigenic relatedness, viruses within each genus are placed in serogroups. Viruses in the genera *Orthobunyavirus*, *Phlebovirus*, *Nairovirus* and *Hantavirus* infect vertebrates; those in the genus *Tospovirus* infect plants. Replication takes place in the cytoplasm of host cells. In the final stages of assembly, virions acquire envelopes by budding into the Golgi network. They are then transported through the cytoplasm in secretory vesicles and released by exocytosis at the cell surface. The viruses are sensitive to heat, acid pH levels, lipid solvents, detergents and disinfectants.

Clinical infections

With the exception of viruses in the genus *Hantavirus*, bunyaviruses are arthropod-borne. These arboviruses are main-tained in nature in complex life cycles involving replication in both arthropod vectors and vertebrate hosts. Infection of mammalian cells often results in cytolysis, while infection of invertebrate cells is non-cytolytic and persistent. Mosquitoes are the most important vectors. Ticks, sandflies and midges may act as vectors for some bunyaviruses. Arthropod vectors acquire virus from vertebrate hosts during viraemic stages of the disease. Each bunyavirus species replicates in a limited number of vertebrate and invertebrate hosts. In contrast, hantaviruses are maintained in nature by persistent infections in rodents which shed virus in urine, faeces and saliva. Transmission between rodent hosts can occur by aerosols and biting. Individual hantaviruses are associated with particular rodent species.

A number of important ruminant diseases are caused by orthobunyaviruses (Table 68.1). Many bunyaviruses infect humans and frequently cause serious zoonotic diseases including California encephalitis, haemorrhagic fever with renal syndrome, hantavirus pulmonary syndrome and Crimean–Congo haemorrhagic fever. Such human infections are generally considered to be incidental and do not usually result in disease transmission.

Table 68.1 Bunyaviruses of veterinary importance.

Genus	Virus	Hosts	Comments
Phlebovirus	Rift Valley fever virus	Sheep, cattle, goats	Causes high mortality in neonatal animals and abortion in pregnant animals. Endemic in southern and eastern Africa. Transmitted by mosquitoes. Important zoonotic disease
Nairovirus	Nairobi sheep disease virus	Sheep, goats	Causes severe, often fatal disease in susceptible animals. Present in central and eastern Africa. Transmitted by ticks
Orthobunyavirus	Akabane virus, Aino virus, Tinaroo virus, Peaton virus, Schmallenberg virus	Cattle, sheep	Viruses belonging to Simbu serogroup, transmitted by mosquitoes and midges. Associated with congenital defects (arthrogryposis, hydranencephaly) and abortion. Schmallenberg virus first recorded in Europe in 2011
	Cache Valley virus	Sheep	Belongs to the Bunyamwera serogroup; transmitted by mosquitoes. Associated with congenital defects in sheep flocks in North America

Concise Review of Veterinary Microbiology, Second Edition. P.J. Quinn, B.K. Markey, F.C. Leonard, E.S. FitzPatrick and S. Fanning.
© 2016 John Wiley & Sons, Ltd. Published 2016 by John Wiley & Sons, Ltd.
Companion website: www.wiley.com/go/quinn/concise-veterinary-microbiology

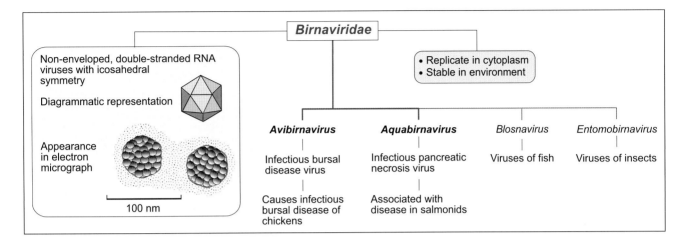

Birnaviruses are so named because their genomes contain two segments of linear, double-stranded RNA. The non-enveloped, icosahedral virions are about 60 nm in diameter. Replication occurs in the cytoplasm of host cells and involves a virion-associated RNA-dependent RNA polymerase. The family *Birnaviridae* contains four genera which infect chickens, fish and insects. Virions are stable over a wide pH range and at a temperature of 60°C for one hour.

Clinical infections

Two economically important diseases associated with birnaviruses are infectious bursal disease of chickens and infectious pancreatic necrosis of salmonids. These diseases occur worldwide and cause considerable losses in poultry units and in farmed salmon.

Infectious bursal disease

This condition is a highly contagious disease of young chickens which is caused by infectious bursal disease virus. The causal agent was first isolated in Gumboro, Delaware and the disease was originally known as Gumboro disease. Two serotypes of the virus are described but only serotype 1 isolates are pathogenic. Isolates of the virus vary in both virulence and antigenicity. Infection, which is usually acquired by the oral route, occurs when maternally-derived antibody levels are waning at two to three weeks of age. Virus is shed in the faeces for up to two weeks after infection and can remain infectious in the environment of a poultry house for several months.

The main target cells of virulent viruses are precursors of B lymphocytes in the cloacal bursa and B lymphocytes. The severity of clinical signs is influenced by the virulence of the virus, the age of chicks at the time of infection, the breed of the chicks and the level of maternally-derived antibody. Chicks develop an acute form of the disease between three and six weeks of age following a short incubation period. Affected birds are depressed and inappetent and show evidence of diarrhoea and vent pecking. Morbidity ranges from 10 to 100% with a mortality rate up to 20% or, occasionally, higher. Many outbreaks are mild, detectable only by impaired weight gains. Although infections before three weeks of age are usually subclinical, severe depression of the humoral antibody response may result. Suboptimal growth, predisposition to secondary infections and poor response to vaccination against other avian pathogens may be encountered.

Viral antigen can be detected in the bursa using immunofluorescence, ELISA or gel diffusion tests. Depopulation, thorough cleaning and effective disinfection programmes are required following an outbreak of disease in a unit. Most commercial units rely on vaccination for control. Because of the emergence of new viral variants, vaccines should contain antigenic material representative of recent outbreaks of disease.

Concise Review of Veterinary Microbiology, Second Edition. P.J. Quinn, B.K. Markey, F.C. Leonard, E.S. FitzPatrick and S. Fanning.
© 2016 John Wiley & Sons, Ltd. Published 2016 by John Wiley & Sons, Ltd.
Companion website: www.wiley.com/go/quinn/concise-veterinary-microbiology

SECTION IV

70 *Picornaviridae*

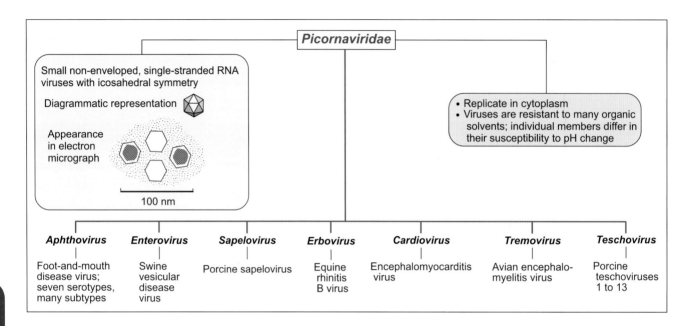

Picornaviridae

Small non-enveloped, single-stranded RNA viruses with icosahedral symmetry

Diagrammatic representation

Appearance in electron micrograph

100 nm

- Replicate in cytoplasm
- Viruses are resistant to many organic solvents; individual members differ in their susceptibility to pH change

Aphthovirus
Foot-and-mouth disease virus; seven serotypes, many subtypes

Enterovirus
Swine vesicular disease virus

Sapelovirus
Porcine sapelovirus

Erbovirus
Equine rhinitis B virus

Cardiovirus
Encephalomyocarditis virus

Tremovirus
Avian encephalo-myelitis virus

Teschovirus
Porcine teschoviruses 1 to 13

Picornaviruses (Spanish *pico*, very small), which are icosahedral and non-enveloped, contain a molecule of single-stranded RNA. Virions are 30 nm in diameter. The capsid is composed of 60 identical subunits, each containing four major proteins, VP1, VP2, VP3 and VP4. The VP4 protein is located on the inner surface of the capsid. Viral replication occurs in the cytoplasm in membrane-associated complexes and infection is usually cytolytic. The family has expanded greatly in recent years and now comprises 29 genera. Viruses of veterinary importance are contained in the genera *Enterovirus*, *Cardiovirus*, *Aphthovirus*, *Avihepatovirus, Erbovirus, Sapelovirus, Tremovirus* and *Teschovirus*. Several enteroviruses of pigs and poultry have been reassigned: porcine enteroviruses 1 to 7 and 11 to 13, which are associated with nervous disease and reproductive problems in pigs, have been reassigned to the genus *Teschovirus* while avian encephalomyelitis virus has been placed in the newly created genus *Tremovirus*. The genus *Rhinovirus* has been removed and human rhinoviruses have been placed in the genus *Enterovirus*.

Viruses of veterinary importance in the family *Picornaviridae* are presented in Table 70.1. Important human pathogens in the family include hepatitis A virus (genus *Hepatovirus*) and enterovirus C (genus *Enterovirus*) the cause of poliomyelitis, a serious neurological disease in humans. Picornaviruses are resistant to ether, chloroform and non-ionic detergents. Individual genera differ in their thermal lability and pH stability. Aphthoviruses are unstable at pH values below 6.5. Viruses in the other genera are stable at acid pH values.

Clinical infections

With the exception of foot-and-mouth disease virus and encephalomyocarditis virus, picornaviruses typically infect a single, or a limited number of, host species. Transmission usually occurs by the faecal–oral route but may also occur by fomites or by aerosols. Some picornaviruses, notably foot-and-mouth disease virus and swine vesicular disease virus, can produce persistent infections. Antigenic variation, which may contribute to the development of persistent infection, has been attributed to a number of molecular mechanisms including genetic recombination. Mixed infections with different serotypes of foot-and-mouth disease virus are known to occur in individual animals, particularly in African Cape buffaloes. Porcine teschovirus infections are widespread in pig populations and frequently subclinical in nature but may result in encephalomyelitis, diarrhoea, pneumonia, pericarditis/myocarditis and reproductive disorders.

Foot-and-mouth disease

This highly contagious disease of even-toed ungulates is characterized by fever and the formation of vesicles on epithelial surfaces. Foot-and-mouth disease (FMD) is a listed disease of the OIE. It is of major importance internationally on account of its rapid spread and the dramatic economic losses which it causes in susceptible animals. Isolates of foot-and-mouth disease virus (FMDV) are grouped in seven serotypes with differing geographical distributions. Infection with one serotype does not

Concise Review of Veterinary Microbiology, Second Edition. P.J. Quinn, B.K. Markey, F.C. Leonard, E.S. FitzPatrick and S. Fanning.

© 2016 John Wiley & Sons, Ltd. Published 2016 by John Wiley & Sons, Ltd.

Companion website: www.wiley.com/go/quinn/concise-veterinary-microbiology

SECTION IV

Table 70.1 Picornaviruses of veterinary importance.

Genus	Virus	Comments
Enterovirus	Swine vesicular disease virus (porcine variant of enterovirus B)	Produces mild vesicular disease in pigs, clinically indistinguishable from foot-and-mouth disease
	Enterovirus E, F (bovine enteroviruses group A, group B)	Isolated from both normal cattle and animals with enteric, respiratory and reproductive disease
Teschovirus	Porcine teschovirus	Thirteen serotypes. Virulent strains of PTV-1 which occur in eastern Europe and Madagascar cause severe encephalomyelitis (Teschen disease); mild strains of PTV-1 are more widely distributed and cause endemic posterior paresis (Talfan disease). Infections with other serotypes of PTV are often asymptomatic but may be associated with encephalomyelitis, SMEDI, pneumonia and diarrhoea
Sapelovirus	Porcine sapelovirus (porcine enterovirus A, porcine enterovirus 8)	Usually an asymptomatic infection but may be associated with SMEDI
Tremovirus	Avian encephalomyelitis virus	Avian encephalomyelitis is of considerable economic importance in chickens. Horizontal and vertical transmission occurs. Nervous signs seen in birds at 1 to 2 weeks of age. Control is achieved by vaccination of breeding flocks
Aphthovirus	Foot-and-mouth-disease virus	Seven serotypes are recognized: A, O, C, Asia 1, SAT 1, SAT 2, SAT 3. Economically important, highly contagious vesicular disease of even-toed ungulates
	Equine rhinitis A virus	Systemic infection, often subclinical but may be associated with respiratory signs
	Bovine rhinitis B virus	Widely distributed. Capable of causing mild respiratory disease
Cardiovirus	Encephalomyocarditis virus	Wide host range; rodents are considered to be the natural hosts. Infection in pigs is often subclinical but sporadic deaths and minor outbreaks may occur
Erbovirus	Equine rhinitis B virus	Considered a minor respiratory pathogen of horses
Avihepatovirus	Duck hepatitis A virus	Severe, fatal disease of young ducklings

confer immunity against the other serotypes. A large number of subtypes is recognized within each serotype.

Cattle, sheep, goats, pigs and domesticated buffaloes are susceptible to FMD. Several wildlife species including African buffaloes, elephants, hedgehogs, deer and antelopes are also susceptible. Large numbers of virus particles are shed in the secretions and excretions of infected animals. Transmission can occur by direct contact, by aerosols, by mechanical carriage by humans or vehicles, on fomites and through animal products. Infected groups of animals, particularly pigs, shed large quantities of virus in aerosols. Under favourable conditions of low temperature, high humidity and moderate winds, virus in aerosols may spread up to 10 km over land. Turbulence is generally less marked over water than over land. In 1981, virus was carried a distance of more than 200 km from France to the south coast of England. Foot-and-mouth virus can persist in the pharyngeal region of carrier animals which have recovered from FMD.

The incubation period ranges from 2 to 14 days, but is generally shorter than a week. Infected cattle develop fever, inappetence and a drop in milk production. Profuse salivation, with characteristic drooling and smacking of lips, accompanies the formation of oral vesicles which rupture, leaving raw, painful ulcers. Ruptured vesicles in the interdigital cleft and on the coronary band lead to lameness. Vesicles may also appear on the skin of the teats and udders of lactating cows. Although the ulcers tend to heal rapidly, there may be secondary bacterial infection which exacerbates and prolongs the inflammatory process. Infected animals lose condition. Mature animals seldom die. Young animals, especially calves and lambs, may die from acute myocarditis. In pigs, foot lesions are severe and the hooves may slough. Marked lameness is the most prominent sign in this species. The disease in sheep, goats and wild ruminants is generally mild, presenting as fever accompanied by lameness which spreads rapidly through groups of animals.

Foot-and-mouth disease clinically resembles other vesicular diseases of domestic animals, including vesicular stomatitis in cattle and pigs, swine vesicular disease and vesicular exanthema in pigs. Consequently, FMD requires laboratory confirmation. Diagnosis is based on the demonstration of FMDV antigen in samples of tissue or in vesicular fluid by ELISA, CFT, RT-PCR or virus isolation. Demonstration of specific antibody by virus neutralization or ELISA can be used to confirm a diagnosis in unvaccinated animals. In endemic areas, interpretation of antibody titres may prove difficult.

In countries which are free from FMD, it is a notifiable disease and affected and in-contact animals are usually slaughtered. Following an outbreak, movement restrictions are applied and infected premises must be thoroughly cleaned and disinfected. Mild acids, such as citric acid and acetic acid, and alkalis such as sodium carbonate are effective disinfectants. Reserves of inactivated virus are maintained in several countries to provide an adequate supply of vaccine at short notice in the event of a major outbreak of the disease. Although ring vaccination around an affected premises may help to limit the spread of the disease, it may also allow the development of the carrier state in animals subsequently exposed to the virus. In countries where FMD is endemic, efforts are generally directed at protecting high-yielding dairy cattle by a combination of vaccination and control of animal movement. Vaccines for FMD, incorporating adjuvant, are derived from tissue culture-propagated virus which has been chemically inactivated. They are usually multivalent, containing three or more virus strains. Protection against antigenically similar strains of virus is satisfactory and lasts for up to six months.

71 Caliciviridae

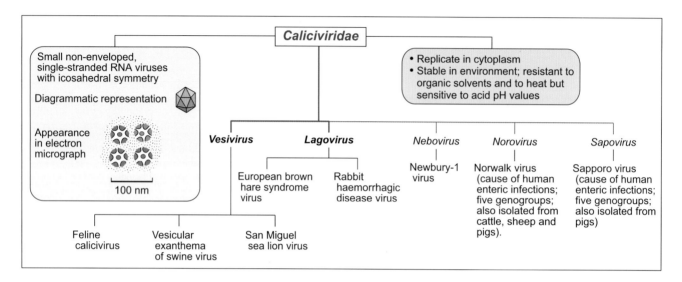

Caliciviruses (Latin *calix*, cup) have cup-shaped depressions on the surface of virions, demonstrable by electron microscopy. The virions, 27 to 40 nm in diameter, are icosahedral and non-enveloped. The genome consists of a single molecule of linear, positive-sense, single-stranded RNA. Replication takes place in the cytoplasm of infected cells and virions are released by cell lysis. Many caliciviruses have not yet been cultured. The virions are resistant to ether, chloroform and mild detergents. They are relatively resistant to heat but are sensitive to acid pH values.

The family *Caliciviridae* is divided into five genera: *Vesivirus, Lagovirus, Nebovirus, Sapovirus* and *Norovirus*. Caliciviruses belonging to the *Norovirus* and *Sapovirus* genera include viruses which cause acute gastroenteritis in humans.

Clinical infections

Caliciviruses have been recovered from many species including humans, cats, pigs, marine mammals, fish, rabbits, hares, cattle, dogs, reptiles, amphibians, shellfish and insects. They are associated with a wide range of conditions including respiratory disease, vesicular lesions, necrotizing hepatitis and gastroenteritis (Table 71.1). Infections with caliciviruses, which are frequently persistent, may be inapparent, mild or acute. Transmission occurs directly or indirectly without vector involvement. However, mechanical transmission of rabbit haemorrhagic disease virus by mosquitoes and fleas has been described.

Feline calicivirus infection

Infections caused by feline calicivirus (FCV) account for about 40% of upper respiratory tract inflammatory disease in cats worldwide. All species of *Felidae* are considered to be susceptible but natural disease tends to be confined to domestic cats and to cheetahs in captivity. There is a high degree of antigenic heterogeneity among FCV isolates. Sequence analysis studies have shown that individual isolates of FCV exist as quasispecies which evolve and exhibit antigenic drift. Significant alterations in the antigenic profiles of sequential virus isolates from carrier cats are thought to be influenced by immune selection and this may play an important part in viral persistence.

Virus replication occurs primarily in the oropharynx with rapid spread throughout the upper respiratory tract and to the conjunctivae. A transient viraemia occurs. Infections range from subclinical to severe, reflecting differences in strain virulence and host immunity. Virulent strains of FCV can cause interstitial pneumonia in young kittens. The virus has been recovered from the joints of lame cats. Highly virulent strains of the virus associated with virulent systemic disease (VSD) have been reported periodically.

The incubation period is up to five days. Clinical signs, which are usually confined to the upper respiratory tract and the conjunctivae, are often less severe than those caused by feline herpesvirus 1 infection. Fever, oculonasal discharge and conjunctivitis are accompanied by the development of characteristic vesicles on the tongue and oral mucosa. These vesicles rupture leaving shallow ulcers. Morbidity may be high but mortality is usually low. Stiffness and shifting lameness, which usually resolve within a few days, are sometimes seen during the acute phase of FCV infection or following inoculation with FCV vaccine. The VSD form of FCV infection is characterized by severe upper respiratory tract disease, facial oedema, ulceration of the skin, vasculitis, multi-organ involvement and high mortality.

Although cats of all ages are susceptible to infection with FCV, acute disease occurs most commonly in kittens as maternally derived antibody wanes between two and three months

Concise Review of Veterinary Microbiology, Second Edition. P.J. Quinn, B.K. Markey, F.C. Leonard, E.S. FitzPatrick and S. Fanning.
© 2016 John Wiley & Sons, Ltd. Published 2016 by John Wiley & Sons, Ltd.
Companion website: www.wiley.com/go/quinn/concise-veterinary-microbiology

SECTION IV

Table 71.1 Caliciviruses of veterinary importance.

Virus	Hosts	Comments
Vesicular exanthema of swine virus	Pigs	Acute, contagious vesicular disease, clinically similar to foot-and-mouth disease. Occurred in the USA before 1956. May have arisen from feeding sea lion and seal meat contaminated with San Miguel sea lion virus
San Miguel sea lion virus	Marine mammals, opal eye fish	Associated with cutaneous vesicles and premature parturition in pinnipeds; when inoculated into pigs, causes vesicular exanthema
Feline calicivirus	Domestic and wild cats	Important cause of upper respiratory tract infection in cats worldwide. Virulent systemic disease described in some outbreaks
Rabbit haemorrhagic disease virus	European rabbits	Acute fatal disease in European rabbits over 2 months of age
European brown hare syndrome virus	European brown hares	Related to rabbit haemorrhagic disease virus. Causes hepatic necrosis and widespread haemorrhages with high mortality
Canine calicivirus	Dogs	Occasionally associated with diarrhoea
Newbury-1 virus	Cattle	Has been linked to diarrhoea in calves

of age. Infected cats excrete large amounts of virus in oronasal secretions. Many cats continue to shed virus continuously from the oropharynx for weeks after recovery from acute infection or following subclinical infection while protected by maternally derived antibody or by response to vaccination. A minority of cats shed virus for months and, occasionally, for years. Infection is maintained in the cat population by these asymptomatic FCV carriers. The highest prevalence of infection is seen in large groups of cats living in colonies or shelters.

Due to the similarity of clinical signs caused by infection with feline herpesvirus 1 and FCV, laboratory tests are required to differentiate these two diseases. Feline calicivirus can be isolated in feline cell lines from oropharyngeal swabs or from lung tissue. Viral RNA can be detected in clinical specimens using RT-PCR. However, detection of FCV may not be aetiologically significant in every instance because of the presence of carrier animals in cat populations. Demonstration of a rising antibody titre in paired serum samples is required for laboratory confirmation.

Vaccination and management practices aimed at reducing exposure to the virus are the main methods of control. Inactivated vaccines for parenteral administration and modified live vaccines for either parenteral or intranasal administration are available. Although vaccination protects effectively against clinical disease in most instances, it does not prevent subclinical infection or the development of a carrier state. Vaccines are based on a limited number of FCV isolates which cross-react with a broad spectrum of field isolates. Live vaccines, for administration by injection, may cause clinical signs of disease if given by other routes.

Rabbit haemorrhagic disease

This is a highly contagious, acute and often fatal disease of European rabbits (*Oryctolagus cuniculus*). Rabbit haemorrhagic disease (RHD) was first reported in China in 1984 and has since been encountered in many parts of the world. This virus is considered to be a mutant form of a non-pathogenic virus, termed rabbit calicivirus, which has been endemic in commercial and wild rabbits in Europe for many years. Rabbit haemorrhagic disease virus (RHDV) has been used for biological control of rabbits in Australia and New Zealand.

Virus is shed in all excretions and secretions. Among rabbits in close contact, transmission is mainly by the faecal–oral route. Infection may also occur by inhalation or through the conjunctiva. Mechanical transmission by a variety of insects, including mosquitoes and fleas, has been demonstrated. The virus survives in the environment and indirect transmission through contaminated foodstuffs or fomites may occur.

Cells of the mononuclear phagocyte lineage are considered to be the major targets of the virus. Rabbits under two months of age do not develop clinical signs. The reason for this resistance is unclear, but it may have a physiological basis. Severe hepatic necrosis is the most obvious lesion in affected rabbits. In addition, there may be evidence of disseminated intravascular coagulation.

The incubation period is up to three days. The disease is characterized by high morbidity and high mortality. The course is short, with death occurring within 36 hours of the onset of clinical signs. Rabbits may be found dead or die in convulsions. A few rabbits may present with milder, subacute signs during the later stages of a major outbreak.

High mortality in rabbits along with characteristic gross lesions including necrotic hepatitis and congestion of spleen and lungs are suggestive of RHD. Culture of RHDV has been unsuccessful. High concentrations of virus are present in affected livers. Confirmation is based on detection of virus by electron microscopy or of viral antigen by ELISA, immunofluorescence or haemagglutination using human erythrocytes. Reverse transcriptase PCR has been developed for the detection of RHDV nucleic acid. Suitable serological tests for the detection of specific antibodies to the virus include haemagglutination-inhibition and ELISA.

In countries where RHD is endemic, control is achieved by vaccination. Inactivated and adjuvanted vaccines are available. A live myxoma virus expressing the capsid protein gene of RHDV is available for the vaccination and protection of rabbits against both viruses.

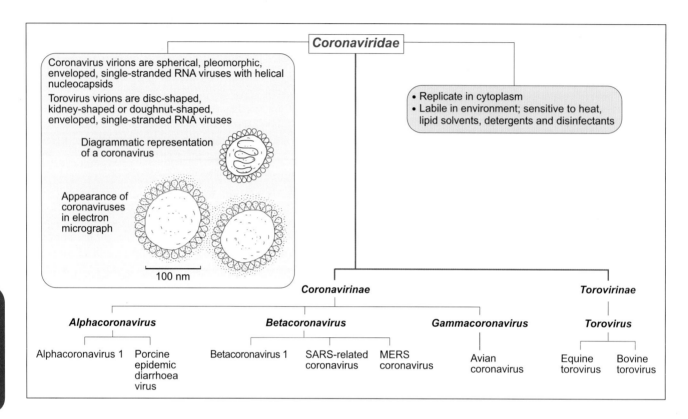

Coronaviridae

Coronavirus virions are spherical, pleomorphic, enveloped, single-stranded RNA viruses with helical nucleocapsids

Torovirus virions are disc-shaped, kidney-shaped or doughnut-shaped, enveloped, single-stranded RNA viruses

Diagrammatic representation of a coronavirus

Appearance of coronaviruses in electron micrograph

100 nm

• Replicate in cytoplasm
• Labile in environment; sensitive to heat, lipid solvents, detergents and disinfectants

Coronavirinae

Torovirinae

Alphacoronavirus

Betacoronavirus

Gammacoronavirus

Torovirus

Alphacoronavirus 1 | Porcine epidemic diarrhoea virus

Betacoronavirus 1 | SARS-related coronavirus | MERS coronavirus

Avian coronavirus

Equine torovirus | Bovine torovirus

Members of the family *Coronaviridae* (Latin *corona*, crown) are large, pleomorphic, enveloped viruses. They contain a single molecule of linear, positive-sense, single-stranded RNA. Club-shaped glycoprotein peplomers projecting from the envelope impart a crown-like appearance to the virus. Each peplomer is composed of a large viral glycoprotein (spike or S protein) which is responsible for attachment to cells. The S protein is the main antigenic component which induces the production of neutralizing antibodies during natural infection. Hypervariable domains in the S protein facilitate the production of virus escape mutants, capable of evading the host immune response. There are two subfamilies in the family, *Coronavirinae* and *Torovirinae*. Coronaviruses, which are almost spherical with a diameter of 120 to 160 nm, have helical nucleocapsids. Toroviruses, which have a tubular nucleocapsid, may be disc-shaped, kidney-shaped or rod-shaped and are 120 to 140 nm in length. The *Coronavirinae* subfamily comprises four genera: *Alphacoronavirus*, *Betacoronavirus*, *Deltacoronavirus* and *Gammacoronavirus*. A number of closely related virus species, which were formerly listed separately, have been grouped together and renamed as follows: alphacoronavirus 1 (comprising feline coronavirus, canine coronavirus and transmissible gastroenteritis virus); betacoronavirus 1 (comprising human coronavirus OC43, bovine coronavirus, porcine haemag-

glutinating encephalomyelitis virus, equine coronavirus and canine respiratory coronavirus); and avian coronavirus (comprising infectious bronchitis virus, turkey coronavirus, pheasant coronavirus, duck coronavirus, goose coronavirus and pigeon coronavirus). The subfamily *Torovirinae* comprises two genera, *Torovirus* and the newly created *Bafinivirus*, which contains a virus of fish.

Coronaviruses replicate in the cytoplasm of cells. Genetic recombination can occur at high frequency between related coronaviruses. The virions are sensitive to heat, lipid solvents, formaldehyde, oxidizing agents and non-ionic detergents. The stability of coronaviruses at low pH values is variable.

Clinical infections

Coronaviruses infect a number of mammalian and avian species and many display tropisms for respiratory and intestinal epithelium. The coronaviruses of veterinary importance and the clinical consequences of infection are indicated in Table 72.1. Coronaviral infections are usually mild or inapparent in mature animals but may be severe in young animals. Coronaviruses are aetiologically important in humans as a cause of the common cold and as a cause of emerging viral diseases including severe acute respiratory syndrome (SARS) and Middle Eastern respiratory syndrome (MERS).

Concise Review of Veterinary Microbiology, Second Edition. P.J. Quinn, B.K. Markey, F.C. Leonard, E.S. FitzPatrick and S. Fanning.
© 2016 John Wiley & Sons, Ltd. Published 2016 by John Wiley & Sons, Ltd.
Companion website: www.wiley.com/go/quinn/concise-veterinary-microbiology

SECTION IV

Table 72.1 Coronaviruses of veterinary significance.

Virus species	Strain	Consequences of infection
Alphacoronavirus 1	Feline coronavirus (FCoV)	Replicates in enterocytes; subclinical infection common. May produce mild gastroenteritis in young kittens; also referred to as feline enteric coronavirus (FECV). Feline infectious peritonitis virus (FIPV) arises through mutation and selection from strains of FCoV which initially replicated in enterocytes and subsequently developed a tropism for macrophages; causes sporadic fatal disease of young cats, often presenting clinically as an effusive peritonitis
	Transmissible gastroenteritis virus (TGEV)	Highly contagious infection with vomiting and diarrhoea in piglets; high mortality in newborn piglets. A deletion mutant of TGEV, porcine respiratory coronavirus, is widely distributed and induces partial immunity to TGEV
	Canine coronavirus	Asymptomatic infection or diarrhoea in dogs characterized by high morbidity and low mortality
Porcine epidemic diarrhoea virus (PEDV)		Causes enteric infection similar to that caused by TGEV but with lower neonatal mortality. Present for many years in Europe and Asia with spread to North America in 2013. Both PEDV and porcine delta coronavirus, referred to as swine enteric coronavirus diseases (SECD), can cause significant morbidity and mortality in piglets
Betacoronavirus 1	Porcine haemagglutinating encephalomyelitis virus	Nervous disease or vomiting and emaciation (vomiting and wasting disease) in young pigs. Infection is widespread but clinical disease is uncommon
	Equine coronavirus	Enteric infection reported in both foals and adult horses
	Bovine coronavirus	Diarrhoea in calves; associated with winter dysentery in adult cattle
	Canine respiratory coronavirus	Associated with respiratory disease in kennelled dogs
Avian coronavirus	Infectious bronchitis virus	Acute, highly contagious respiratory infection in young birds; causes a drop in egg production in layers. Spread of infection occurs rapidly among susceptible birds and mortality may reach 100%
	Turkey coronavirus	Infectious enteritis (bluecomb disease)

Although evidence of torovirus infection has been found in pigs, sheep, goats and cats, the clinical significance of these infections has not been determined. Two toroviruses have been implicated in enteric diseases of domestic animals, equine torovirus (Berne virus) and bovine torovirus (Breda virus).

Feline infectious peritonitis

A sporadic disease of domestic cats and other *Felidae*, feline infectious peritonitis (FIP), which is caused by certain strains of feline coronavirus, occurs worldwide and is invariably fatal. Strains of feline coronavirus vary in pathogenicity. The term 'feline enteric coronavirus' (FECV) has been used to describe strains that cause mild or inapparent enteritis, while the term 'feline infectious peritonitis virus' (FIPV) is applied to those strains aetiologically implicated in FIP. It is believed that FIPV occurs as a mutant of the widely distributed FECV, resulting in an alteration in tropism from exclusively enteric epithelial cells to myeloid cells, particularly macrophages. The term 'feline coronavirus' (FCoV), as currently used, includes strains of varying virulence which can be grouped into two biotypes, enteric and FIP-associated.

Feline infectious peritonitis occurs sporadically in catteries or multi-cat households. The incidence is reported to be higher in pedigree cats. Although cats of any age may be affected, those less than one year of age appear to be most susceptible. Infected cats shed FECV in faeces and oronasal secretions. Transmission is mainly by ingestion or inhalation. Infection is acquired by young kittens from their mothers or from other adult cats. Persistently infected FECV carrier cats occur and play a key role in the epidemiology.

Infection with FIPV does not always result in clinical disease. Factors which may influence the development of the disease include the age, immune status and genetic characteristics of the host and the emergence of virulent virus strains. In most infected kittens, the development of effective cell-mediated immunity (CMI) restricts viral replication and ultimately eliminates infection. Some individual animals with less effective CMI may shed virus intermittently while remaining clinically normal. When CMI is severely impaired or defective, virus replication continues, leading to B-cell activation and the production of non-protective antibodies. The immune complexes, formed from these antibodies combined with FIPV, activate complement and contribute to the characteristic lesions of vasculitis.

The incubation period ranges from weeks to months. The onset of clinical signs may be either sudden or slow and insidious.

Currently, histological examination of affected tissues is the only procedure available for the definitive diagnosis of FIP. A serum hyperproteinaemia is frequently present in affected cats due to hypergammaglobulinaemia. Diagnostic serological tests, including IFA and ELISA, do not distinguish between cats infected with FCoV and FIPV. An intranasal vaccine employing a temperature-sensitive mutant strain of FIPV is available.

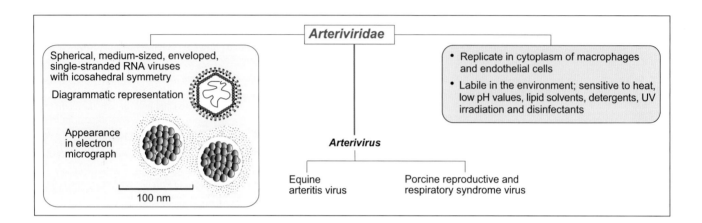

Arteriviridae

Spherical, medium-sized, enveloped, single-stranded RNA viruses with icosahedral symmetry

Diagrammatic representation

Appearance in electron micrograph

100 nm

- Replicate in cytoplasm of macrophages and endothelial cells
- Labile in the environment; sensitive to heat, low pH values, lipid solvents, detergents, UV irradiation and disinfectants

Arterivirus

Equine arteritis virus

Porcine reproductive and respiratory syndrome virus

Arteriviruses, formerly classified as members of the family *Togaviridae*, have been assigned to the family *Arteriviridae* which contains a single genus, *Arterivirus*. The name of the genus derives from the disease, equine arteritis, which is caused by the type species. Arteriviruses are spherical, 50 to 74 nm in diameter and possess a lipid-containing envelope which has small surface projections. The icosahedral nucleocapsid contains a molecule of linear, positive-sense, single-stranded RNA. Replication takes place in the cytoplasm of infected cells. Arteriviruses, which are relatively labile, are sensitive to heat, low pH, lipid solvents, detergent treatment, UV irradiation and many disinfectants.

Clinical infections

Members of the genus are host-specific. Infections have been described in horses, pigs, mice and monkeys. The primary target cells are macrophages. These viruses, which frequently persist in infected animals, can be spread horizontally by aerosols, by biting and also by venereal transmission.

Equine viral arteritis

Although infection with equine arteritis virus occurs worldwide, outbreaks of clinical disease are comparatively rare. Conjunctivitis, upper respiratory tract infection, ventral oedema and abortion are prominent clinical features. Close contact facilitates spread of infection. Virus is usually eliminated from mares and geldings within one to two months but may persist in about 35% of infected stallions. Carrier stallions are asymptomatic and shed virus continuously in semen. Mares infected venereally may spread virus horizontally to in-contact susceptible animals. Abortion or infection of the foal may occur when pregnant mares are infected.

Diagnosis requires laboratory confirmation. Virus isolation should be carried out in appropriate cell lines such as rabbit or equine kidney cells. Viral RNA can be detected in semen and other specimens using RT-PCR. Acute and convalescent blood samples should be submitted for serology. Seropositive stallions should be tested for virus in their semen and the breeding activities of carrier stallions confined to seropositive or vaccinated mares. In order to reduce the risk of colt foals becoming carriers, vaccination at six to twelve months of age is recommended.

Porcine reproductive and respiratory syndrome

This economically important condition is characterized by reproductive failure in sows and pneumonia in young pigs. The syndrome was first described in the USA in 1987. Despite attempts at controlling spread, the disease is now endemic in many countries. Natural infection occurs in pigs and wild boars. Significant antigenic and genomic differences between European and American isolates of the virus are evident, referred to as type 1 and type 2 genotypes, respectively. A variant of type 2 has been the cause of severe disease in China and south-east Asia. Nose-to-nose contact is considered to be the most likely route of transmission. Introduction of virus to a breeding herd is usually followed by reproductive failure. In some cases, cyanosis of the ears and vulva along with erythematous plaques on the skin ('blue-ear disease') have been described. Respiratory distress and increased pre-weaning mortality are important features of the disease in neonatal pigs. Severe outbreaks of other infections such as enzootic pneumonia or *Streptococcus suis* meningitis are frequently reported in infected herds. Subclinical infection occurs in some herds.

Serology is the most widely used diagnostic method. However, these tests do not distinguish carrier from vaccinated animals. The presence of PRRSV may be demonstrated by virus isolation, immunohistochemical staining or RT-PCR. Vaccination, combined with effective hygiene and health management are important measures for preventing disease transmission.

74 *Togaviridae*

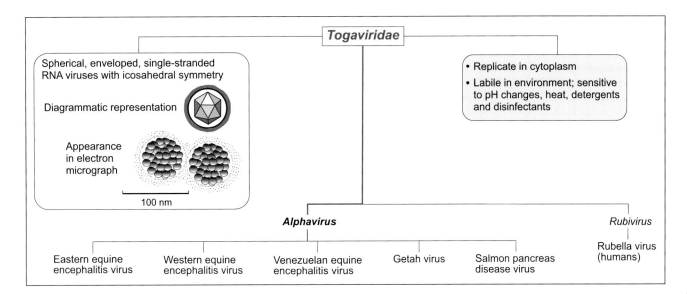

Viruses in the family *Togaviridae* (Latin *toga*, cloak) are enveloped RNA viruses, approximately 70 nm in diameter, with icosahedral symmetry. The envelope, which contains glycoprotein spikes, is closely bound to an icosahedral capsid. There are two genera, *Alphavirus* and *Rubivirus*, in the family. The sole member of the genus *Rubivirus* is rubella virus, which causes German measles in children and young adults and anomalies in the developing foetus when mothers are not vaccinated.

The genus *Alphavirus* includes more than 30 species, a number of which are important animal pathogens. Replication of alphaviruses, which contain positive-sense single-stranded RNA, occurs in the cytoplasm. In vertebrates, alphavirus infection results in cytolysis. Viral infection of invertebrate cells is usually non-cytolytic and persistent.

Alphaviruses, in common with certain members of the *Flaviviridae*, *Reoviridae*, *Rhabdoviridae* and *Bunyaviridae*, are termed arboviruses indicating that they are arthropod-borne and maintained in nature through biological transmission by haematophagous arthropods between vertebrate hosts. This term has no taxonomic significance. Alphaviruses usually have a principal invertebrate vector and an amplifying or reservoir vertebrate host. It is this enzootic cycle of infection that tends to determine the geographical distribution of these viruses.

Clinical infections

Domestic animals and humans are usually considered to be incidental, 'dead-end' hosts of alphaviruses because they do not develop a sufficiently high titre of circulating virus to act as reservoir hosts. A number of important equine diseases are caused by infection with members of the genus *Alphavirus* (Table 74.1).

Table 74.1 Alphaviruses of veterinary significance.

Virus	Vector	Comments
Eastern equine encephalitis virus	Mosquito (*Culiseta melanura*, *Aedes* species)	Infection endemic in passerine birds which frequent freshwater swamps of eastern North America, Caribbean islands and parts of South America. Causes disease in horses, humans and pheasants
Venezuelan equine encephalitis virus	Mosquito (*Culex* species)	Infection endemic in small mammals in Central and South America. Causes outbreaks of disease in horses, donkeys and humans in endemic regions, occasionally spreading to southern USA
Western equine encephalitis virus	Mosquito (*Culex tarsalis* and other *Culex* species, *Aedes* species)	Infection of passerine birds widespread in the Americas. Causes mild disease in horses and humans
Getah virus	Mosquito	Causes sporadic disease in horses in south-east Asia and Australia characterized by fever, urticaria and oedema of the limbs. Subclinical infection occurs in pigs

Concise Review of Veterinary Microbiology, Second Edition. P.J. Quinn, B.K. Markey, F.C. Leonard, E.S. FitzPatrick and S. Fanning.
© 2016 John Wiley & Sons, Ltd. Published 2016 by John Wiley & Sons, Ltd.
Companion website: www.wiley.com/go/quinn/concise-veterinary-microbiology

75 *Flaviviridae*

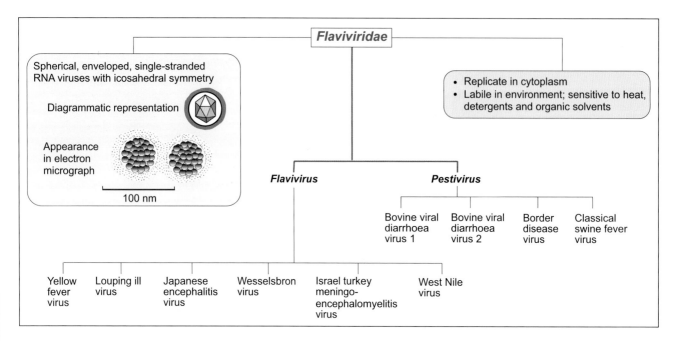

The family name of the *Flaviviridae* (Latin *flavus*, yellow) is derived from yellow fever, a disease of humans caused by a flavivirus, with jaundice as a major clinical feature. Members of the family are 40 to 60 nm in diameter with icosahedral capsids and tightly adherent envelopes which contain either two or three virus-encoded proteins, depending on the genus. The genome is composed of positive-sense single-stranded RNA. Replication of virus occurs in the cytoplasm with maturation in cytoplasmic vesicles and release by exocytosis. The mature virions, which are generally labile, are sensitive to heat, detergents and organic solvents. The family comprises four genera. Two genera, *Flavivirus* and *Pestivirus*, contain viruses of veterinary importance. The genus *Flavivirus* contains more than 50 members assigned to several serologically defined groups. Most members of the genus are arboviruses, which require either mosquitoes or ticks as vectors. The genus *Pestivirus* contains viruses of veterinary importance, namely bovine viral diarrhoea virus 1 and 2, border disease virus and classical swine fever virus. The sole member of the *Hepacivirus* genus, hepatitis C virus, causes hepatitis in humans. The genus *Pegivirus* contains viruses isolated from primates (pegivirus A, which is also known as hepatitis G virus) and from fruit bats (pegivirus B).

Clinical infections

In the genera *Flavivirus* and *Pestivirus* there are several viruses of particular veterinary importance (Table 75.1). Four members of the genus *Flavivirus*, louping ill virus, Japanese encephalitis virus, Israel turkey meningoencephalitis virus and Wesselsbron virus, cause disease in domestic animals. In addition, infection with West Nile virus, an important human pathogen, causes fatal disease in birds and horses. Other members of the genus which are important human pathogens include yellow fever virus, dengue virus, Japanese encephalitis virus, tick-borne encephalitis virus and St Louis encephalitis virus.

The four recognized members of the *Pestivirus* genus which infect domestic species are closely related antigenically. Infections with these pestiviruses may be inapparent, acute or persistent and are economically important worldwide. An additional four viruses have been proposed but are not yet officially recognized, namely atypical pestivirus (isolates from cattle, sheep and pigs, also referred to as HoBi-like virus), Bungowannah virus, pronghorn antelope pestivirus and giraffe pestivirus.

Bovine viral diarrhoea and mucosal disease

Infection with bovine viral diarrhoea virus (BVDV) is common in cattle populations throughout the world. The virus can cause both acute disease, bovine viral diarrhoea (BVD), and a protracted form of illness, mucosal disease, arising from persistent infection. Using cell culture, cytopathic and non-cytopathic biotypes are recognized. The biotype most often isolated from cattle populations is non-cytopathic. Cytopathic isolates can arise from non-cytopathic BVDV as a result of recombination events, including incorporation of host RNA and duplication of viral RNA sequences in the *NS2-3* gene resulting in cleavage of NS2-3 and increased production of NS3. Two genotypes, now considered separate species, BVDV 1 (classical BVDV isolates) and

Concise Review of Veterinary Microbiology, Second Edition. P.J. Quinn, B.K. Markey, F.C. Leonard, E.S. FitzPatrick and S. Fanning.
© 2016 John Wiley & Sons, Ltd. Published 2016 by John Wiley & Sons, Ltd.
Companion website: www.wiley.com/go/quinn/concise-veterinary-microbiology

Table 75.1 Viruses of veterinary importance in the genera *Flavivirus* and *Pestivirus*.

Genus	Virus	Hosts	Comments
Flavivirus	Louping ill virus	Sheep, cattle, horses, red grouse, humans	Present in defined regions of Europe. Transmitted by the tick *Ixodes ricinus*; produces encephalitis in sheep and other species
	Japanese encephalitis virus	Waterfowl, pigs, horses, humans	Widely distributed in Asia. Transmitted by mosquitoes. Waterfowl are reservoir hosts. Infection in pigs results in abortion and neonatal mortality
	Wesselsbron virus	Sheep	Occurs in parts of sub-Saharan Africa. Transmitted by mosquitoes. Produces generalized infection, hepatitis and abortion
	Israel turkey meningo-encephalomyelitis virus	Turkeys	Reported in Israel and South Africa. Transmitted by mosquitoes. Progressive paresis and paralysis
	West Nile virus	Birds, humans, horses	Birds are the natural hosts. Transmitted by mosquitoes. Serious nervous disease reported sporadically in humans and horses. Has become widespread in North America since first appearance in 1999
Pestivirus	Bovine viral diarrhoea virus 1 and 2	Cattle (sheep, pigs)	Occur worldwide. Cause inapparent infection, bovine viral diarrhoea and mucosal disease. Congenital infection may result in abortion, congenital defects and persistent infection due to immunotolerance
	Border disease virus	Sheep	Occurs worldwide. Infection of pregnant ewes may result in abortion, congenital abnormalities or persistent infection
	Classical swine fever (hog cholera) virus	Pigs	Highly contagious, economically important disease with high mortality. Generalized infection with nervous signs and abortion; congenital tremors in piglets

BVDV 2 (atypical BVDV isolates), are recognized on the basis of differences in the 5′-untranslated region of the viral genome. Both genotypes contain cytopathic and non-cytopathic isolates and produce similar clinical syndromes in cattle. However, only type 2 isolates have been associated with thrombocytopenia and a haemorrhagic syndrome, first described in North America.

Persistently infected (PI) animals, which shed virus in secretions and excretions, are particularly important sources of infection. Persistent infection develops when infection of the foetus with a non-cytopathic strain occurs before day 120 of gestation. About 1% of animals in an infected population are persistently infected and viraemic. The presence of cattle with persistent infection in a herd results in constant exposure of the other cattle to virus, producing a high level of herd immunity. The outcome of transplacental spread depends on the age of the foetus at the time of infection. During the first 30 days of gestation, infection may result in embryonic death with return of the dam to oestrus. The effects of foetal infection between 30 and 90 days of gestation include abortion, mummification and congenital abnormalities of the CNS, often cerebellar hypoplasia. Foetuses which become infected after day 120 of gestation can mount an active immune response and are usually normal at birth. If virus invades the foetus before development of immune competence, immunotolerance to the agent results, with persistent infection for the lifetime of the animal. The virus involved in this persistent infection is non-cytopathic. Later, usually between six months and two years of age, a cytopathic biotype emerges

as a consequence of mutation of the non-cytopathic virus or of recombination with nucleic acid of the host cell or other non-cytopathic biotypes. Cytopathic isolates have a particular tropism for gut-associated lymphoid tissues. These molecular changes in BVDV may lead to the development of mucosal disease in some animals.

Most BVDV infections are subclinical. Outbreaks of BVD are usually associated with high morbidity and low mortality. When present, clinical signs include inappetence, depression, fever and diarrhoea. Although a significant proportion of PI animals are clinically normal, some are born undersized and exhibit growth retardation and decreased viability. Mucosal disease is usually sporadic in occurrence. Clinical signs include depression, fever, profuse watery diarrhoea, nasal discharge, salivation and lameness. Ulcerative lesions are present in the mouth and interdigital clefts. The case fatality rate is 100%.

A tentative diagnosis may be possible on the basis of clinical signs and pathological findings. Laboratory confirmation requires demonstration of antibody, viral antigen or viral RNA. Seroconversion and the presence of viraemic animals are necessary for confirmation of established infection in a herd. Most losses arising from BVDV infections in herds result from the effects of prenatal infections and mucosal disease. Control strategies are directed at preventing infections which can lead to the birth of PI animals. Killed, attenuated live and temperature-sensitive mutant virus vaccines have been developed. The elimination of BVDV from a herd requires the identification and

SECTION IV

removal of PI animals. Testing to detect viral antigen or viral RNA in blood or ear notch samples is used to identify PI animals. In national eradication programmes, herds containing PI animals can be detected by testing bulk milk or pooled blood samples for antibodies to BVDV.

Border disease

This congenital disease of lambs, also known as hairy shaker disease, occurs worldwide. Border disease, which was first reported from the Welsh–English border, is caused by infection of the foetus with a pestivirus which is non-cytopathic. Pestivirus isolates from sheep can infect other domestic ruminants and pigs. Moreover, pestivirus isolates from a number of domestic species can infect pregnant sheep causing border disease in their offspring.

Persistently infected animals shed virus continuously in excretions and secretions. These animals tend to have a low survival rate under field conditions, although some may survive for several years without developing clinical signs. Persistently infected ewes may give birth to persistently infected lambs. Acute infections in susceptible sheep are transient and result in immunity to challenge with homologous strains of border disease virus (BDV).

Virus is probably acquired by the oronasal route. In susceptible pregnant ewes, infection results in placentitis and invasion of the foetus. The immune response of the ewe does not protect the developing foetus. The age of the foetus at the time of infection ultimately determines the outcome. The foetus develops immune competence between 60 and 80 days of gestation. Foetal death may follow infection prior to the development of immune competence, the outcome being resorption, abortion or mummification. Foetuses which survive infection become immunotolerant and remain persistently infected. These animals may be clinically normal at birth or may display tremors and hairy birthcoat, consequences of viral interference with organogenesis. Congenital defects in affected lambs include skeletal growth retardation, hypomyelinogenesis and enlarged primary hair follicles with reduced numbers of secondary follicles. Infection after day 80 of gestation induces an immune response with elimination of the virus and the birth of a healthy lamb. Foetal infection during mid-gestation when the immune system is developing may result in lesions in the CNS including cerebral cavitation and cerebellar dysplasia.

In flocks infected with BDV, there may be an increase in the number of abortions and weak neonatal lambs. Characteristic signs of infection in newborn lambs include altered body conformation, changes in fleece quality and tremors. Affected lambs are often small and their survival rate is poor. In well-nursed lambs, the neurological signs may gradually abate and such animals may eventually become clinically normal.

The characteristic clinical signs are diagnostic. Dysmyelination may be demonstrable histologically in the CNS. Immunocytochemical staining can be used to demonstrate virus in brain tissue. Serological testing, employing methods such as serum neutralization and ELISA, can be used to determine the extent of infection in a flock.

Control should be based on identification and removal of persistently infected animals and precautions to avoid introduction of infected animals into a flock. Where such a policy is not feasible, breeding stock should be deliberately mixed with persistently infected animals at least two months before mating.

Classical swine fever (hog cholera)

This highly contagious, potentially fatal OIE-listed disease of pigs, although still present in many countries, has been eradicated from North America, Australia and most European countries. Infected animals occur in the wild boar populations in Europe, which act as reservoirs of infection. Direct contact between infected and susceptible animals is the main means of transmission. In endemic areas, the disease is spread principally by movement of infected pigs. Shedding of virus may begin before clinical signs become evident. Virulent virus is shed in all excretions and secretions. Virus strains of moderate virulence may result in chronic infection with continuous or intermittent shedding by infected pigs. In addition, congenital infections with strains of low virulence may result in the birth of persistently-infected piglets. Spread between premises can occur indirectly, particularly in regions with a high density of pig farms. The virus, which is relatively fragile and does not persist in the environment, is not spread over long distances by air movement. However, it can be transmitted mechanically by personnel, vehicles and biting arthropods. Despite its lability, classical swine fever virus (CSFV) can survive for long periods in protein-rich biological materials such as meat or body fluids, particularly if chilled or frozen. Although legislation is in place in most European countries prohibiting the feeding of uncooked swill, outbreaks of classical swine fever can still be traced to waste food fed to pigs.

Pigs are usually infected by the oronasal route. The tonsil is the primary site of viral multiplication. Virus spreads to regional lymph nodes and viraemia develops after further viral multiplication. Virus, which has an affinity for vascular endothelium and reticuloendothelial cells, can be isolated from all major organs and tissues. In acute swine fever, vascular damage in conjunction with severe thrombocytopenia results in widespread petechial haemorrhages. A non-suppurative encephalitis with prominent perivascular cuffing is present in most CSFV-infected pigs. Virus strains of reduced virulence can cause a mild form of the disease. In pregnant sows, infection may result in stillbirths, weak newborn piglets with congenital tremors and, occasionally, clinically normal piglets.

Following an incubation period of up to 10 days, affected animals develop high fever and become inappetent and depressed. Sick pigs are inclined to huddle together. Vomiting and constipation are followed by diarrhoea. Some animals may die soon after developing convulsions. A swaying gait usually precedes posterior paresis. Most cases of acute classical swine fever succumb within 20 days after infection. Signs of disease are milder in infections caused by strains of low virulence.

Although clinical signs and history may provide evidence for a tentative diagnosis, laboratory confirmation is essential, particularly with infections caused by strains of reduced virulence. In acute disease, haemorrhages are present in many internal organs and on serosal surfaces. Petechiae are often present on kidney surfaces and in lymph nodes. Other gross pathological features of diagnostic significance are splenic infarction and 'button' ulcers in the mucosa of the terminal ileum near the ileocaecal valve. Rapid confirmation is possible using direct immunofluorescence on frozen sections of tonsillar tissue, kidney, spleen, distal ileum and lymph nodes. Antigen-capture ELISAs are available commercially and suitable for detection of viral antigen in blood or organ suspensions. The RT-PCR assays for detection of CSFV RNA are sensitive and rapid, replacing most other methods used for virus detection. Serological testing is useful on farms infected with strains of low virulence or for serological surveys.

The disease is notifiable in many countries which have adopted slaughter policies and banned vaccination. Pigs and pig products should not be imported from countries where infection with CSFV is present. Swill must be boiled before being fed to pigs. In countries where the disease is endemic or during the early stages of an eradication programme, vaccination may be used. Live vaccines attenuated either by serial passage in rabbits or in tissue culture are currently used. These vaccines are safe and effective. The use of recombinant E2 glycoprotein marker vaccine in conjunction with a specific ELISA capable of detecting antibodies to the other main envelope glycoprotein, E^{rns}, offers a means of distinguishing vaccinated from naturally infected pigs.

Louping ill
The name 'louping ill' derives from the Scottish vernacular for 'leaping' or 'bounding', an allusion to the abnormal gait of some affected animals. Although primarily a disease of sheep, louping ill can occur in other animals and also in humans. The disease, which is largely confined to Britain and Ireland, has also been described in Norway, Spain, Bulgaria and Turkey. Louping ill virus is transmitted by the tick *Ixodes ricinus* and the seasonal incidence and regional distribution of the disease reflect periods of tick activity in suitable habitats such as upland grazing. The host range of *I. ricinus* is wide and infection with louping ill virus can occur in many vertebrate species including sheep, cattle, horses, deer, red grouse and humans. On farms where infection is endemic, losses occur mainly in sheep under two years of age. Following infection, most sheep acquire life-long immunity. Young lambs are protected by colostral antibody.

Viral replication occurs initially in lymph nodes draining sites of inoculation. Viraemia follows, with dissemination to other lymphatic organs and to the brain and spinal cord. The speed and onset of the immune response are important in preventing spread of virus and limiting the degree of damage in the central nervous system. Immunosuppression caused by infection with *Anaplasma phagocytophilum*, the agent of tickborne fever, is considered to be responsible for increased mortality in sheep with louping ill.

A history of neurological signs or unexplained deaths in sheep in endemic areas during periods of tick activity may be indicative of louping ill. Laboratory confirmation is usually required. A non-suppurative encephalomyelitis is usually detectable histologically. Detection of louping ill virus using an RT-PCR protocol has been described. Antibody to the virus can be detected using complement fixation and gel diffusion tests. Inactivated vaccines are protective. Purchased sheep or animals within the flock intended for breeding should be vaccinated at six to 12 months of age. Colostral immunity usually protects lambs for the first six months of life. Measures aimed at clearing grazing land of tick habitats and dipping of sheep decrease the risk of infection with louping ill virus.

West Nile virus
West Nile virus (WNV), a member of the Japanese encephalitis virus serocomplex, is a mosquito-borne flavivirus which infects many species of animals including horses, birds and humans. From its initial detection in New York in 1999, the virus has spread throughout North America and to Central and South America. Mosquito vectors include *Culex* species and also *Aedes* and *Anopheles* species. The virus is transmitted in enzootic cycles involving mosquitoes and birds. Incidental infections occur in humans and domestic animals. Transmission occurs through the bite of insect vectors and horizontal transmission is not described in domestic animals. Migrating birds may carry the virus to new geographical regions. Although some birds may remain asymptomatic, many species including crows, ravens, jays and geese develop high levels of viraemia with high mortality. A proportion of infected horses and humans develop clinical signs. Neurological signs in horses include leg weakness and flaccid paralysis. Virus can be recovered from a wide range of tissues in avian species but brain and spinal cord are the preferred specimens for laboratory diagnosis of disease in horses. Virus isolation can be carried out in cell culture. Infection can be confirmed by detection of viral antigen by immunoassay and immunohistochemistry or by detection of viral RNA by RT-PCR. Suitable serological tests include ELISA and plaque reduction neutralization test. Control is based on vaccination and commercially available vaccines for horses currently include an inactivated whole virus vaccine and a recombinant canarypox-vectored vaccine.

76 Prions

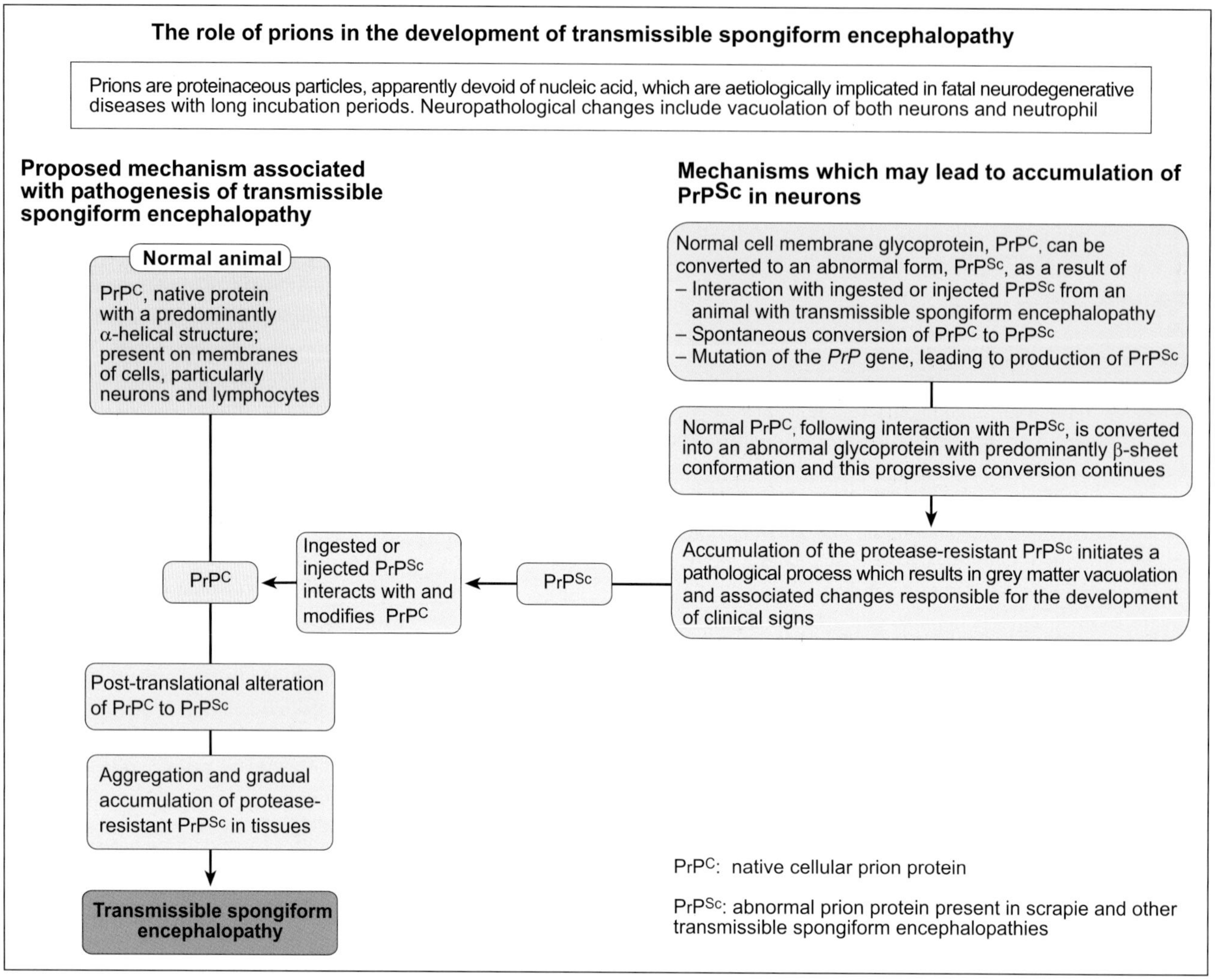
The role of prions in the development of transmissible spongiform encephalopathy
Prions are proteinaceous particles, apparently devoid of nucleic acid, which are aetiologically implicated in fatal neurodegenerative diseases with long incubation periods. Neuropathological changes include vacuolation of both neurons and neutrophil
Proposed mechanism associated with pathogenesis of transmissible spongiform encephalopathy
Normal animal
PrPC, native protein with a predominantly α-helical structure; present on membranes of cells, particularly neurons and lymphocytes
PrPC
Ingested or injected PrPSc interacts with and modifies PrPC
PrPSc
Post-translational alteration of PrPC to PrPSc
Aggregation and gradual accumulation of protease-resistant PrPSc in tissues
Transmissible spongiform encephalopathy
Mechanisms which may lead to accumulation of PrPSc in neurons
Normal cell membrane glycoprotein, PrPC, can be converted to an abnormal form, PrPSc, as a result of
– Interaction with ingested or injected PrPSc from an animal with transmissible spongiform encephalopathy
– Spontaneous conversion of PrPC to PrPSc
– Mutation of the PrP gene, leading to production of PrPSc
Normal PrPC, following interaction with PrPSc, is converted into an abnormal glycoprotein with predominantly β-sheet conformation and this progressive conversion continues
Accumulation of the protease-resistant PrPSc initiates a pathological process which results in grey matter vacuolation and associated changes responsible for the development of clinical signs
PrPC: native cellular prion protein
PrPSc: abnormal prion protein present in scrapie and other transmissible spongiform encephalopathies

Prions are infectious proteinaceous particles that have been described in fungi and in a number of mammalian species. They are responsible for a unique group of neurodegenerative diseases in mammals known as transmissible spongiform encephalopathies (TSEs). Prions are 'unconventional' infectious agents because they appear to be devoid of nucleic acid, unlike viruses and other microbial agents. In addition, they are non-immunogenic and are extremely resistant to inactivation by heating, exposure to chemicals and irradiation. Prions of vertebrates are derived through a post-translational process from a native glycoprotein PrP^C, with a predominantly α-helical structure (cellular isoform of the prion protein), associated with the plasma membrane of many cell types. Following exposure to the abnormal, pathogenic isoform of the prion protein PrP^{Sc} (named after scrapie, the prototypic prion disease), PrP^C is altered post-translationally to a conformational structure similar to that of PrP^{Sc} which is folded mainly into β-sheets, has increased resistance to proteases and a strong propensity to aggregate. As more PrP^C is converted to PrP^{Sc}, this protease-resistant molecule gradually accumulates, especially in the long-lived cells of the CNS. The formation of PrP^{Sc} from PrP^C in TSEs may be initiated following exposure to an external source of PrP^{Sc}, usually by ingestion as occurred in kuru following ritualistic cannibalism in the Fore peoples of Papua New Guinea. Rarely, random spontaneous conversion of native PrP^C to PrP^{Sc} may initiate the process in an individual, as occurs in sporadic Creutzfeldt–Jakob disease (CJD) in humans. A third mechanism which predisposes to conformational change in PrP^C relates to mutation in the *PrP* gene,

Concise Review of Veterinary Microbiology, Second Edition. P.J. Quinn, B.K. Markey, F.C. Leonard, E.S. FitzPatrick and S. Fanning.

Companion website: www.wiley.com/go/quinn/concise-veterinary-microbiology

Table 76.1 Transmissible spongiform encephalopathies of animals.

Disease	Comments
Scrapie	Recognized in sheep in parts of Europe for 300 years; apart from Australia and New Zealand, now occurs worldwide. Occurs in goats also
Bovine spongiform encephalopathy	First reported in England in 1986; developed into a major epidemic over a 10-year period. Prevalence sharply declined with the implementation of effective control measures. Occurred at low frequency in many other European countries. Cases also described in USA, Japan and Canada
Chronic wasting disease	First observed in captive mule deer in Colorado in 1967. Occurs in North American deer and elk populations in the wild. Horizontal transmission occurs with shedding of prions in saliva. Clinical signs include severe generalized wasting, trembling and ataxia
Transmissible mink encephalopathy	First recognized in caged mink in Wisconsin in 1947; attributed to the feeding of scrapie-infected sheep meat
Feline spongiform encephalopathy	First recorded during the BSE epidemic in the early 1990s. Most cases occurred in the UK and were attributed to the consumption of BSE-infected meat
Exotic ungulate encephalopathy	First recorded during the BSE epidemic in 1986. Reported in greater kudu, nyala, oryx and some other captive ruminants in zoological collections. Attributed to the feeding of prion-contaminated meat-and-bone meal

as occurs in the Gerstmann–Sträussler–Scheinker syndrome and familial CJD in humans.

The *PrP* gene of an infected animal determines the primary amino acid sequence of the prion protein in that animal. The resistance of some species to infection by prions derived from another species is termed the 'species barrier'. This barrier is attributed to differences between the amino acid sequences of the prion proteins in the two species. On initial transfer of PrP^{Sc} between species, the incubation period tends to be relatively long. Subsequent transfer between members of the recipient species leads to shorter incubation periods. The presence of a 'species barrier' may explain the resistance of humans to infection with PrP^{Sc} in meat derived from sheep with scrapie.

Diseases attributed to prions occur sporadically and are significantly influenced by the genome of the affected animal. These slowly progressive neurodegenerative diseases, which are characterized by long incubation periods and spongiform changes in the brain, have been described in many animal species and in humans. Transmissible spongiform encephalopathies have been recognized in both ruminants and carnivores (Table 76.1). In scrapie, there is convincing evidence for the importance of the genetic constitution of certain breeds of sheep in determining susceptibility to the disease. Distinct disease phenotypes are described associated with defined prion strains.

Prions can exist in multiple molecular forms and such strains are believed to arise due to differences in conformation and glycosylation patterns.

Scrapie

This insidious, fatal, neurological disease of adult sheep and goats occurs worldwide, except in Australia and New Zealand. The mode of transmission of scrapie is not clearly understood. The disease has a long incubation period. Neurological signs develop predominantly in sheep of breeding age with a peak incidence between three and four years of age. Initially, affected animals may present with restlessness or nervousness, particularly after sudden noise or movement. Pruritis may result in loss of wool. Progression of the disease leads to emaciation. Death usually occurs within six months from the onset of clinical signs. Diagnosis is based on characterisitic clinical signs and histopathological examination of the CNS. Distinctive microscopic changes include neuronal vacuolation and degeneration, vacuolar change in the neuropil and astrocytosis, particularly in the medulla. No obvious inflammatory response is evident. Confirmatory methods include immunohistochemical staining for PrP^{Sc}, immunoblotting for detection of proteinase-K-resistant PrP^{Sc} and electron microscopy for demonstration of scrapie-associated fibrils in detergent-treated extracts of brain.

In the EU, scrapie has been designated a notifiable disease. Slaughter policies have been enforced with different degrees of success in several countries. In Australia and New Zealand an eradication policy, implemented soon after the introduction of the disease, was successful. Eradication was abandoned in the USA because of the cost and difficulties involved in its implementation. Breeding scrapie-resistant sheep may be a realistic method for reducing the frequency of the disease.

Bovine spongiform encephalopathy

This condition is a progressive neurodegenerative disease of adult cattle, first recognized in England in 1986. More than 180,000 cases of the disease were subsequently confirmed and an estimated one million animals were infected. Following importation of cattle from Great Britain, the disease was reported in several countries. In addition, indigenous cattle in a number of European countries, including Switzerland, Ireland, France and Portugal, have developed the disease.

The prion strain causing bovine spongiform encephalopathy (BSE) is not considered to be species-specific. In 1996, a novel form of human prion disease, termed variant Creutzfeldt–Jakob disease (vCJD) was recognized in Great Britain. Molecular strain-typing studies and experimental transmission in transgenic and conventional mice indicated that vCJD and BSE are caused by indistinguishable prion strains. The BSE epidemic in Great Britain was attributed to contaminated meat-and-bone meal (MBM) prepared from slaughterhouse offal and fed as a protein dietary supplement to cattle. It is postulated that the scrapie agent crossed the species barrier into cattle in the early 1980s, following changes in the rendering process which allowed survival of increased amounts of scrapie PrP (PrP^{Sc}) in MBM. As a result of the banning of ruminant-derived MBM in 1988, there was a marked decline in the prevalence of BSE in Great Britain after 1993. Horizontal transmission of BSE does not appear to occur. The mean incubation period is about five years. Neurological signs, which are highly variable, include changes in behaviour and deficits in posture and movement. Ataxia, hypermetria and a tendency to fall become increasingly evident in the later stages of the disease. The clinical course may extend over many days or months.

Bovine spongiform encephalopathy can be confirmed by histopathological examination of brain tissue and specific immunological confirmatory methods. Bovine spongiform encephalopathy is a notifiable disease in countries of the EU. Control is based on slaughter of affected animals and exclusion of ruminant-derived protein from ruminant rations.

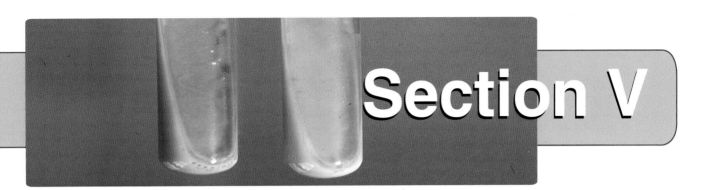

Section V

Prevention and Control
of Infectious Disease

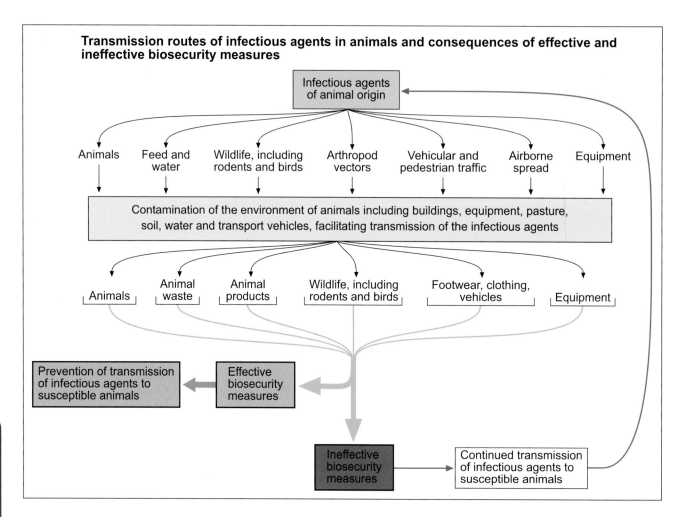

Transmission routes of infectious agents in animals and consequences of effective and ineffective biosecurity measures

Infectious agents of animal origin

Animals | Feed and water | Wildlife, including rodents and birds | Arthropod vectors | Vehicular and pedestrian traffic | Airborne spread | Equipment

Contamination of the environment of animals including buildings, equipment, pasture, soil, water and transport vehicles, facilitating transmission of the infectious agents

Animals | Animal waste | Animal products | Wildlife, including rodents and birds | Footwear, clothing, vehicles | Equipment

Prevention of transmission of infectious agents to susceptible animals

Effective biosecurity measures

Ineffective biosecurity measures

Continued transmission of infectious agents to susceptible animals

The term 'biosecurity' includes a wide range of measures aimed at preventing or limiting exposure of domesticated animals to microbial pathogens from outside sources or to infectious agents shed by infected animals within the herd. These measures are important for the prevention and control of infectious diseases (Box 77.1). Effective management practices which prevent the spread of pathogens from infected animals to susceptible animals and that prevent the introduction of infected animals or microbial pathogens into a herd or region of a country where a disease does not occur, minimize the risk of such diseases occurring in susceptible livestock. Benefits of an effective biosecurity programme include a high standard of animal health and welfare, freedom from specific pathogens, improved animal production and reduced production costs. An effective biosecurity programme has many components, all aimed at ensuring that the risks of healthy animals acquiring infection are minimized. These include the design, location and environment of farm buildings, policies relating to the purchase of replacement

animals, feed supplies, regulation of employees, transport vehicles, service personnel and people visiting the farm with or without prior appointments (Table 77.1). The larger the operation, the greater the need for effective biosecurity measures.

Ensuring that the domestic animal population within a country remains free of major infectious diseases is a constant challenge for national and local veterinary personnel and staff in diagnostic laboratories. Exclusion of suspect animals from a country, quarantine at point of entry, isolation of infected and in-contact animals on the farm, followed by diagnostic testing and, if necessary, slaughter are widely applied measures for the control of exotic infectious diseases in animal populations. Free movement of animals between countries or within a country also invariably leads to free movement of microbial pathogens. Because movement of vehicles and animals is an unavoidable feature of stud farms, it is important to ascertain the health status of mares and stallions used for breeding purposes. There are inherent risks associated with the movement of breeding mares

Concise Review of Veterinary Microbiology, Second Edition. P.J. Quinn, B.K. Markey, F.C. Leonard, E.S. FitzPatrick and S. Fanning.
© 2016 John Wiley & Sons, Ltd. Published 2016 by John Wiley & Sons, Ltd.
Companion website: www.wiley.com/go/quinn/concise-veterinary-microbiology

SECTION V

Table 77.1 Biosecurity for farm animals.

Component	Considerations	Comments
Animals	Replacement animals should be purchased from reputable sources	Newly purchased animals should be isolated and closely monitored for at least 2 weeks
Feed	Close attention should be given to source and quality of feed	Feed can become contaminated by wild birds and rodents during storage
Water supply	Source and quality of water should be evaluated	Drinkers within buildings and water troughs for grazing animals can become contaminated with faeces or urine
Vehicular and pedestrian traffic	Delivery vehicles should conform to farm's standard of hygiene; staff, service personnel and visitors should wear protective clothing and waterproof footwear and use footbaths provided	Particular care is required with vehicles used for transportation of animals, slurry tankers and vehicles used for disposal of bedding material
Farm equipment	Sharing of farm equipment and vehicles for transportation of animals should be avoided	Equipment used for cleaning farm buildings or spreading animal waste should not be borrowed or loaned
Animal waste	Liquid animal waste should be stored in slurry tanks; solid animal waste should be composted on the farm and spread on arable land	An interval of 2 months should elapse between the application of slurry to pasture and commencement of grazing
Wildlife, including rodents and wild birds	When wildlife and grazing domestic animals live in close association, wildlife can transmit microbial pathogens to domestic animals; rodents can act as reservoirs of microbial pathogens and wild birds can transmit viral and bacterial pathogens to commercial poultry flocks	Wild birds should not have access to poultry houses or feed mills and buildings should be designed to exclude rodents
Cleaning and disinfection	Thorough cleaning followed by disinfection is essential for the elimination of microbial pathogens from farm buildings, transport vehicles and equipment	Although effective cleaning can reduce the number of microbial pathogens in a building, chemical disinfection is required to inactivate residual microbial pathogens

onto a farm. Such animals should have their vaccination status confirmed in advance of acceptance by the stud farm and be certified free of *Taylorella equigenitalis*. *Streptococcus equi* is a constant source of concern when horses are brought together for breeding purposes, for competitive events or for sales. A thorough clinical examination together with a detailed clinical history of each animal may aid in the detection and exclusion of suspect animals at the point of arrival.

Replacement animals should be purchased from reputable sources where the history of the herd or flock from which they derived is known. Imported animals should be quarantined at point of arrival in a country and subjected to thorough clinical examination combined with appropriate laboratory test procedures. A limitation of both quarantine and isolation of animals after purchase relates to diseases with long incubation periods such as paratuberculosis in cattle, scrapie in sheep and rabies in dogs and cats. Because latent viral infections and latent bacterial infections may not be detectable by clinical examination of animals, serological tests and collection of specimens for culture or virus isolation may be required to detect a carrier state in apparently healthy animals.

The harmonious relationship between animals and their environment can be reinforced by good management systems, optimal nutrition, adequate floor space and effective disease control programmes. Factors that can adversely affect animals' wellbeing include overcrowding, uncontrolled environmental temperature, nutritional imbalances and absence of a well designed and implemented disease control programme. Buildings, farm-

yards, paddocks and other grazing areas can be planned so as to promote animal health. Conversely, improper building design, inadequate ventilation and insufficient floor space for the animal population can predispose to stressful environmental conditions for intensively-reared animals. Careful temperature control is a requirement for neonatal pigs and newly hatched chicks. Building design should incorporate features which facilitate cleaning and disinfection at the end of a production cycle or following an outbreak of infectious disease. Floors and walls with a moderately smooth finish facilitate cleaning and minimize trauma to animals without predisposing to slipping. On large farms, consideration should be given to the inclusion of facilities for washing and disinfecting vehicles for transportation of animals. Dusty paddocks and heavily grazed pasture can lead to a build-up of *Rhodococcus equi* which can result in suppurative bronchopneumonia in foals up to four months of age. Rough pastures provide cover for many tick species such as *Ixodes ricinus*. The acquisition of tick-borne diseases such as louping ill and tick-borne fever is usually associated with animals grazing rough pasture.

The source and quality of feed for farm animals requires careful consideration to ensure freedom from microbial pathogens or toxic factors. Feed such as grain can become contaminated during storage with viral or bacterial pathogens before it reaches feed mills. Wild birds and rodents have been implicated in feed contamination and cats shedding oocysts of *Toxoplasma gondii* in their faeces can contaminate grain in feed mills or on farms. Animal-derived protein should be excluded from the diets of ruminants due to the association of BSE in cattle with the feeding of meat-and-bone meal. Crops grown by the owner on the farm are sometimes the source of infectious agents or biological toxins. *Listeria monocytogenes* can replicate in the surface layers of poor-quality silage and produce listeriosis in ruminants. Botulism in farm animals has been associated with feeding baled silage and with the landspreading of poultry litter.

The source and quality of water for farm animals may be influenced by farm location, climatic factors and other environmental influences. Contamination of a clean water supply on a farm can occur due to faecal or urinary shedding of pathogens into drinkers in buildings. For grazing animals, ponds or larger bodies of water may become contaminated by run-off from slurry spreading or overflowing slurry tanks. Wildlife, either resident or migratory, can contaminate ponds with enteric pathogens or leptospires. If poultry houses are located close to lakes or large ponds, migrating waterfowl or seabirds can transmit avian influenza or Newcastle disease to domestic poultry.

Control of vehicles calling at farms requires close surveillance. Particular attention should be paid to vehicles used for collection of animals, slurry tankers and other vehicles used for disposal of animal waste. Staff working on farms, service personnel, veterinarians and others on official business should adhere strictly to wearing protective clothing and footwear at all times. Footbaths, strategically positioned for pedestrians, should be used by all persons entering the farm. To ensure compliance with footbath use, all pedestrians entering the premises should wear clean, waterproof footwear. A secure perimeter fence is an essential component of any biosecurity system. Footbaths should be large enough to accommodate the largest size of footwear worn by workers or visitors. Disinfectants suitable for footbath use include iodophors, phenolic compounds and formalin. If a specific infectious agent is identified as the cause of a disease outbreak, a disinfectant known to be effective against that agent should be used in all footbaths on the premises.

Wheel baths are sometimes positioned at farm entrances as part of a disease control programme. The design of wheel baths should be such that there is adequate contact with the disinfectant for a sufficient time to ensure the inactivation of infectious agents on wheel surfaces. The tyre of the largest vehicle wheel entering the bath should be completely immersed in one revolution. Installation of a properly designed wheel bath is expensive and may impart an unrealistic impression of biosecurity. In many instances, the contents of vehicles including animals, their excretions and secretions, animal feed and bedding pose a greater threat of transferring infectious agents than vehicle wheels.

In buildings with slatted floors, animal waste is stored in slurry tanks. Such tanks should be constructed to high specifications and have ample capacity to ensure that overflowing of contents does not occur. Slurry spreading is usually restricted to defined times of the year when ground conditions are suitable for slurry tankers and when the risk of run-off is low. An interval of two months should elapse between the application of slurry to pasture and the commencement of grazing. Straw used for bedding animals or litter from poultry houses should be composted for at least two months before spreading on land used for tillage.

Control measures for rodents and insects should form part of a biosecurity programme. Rats and mice are often attracted to farm buildings because they provide shelter in cold weather and because of the abundance of food available in such buildings. Rodents can act as reservoirs of *Salmonella* species which they excrete in their faeces. Rats sometimes shed leptospires in their urine and can transmit these virulent pathogens to domestic animals and to humans. To lessen their attraction for rodents, feed bins should be rodent proof and feed spillages should be cleared up promptly. Strategic use of rodenticides in the vicinity of farm buildings is an effective method for controlling rodent populations.

At the end of a production cycle or following an outbreak of disease, cleaning and disinfection is an essential component of a biosecurity programme. If carried out in a competent manner, cleaning alone can reduce substantially the number of pathogens on building surfaces, thereby decreasing the risk of infection to animals introduced into the building. One of the principal reasons for failure of a disinfection procedure is the presence of residual organic matter on surfaces, equipment or transport vehicles due to inadequate cleaning. Food receptacles and drinkers require special attention in this respect. Selection of an effective and economical disinfectant for the terminal disinfection of a farm building requires consideration of the infectious agents likely to be present, the amount of organic matter remaining on surfaces and the antimicrobial spectrum of the compound selected.

Schemes for the diagnosis, control and prevention of important endemic diseases of animals are formulated by national governments and implemented by veterinary personnel at district level and at farm level. In the event of an outbreak of infectious disease subject to government control, a rigorous testing policy, followed by slaughter of infected animals, segregation, monitoring and retesting of in-contact animals usually applies.

Box 77.1 Strategies for the prevention, treatment or control of infectious diseases in animal populations

- Exclusion of animals from a country or continent
- Quarantine of imported animals at point of entry
- Accurate identification of farm animals, especially ruminants, using ear tags or microchip implantation; colour markings can be used for horse identification while dogs and cats may require detailed written descriptions with accompanying photographs
- Isolation of infected or in-contact animals on the farm of origin or on the premises being inspected
- Exclusion of animal-derived food components from the diet of ruminants
- Clinical or laboratory confirmation of exotic infectious disease followed by slaughter and careful disposal of infected carcasses
- Vaccination of susceptible domestic animals before exposure to possible sources of endemic or exotic diseases
- Either vaccination or depopulation of wildlife reservoirs depending on the importance of the disease and the feasibility of implementing control measures
- Chemotherapy for animals with endemic disease
- Chemoprophylaxis for prevention of predictable infectious disease in animal populations when vaccination is either impractical or ineffective

A closed herd or a closed flock is the most effective method for excluding infectious agents from an animal population.

Implementation of a biosecurity programme is dependent on many factors including the size, location and type of farm and the financial resources of the owner. Strategies appropriate for the implementation of a biosecurity programme on a particular farm require a detailed understanding of the enterprise, a positively motivated owner and a realistic estimate of the costs and the likely financial benefits deriving from strict adherence to the measures proposed. In some circumstances, however, biosecurity measures have defined limitations. Close interaction between grazing animals and wildlife can result in the transfer of infectious agents from wild animals to domestic animals. Feral carnivores with rabies can transmit rabies virus not only to domestic animals but also to humans. In these instances, biosecurity measures may be initiated by individual animal owners but ultimately require national government resources for their effective implementation.

78 Vaccination

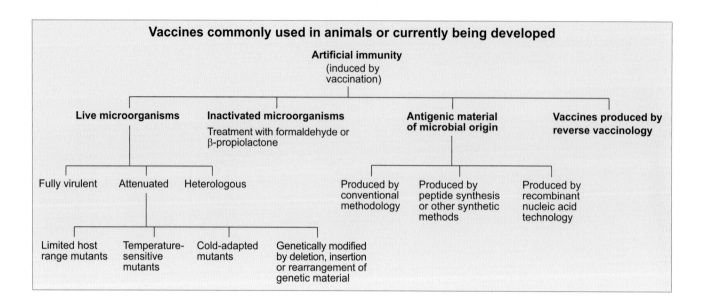

Vaccines commonly used in animals or currently being developed

Artificial immunity
(induced by vaccination)

- Live microorganisms
  - Fully virulent
  - Attenuated
    - Limited host range mutants
    - Temperature-sensitive mutants
    - Cold-adapted mutants
    - Genetically modified by deletion, insertion or rearrangement of genetic material
  - Heterologous
- Inactivated microorganisms
  Treatment with formaldehyde or β-propiolactone
- Antigenic material of microbial origin
  - Produced by conventional methodology
  - Produced by peptide synthesis or other synthetic methods
  - Produced by recombinant nucleic acid technology
- Vaccines produced by reverse vaccinology

The process of stimulating protective immune responses in animals against pathogenic microorganisms by exposing them to non-pathogenic forms or components of microorganisms is referred to as vaccination. A successful vaccine induces an effective long-term adaptive immune response directed at appropriate target antigens on the pathogen without causing disease in the recipient. Among the types of vaccines currently in use or being developed are those composed of inactivated microorganisms, live attenuated microorganisms, microbial products, synthetic peptides and DNA of microbial origin. When feasible, effective and safe, vaccination is one of the most cost-effective measures for controlling infectious disease, not only in companion animals but also in food-producing animals. The duration of protection following vaccination is influenced by many host factors including age, immune competence and the presence of maternal antibodies in the animal's circulation. In common with many disease control measures, however, vaccination has defined limitations. Effective vaccines for controlling equine infectious anaemia and African swine fever are not available at present. Protective immunity against *Staphylococcus aureus* using vaccination cannot be induced in a predictable manner and prevention of fungal infections through vaccination has had limited success.

In a large population of animals of a comparable age and immune status, the response to vaccination is not uniform. The immune response is influenced by many genetic and environmental factors and the outcome of vaccination tends to follow a normal distribution. A small percentage of animals have a weak response to vaccination and if challenged might be susceptible to infection. The majority of the animal population respond adequately and a small percentage respond strongly to vaccination. The addition of appropriate adjuvants to vaccines can enhance and prolong the duration of the immune response, decrease the antigen concentration required for effective immunization and promote the development of cell-mediated immune responses.

Adjuvants

Substances with the ability to increase or modulate the intrinsic immunogenicity of an antigen are referred to as adjuvants. If mixed with antigens before administration, adjuvants boost the immune response to antigens of low immunogenicity. They also enhance the immune response to small amounts of antigenic material. Proposed modes of action of adjuvants include retention and slow release of antigenic material from the site of injection (depot effect), increased immunogenicity of small or antigenically weak synthetic peptides and improved speed of response and persistence of response to effective antigens. Adjuvants may stimulate dendritic cell and macrophage activity and promote T and B lymphocyte responses. A wide range of substances including mineral salts, bacterial derivatives, biodegradable particles, emulsions and cytokines are currently used as adjuvants.

Although aluminium salts have been used as adjuvants for almost 80 years, their modes of action are not clearly defined. Their adjuvant activity is attributed to activation of macrophages and increased uptake of antigen by antigen-presenting cells. The adjuvant effect of bacterial derivatives such as muramyl dipeptides is attributed to their ability to stimulate macrophages and dendritic cells, interferon-γ production and T-helper (T_H)

Concise Review of Veterinary Microbiology, Second Edition. P.J. Quinn, B.K. Markey, F.C. Leonard, E.S. FitzPatrick and S. Fanning.
© 2016 John Wiley & Sons, Ltd. Published 2016 by John Wiley & Sons, Ltd.
Companion website: www.wiley.com/go/quinn/concise-veterinary-microbiology

SECTION V

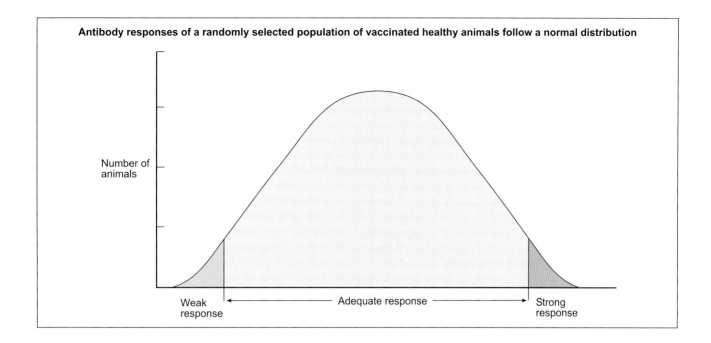

Antibody responses of a randomly selected population of vaccinated healthy animals follow a normal distribution

Number of animals

Weak response

Adequate response

Strong response

cell activity. Antigenic material can be either encapsulated into biodegradable particles or carried on their surfaces through adsorption or covalent linkages. Liposomes are biodegradable particles which are taken up by antigen-presenting cells and their contents are processed via MHC class II-dependent pathways. Cytokines and related substances can be combined with antigenic material and used to direct the immune reaction toward a humoral or cell-mediated response. Immunostimulating complexes (ISCOMs) are saponin-based adjuvants which augment T_H1 and T_H2 cell responses. Their activity is attributed to interactions with macrophages and dendritic cells and activation of $CD4^+$ T cells.

Inactivated vaccines

Infectious agents can be killed without substantially altering the immunogenicity of their antigens which induce protective immunity. Although most inactivating chemicals alter the immunogenicity of infectious agents, some such as formaldehyde cause limited antigenic change. A major limitation of inactivated vaccines is that some protective antigens are not produced readily *in vitro*. Because they are processed as exogenous antigens in the body, many inactivated vaccines can induce high levels of circulating antibody but are less effective at stimulating cell-mediated and mucosal immunity. As inactivated vaccines do not contain agents which can replicate, a greater antigenic mass and a more frequent administration of vaccine (booster injections) are required to achieve results comparable to those obtained with live attenuated vaccines. Advantages of inactivated vaccines include stability at ambient temperatures, safety for recipients due to their inability to revert to a virulent state and a long shelf life.

Live attenuated vaccines

The virulence of living organisms can be reduced by attenuation, a process that involves adapting them to grow under conditions whereby they lose their affinity for their usual host and do not produce disease in susceptible animals. Viruses can be attenuated by growing them in monolayers prepared from

species to which they are not naturally adapted. Chick embryo attenuation has been employed successfully for a number of viruses which infect animals and humans. Live attenuated vaccines have many potential advantages over inactivated vaccines. They can be administered by a number of different routes and present all the relevant antigens required for the induction of protective immunity since they multiply in the recipient. They usually induce a satisfactory level of cell-mediated and humoral immunity at sites where protection is required such as mucosal surfaces. Disadvantages of modified live vaccines include the possibility of reversion to virulence, contamination with infectious agents capable of causing disease in the recipient and neutralization by maternal antibodies in young animals acquired by ingestion of colostrum. A live attenuated viral vaccine has a limited shelf life and should be refrigerated during transportation and storage to ensure its viability.

Vaccines produced by recombinant nucleic acid technology

Recombinant vaccines are classified into three categories: vaccines composed of antigens produced by recombinant nucleic acid technology or genetic engineering, vaccines consisting of genetically attenuated microorganisms and vaccines composed of modified live viruses or bacteria into which DNA encoding protective antigens are introduced by cloning. Vaccines produced by recombinant nucleic acid technology are composed of subunit proteins produced by recombinant bacteria or other microorganisms. DNA encoding the required antigen is cloned in a suitable bacterium or yeast strain in which the recombinant antigen is expressed.

Virulent microorganisms can be rendered less virulent by gene deletion or site-directed mutagenesis. Virulent viruses and bacteria can be modified by deletion of appropriate genes and animals vaccinated with such vaccines can be differentiated from animals infected with a field strain of the pathogen. The failure of some vaccines used in veterinary medicine to induce a protective immune response can result from problems related to delivery. Vaccines composed of modified live organisms called

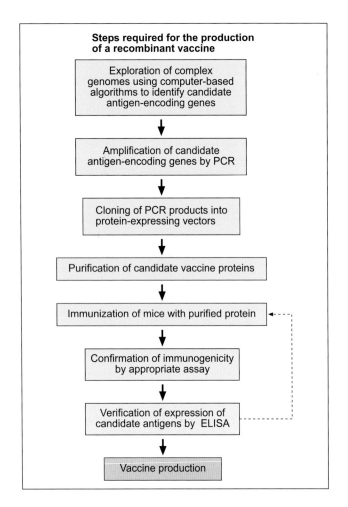

Steps required for the production of a recombinant vaccine

Exploration of complex genomes using computer-based algorithms to identify candidate antigen-encoding genes

↓

Amplification of candidate antigen-encoding genes by PCR

↓

Cloning of PCR products into protein-expressing vectors

↓

Purification of candidate vaccine proteins

↓

Immunization of mice with purified protein

↓

Confirmation of immunogenicity by appropriate assay

↓

Verification of expression of candidate antigens by ELISA

↓

Vaccine production

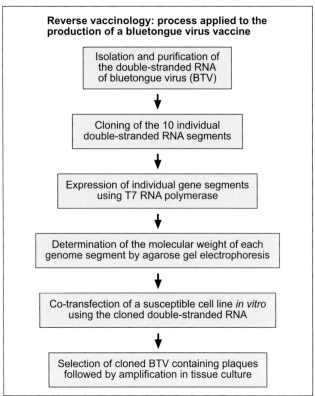

Reverse vaccinology: process applied to the production of a bluetongue virus vaccine

Isolation and purification of the double-stranded RNA of bluetongue virus (BTV)

↓

Cloning of the 10 individual double-stranded RNA segments

↓

Expression of individual gene segments using T7 RNA polymerase

↓

Determination of the molecular weight of each genome segment by agarose gel electrophoresis

↓

Co-transfection of a susceptible cell line *in vitro* using the cloned double-stranded RNA

↓

Selection of cloned BTV containing plaques followed by amplification in tissue culture

vectors, into which a gene encoding an antigenic determinant is introduced, can be used as a delivery system. Currently a small number of viral vectored vaccines have been approved for use in animals. A vaccinia vaccine vector carrying the rabies G glycoprotein has been used successfully as an oral vaccine administered to wild carnivores in bait. The G glycoprotein induces virus-neutralizing antibodies in vaccinated animals which protect against rabies. Other examples include a canarypox virus-vectored vaccine against canine distemper virus in dogs and a fowlpox virus-vectored vaccine designed to protect against avian influenza in poultry.

Synthetic peptide vaccines

If the structure of epitopes that can induce a protective immune response is known, it is possible to chemically synthesize peptides corresponding to these antigenic determinants. Only a small portion of antigenic molecules interact with specific receptors on B cells and T cells. For B cells, an antibody interacts with up to five amino acids in its antigen-binding site. Epitopes for T-cell receptors can be composed of 12 to 15 amino acids.

The general approach with synthetic peptide vaccines is to identify appropriate epitopes in protein components of the infectious agent and to synthesize a series of peptides corresponding to the amino acid sequences. Limited progress has been made with synthetic peptides for the induction of protective immune responses against infectious agents.

DNA vaccines

One of the most important developments in vaccine production in recent years involves the use of DNA, encoding microbial antigens cloned in a bacterial plasmid, for immunization. The procedure involves injection of a plasmid containing the DNA sequence for a protective antigen whose expression is controlled by a strong mammalian promoter. For an infectious agent expressing that antigen, injection of this recombinant plasmid into the skin or muscles of animals may result in the production of protein inducing immunity against that infectious agent. This leads to the expression in host cells of encoded genes, with the development of a significant immune response to the gene products in the recipient. Unlike viral vectors, the recombinant plasmid cannot replicate in the mammalian cells, but transfected host cells express the vaccine antigen. Although transfection rates appear to be low, antigen production has been detected in animals vaccinated with DNA intramuscularly for up to six months after injection. Because DNA vaccination induces intracellular processing of antigen, it seems to mimic a natural infection and is, therefore, an effective method of inducing T cell responses. Humoral responses, however, may not be as high as those obtained by injection of a purified antigen. Although immune response may be delayed following DNA vaccination, a persistent response may occur. In contrast to live viral vaccines, maternal antibody does not appear to affect the immune response in young animals.

Questions related to the safety of DNA vaccines remain unresolved. The possibility that foreign DNA could integrate into the host chromosome and induce neoplastic changes or other cellular alterations has been suggested. It has also been suggested that DNA introduced into the body by this method of

Factors associated with vaccination failure

Vaccination Failure

Animal-related factors
- Infection (incubating the disease)
- Immunosuppression caused by drugs or infectious agents
- Genetic influences on immune responsiveness
- Passive protection by colostral antibodies (neutralization of live viral vaccines)
- Immunodeficient state due to developmental defects
- Exposure to a heavy challenge dose of infectious agent shortly after vaccination

Vaccine-related factors

Characteristics of vaccine
- Out-of-date
- Stored at incorrect temperature, loss of potency
- Exposed to sunlight with resultant partial inactivation
- Ineffective vaccine, incapable of inducing protective immunity
- Wrong strain or serotype of pathogen
- Death of live vaccine

Vaccine reconstitution and administration
- Lyophilized vaccine reconstituted with inappropriate diluent
- Incorrect route of administration
- Aerosolized vaccine not distributed properly among animals
- Contamination of multi-dose containers by non-sterile equipment

vaccination might induce anti-DNA antibodies to the recipient's own DNA.

Reverse vaccinology

The availability of genome sequences for many infectious agents offers the possibility of identifying target genes that can code for relevant proteins, thereby providing an opportunity for the rational selection of vaccine candidates. This novel approach, termed reverse vaccinology, can be combined with immunological procedures to optimize epitope prediction, leading to the development of DNA vaccines. A limitation of reverse vaccinology is that the strain of organism selected may not be representative of the genetic diversity of the species. Comparison of the genomes of several different strains of bacteria indicates that important differences exist among different strains of the same bacterial species. Accordingly, it may be necessary to evaluate genome sequences from multiple strains of a microbial pathogen to identify appropriate targets for vaccine production.

Adverse reactions following vaccination

Undesirable reactions to vaccination may occur as a consequence of contamination of the vaccine during manufacture, reconstitution or administration. These adverse reactions may include allergic responses to vaccine components, especially protein from tissue culture fluids or chick embryo sources. Reactions at the injection site may follow introduction of pyogenic bacteria into the tissues. Granulomas at the injection site may result from the type of adjuvant present in a vaccine. There may be a risk of immunosuppression following administration of some live vaccines to particular breeds of animals (Box 78.1).

Box 78.1 Potential adverse reactions following vaccination

- Local or systemic infection caused by contamination of live vaccine with extraneous agents
- Disease produced by the survival of infectious agents in a supposedly killed vaccine
- Disease produced by resistant infectious agents such as prions surviving in inactivated vaccines
- Disease production by live vaccine in immunosuppressed animals
- There may be a risk of congenital defects if particular live vaccines are administered to pregnant animals
- Vaccine-induced immunosuppression
- Development of hypersensitivity reactions to vaccine components (immediate or delayed responses)
- Adjuvants containing mineral oil may induce a granulomatous reaction at the injection site
- Induction of neoplastic changes due to the presence of oncogenic infectious agents or from the action of particular adjuvants

Vaccination failure

The outcome of vaccination is determined by many factors, some related to vaccine composition and others related to characteristics of the animals receiving the vaccine. Vaccine-related factors that can contribute to vaccination failure include inherent characteristics of the vaccine and problems with reconstitution and administration. Animal-related factors include the possibility of animals incubating the disease at time of vaccination, neutralization of live viral vaccines by colostral antibodies and immunosuppression caused by drugs or infectious agents.

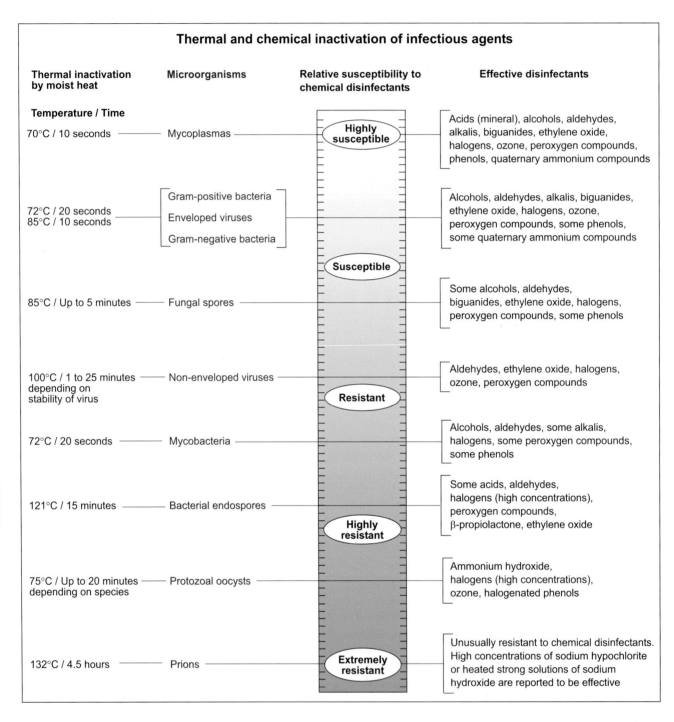

Thermal and chemical inactivation of infectious agents

Thermal inactivation by moist heat	Microorganisms	Relative susceptibility to chemical disinfectants	Effective disinfectants
Temperature / Time			
70°C / 10 seconds	Mycoplasmas	Highly susceptible	Acids (mineral), alcohols, aldehydes, alkalis, biguanides, ethylene oxide, halogens, ozone, peroxygen compounds, phenols, quaternary ammonium compounds
72°C / 20 seconds 85°C / 10 seconds	Gram-positive bacteria / Enveloped viruses / Gram-negative bacteria	Susceptible	Alcohols, aldehydes, alkalis, biguanides, ethylene oxide, halogens, ozone, peroxygen compounds, some phenols, some quaternary ammonium compounds
85°C / Up to 5 minutes	Fungal spores		Some alcohols, aldehydes, biguanides, ethylene oxide, halogens, peroxygen compounds, some phenols
100°C / 1 to 25 minutes depending on stability of virus	Non-enveloped viruses	Resistant	Aldehydes, ethylene oxide, halogens, ozone, peroxygen compounds
72°C / 20 seconds	Mycobacteria		Alcohols, aldehydes, some alkalis, halogens, some peroxygen compounds, some phenols
121°C / 15 minutes	Bacterial endospores	Highly resistant	Some acids, aldehydes, halogens (high concentrations), peroxygen compounds, β-propiolactone, ethylene oxide
75°C / Up to 20 minutes depending on species	Protozoal oocysts		Ammonium hydroxide, halogens (high concentrations), ozone, halogenated phenols
132°C / 4.5 hours	Prions	Extremely resistant	Unusually resistant to chemical disinfectants. High concentrations of sodium hypochlorite or heated strong solutions of sodium hydroxide are reported to be effective

Infectious agents shed in the excretions or secretions of animals, or present in products of animal origin, may remain viable for long periods in the environment. Buildings, equipment, transport vehicles, soil, pasture, water and fomites may become contaminated by faeces or urine containing bacterial, viral or protozoal pathogens. Fungal pathogens such as dermatophytes may contaminate tables, building surfaces and grooming equipment. Respiratory secretions of sick animals may contain viral or bacterial pathogens and, following abortion caused by *Brucella abortus*, high numbers of brucellae may be present in foetal

Concise Review of Veterinary Microbiology, Second Edition. P.J. Quinn, B.K. Markey, F.C. Leonard, E.S. FitzPatrick and S. Fanning.
© 2016 John Wiley & Sons, Ltd. Published 2016 by John Wiley & Sons, Ltd.
Companion website: www.wiley.com/go/quinn/concise-veterinary-microbiology

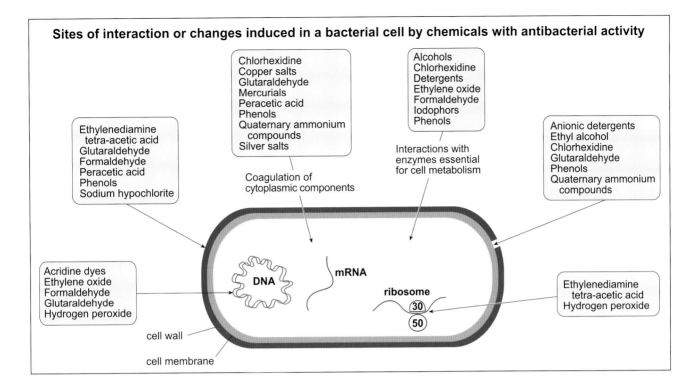

Sites of interaction or changes induced in a bacterial cell by chemicals with antibacterial activity

Chlorhexidine
Copper salts
Glutaraldehyde
Mercurials
Peracetic acid
Phenols
Quaternary ammonium
    compounds
Silver salts

Alcohols
Chlorhexidine
Detergents
Ethylene oxide
Formaldehyde
Iodophors
Phenols

Ethylenediamine
    tetra-acetic acid
Glutaraldehyde
Formaldehyde
Peracetic acid
Phenols
Sodium hypochlorite

Interactions with
enzymes essential
for cell metabolism

Coagulation of
cytoplasmic components

Anionic detergents
Ethyl alcohol
Chlorhexidine
Glutaraldehyde
Phenols
Quaternary ammonium
    compounds

Acridine dyes
Ethylene oxide
Formaldehyde
Glutaraldehyde
Hydrogen peroxide

Ethylenediamine
    tetra-acetic acid
Hydrogen peroxide

DNA

mRNA

ribosome

30

50

cell wall

cell membrane

fluids. Disinfection is an essential part of disease control programmes for both endemic and exotic diseases. It is also used to lessen the risk of disease transmission from animals to humans not only during the production stage but also at the processing stages in meat plants and dairies.

Disinfection implies the use of physical and chemical methods for the destruction of microorganisms, especially potential pathogens, on surfaces of inanimate objects or in the environment. There is wide variation in the susceptibility of infectious agents to thermal inactivation. Although both moist heat and dry heat can be used for the inactivation of microorganisms, moist heat is more effective and requires less time to achieve inactivation than dry heat. At temperatures above 80°C most vegetative bacteria are killed within seconds. Bacterial endospores are exceptionally thermoresistant and moist heat at 121°C for at least 15 minutes is required for their inactivation. Many enveloped viruses are labile at temperatures above 70°C. Non-enveloped viruses such as foot-and-mouth disease virus are thermostable and temperatures close to 100°C for more than 20 minutes may be required to inactivate such resistant viruses. The prions which cause transmissible spongiform encephalopathies are extremely resistant to thermal inactivation. Dry heat at 160°C does not inactivate these agents and traces of infectivity were detected following treatment in a muffle furnace at 600°C for 15 minutes. Autoclaving at 132°C for at least 4.5 hours is required for their inactivation.

Infectious agents vary widely in their susceptibility to chemical disinfectants. Most vegetative bacteria and enveloped viruses are readily inactivated by disinfectants. However, biofilm formation on equipment surfaces, especially in inaccessible locations, confers protection on microorganisms against chemical inactivation. Fungal spores and non-enveloped viruses are moderately resistant to chemical inactivation. Mycobacteria and bacterial endospores are resistant to many commonly used disinfectants. Prions are extremely resistant to chemical inactivation. High

concentrations of sodium hypochlorite or autoclaving at 121°C for 30 minutes in 2 mol/L sodium hydroxide inactivated the prion agents tested.

Chemical compounds with antibacterial activity may react with the cell wall, cell membrane, nucleic acid or other cytoplasmic constituents. The targets of chemicals with sporicidal activity include the outer coat, the inner coat, the spore cortex and the small acid-soluble DNA-binding proteins in the endospore core. Virucidal disinfectants may react with nucleic acids, structural or functional proteins, glycoproteins and, in the case of enveloped viruses, with the lipid envelope.

In addition to the intrinsic resistance of bacterial endospores, mycobacteria and some Gram-negative bacteria to particular chemical compounds, the ability of a number of pathogenic bacteria to acquire resistance to chemical disinfectants has been observed in recent years. In a number of instances, there is evidence that resistance to disinfectants and antibiotics is genetically linked.

For the success of a disinfection programme, thorough cleaning should precede the application of disinfectant. The disinfectant selected should be active against the infectious agents present and it should be diluted to yield the correct concentration. Most disinfectants require several hours to inactivate infectious agents on surfaces. The presence of organic matter such as faeces, exudates, body fluids, bedding or food residues interferes with the antimicrobial activity of disinfectants and slows their action. Failure to inactivate infectious agents present in buildings, on equipment or in transport vehicles may be due to the selection of an inappropriate disinfectant, careless use of a potentially effective disinfectant or environmental factors. As no residual antimicrobial activity persists after disinfection, infectious agents may be reintroduced by infected domestic animals, fomites, food, on the footwear or clothing of personnel or by rodents.

Appendix: relevant websites

General topics

American Society for Microbiology (ASM):
   http://www.asm.org

American Tissue Culture Collection (ATCC):
   http://www.atcc.org

Animal diseases: http://www.oie.int

Antimicrobial susceptibility testing: http://www.clsi.org

Centers for Disease Control and Prevention:
   http://www.cdc.gov

Society for Applied Microbiology: http://www.sfam.org.uk

Society for General Microbiology: http://www.sgm.ac.uk

Genomic analysis

Bacterial genome listing: http://www.ncbi.nlm.nih.gov/genome

BLAST alignment tool: http://www.ncbi.nlm.nih.gov/BLAST

In silico simulation of molecular biology experiments:
   http://insilico.ehu.es

J. Craig Venter Institute (formerly TIGR): http://www.jcvi.org/

Kyoto Encyclopedia of Genes and Genomes:
   http://www.genome.jp/kegg

Multi-locus sequence typing (MLST): http://www.mlst.net

Ribosomal Database Project: http://rdp.cme.msu.edu

Bacteriology

American Society for Microbiology, Approved Lists of
   Bacterial Names:
   http://www.ncbi.nlm.nih.gov/books/NBK815

Collection of bacterial taxonomic and genomic information at
   PathoSystems Resource Integration Center:
   http://patricbrc.vbi.vt.edu/portal/portal/patric/Home

List of prokaryotic names with standing in nomenclature:
   http://www.bacterio.net/

Up-to-date information on prokaryotic nomenclature:
   http://www.dsmz.de/microorganisms/pnu/bacterial_
   nomenclature_mm.php

Taxonomic outlines for *Bergey's Manual*, Volumes 3, 4 and 5:
   http://www.bergeys.org/outlines.html

European platform for the responsible use of medicines in
   animals: http://www.epruma.eu/

The European Committee for Antimicrobial Susceptibility
   testing: http://www.eucast.org/

Mycology

Index Fungorum, names of fungi:
   http://www.indexfungorum.org/

MycoBank, fungal database with a remit to document
   mycological nomenclatural novelties and their associated
   descriptions and illustrations: http://www.mycobank.org/

ViralZone: http://viralzone.expasy.org/

Virology

European Advisory Board on Cat Diseases (ABCD) with
   useful review articles on infectious diseases of cats:
   http://www.abcd-vets.org/

International Committee on Taxonomy of Viruses (ICTV) with
   latest information on viral nomenclature: http://ictvonline.
   org/virusTaxonomy.asp?bhcp=1

Infectious diseases

Department for Environment, Food and Rural Affairs
   (DEFRA): https://www.gov.uk/government/organisations/
   department-for-environment-food-rural-affairs

European Food Safety Authority, Biohazard Panel. Many
   useful documents on selected zoonoses:
   http://www.efsa.europa.eu/en/panels/biohaz.htm

Fact files on infectious diseases of animals at Center for Food
   Security and Public Health, Iowa State University:
   http://www.cfsph.iastate.edu/DiseaseInfo/index.php

Food and Agriculture Organization of the United Nations
   (UN-FAO): http://www.fao.org/

Material safety data sheets, Canadian Laboratory Center for
   Disease Control: http://www.phac-aspc.gc.ca/id-mi/
   index-eng.php

ProMED mail, a global electronic reporting system for
   outbreaks of emerging infectious diseases, maintained by the
   International Society for Infectious Diseases (ISID):
   http://www.promedmail.org

World Organization for Animal Health (OIE)

Useful information on infectious disease occurrence:
   http://www.oie.int/wahis_2/public/wahid.php/Wahidhome/
   Home

Online manual of diagnostic tests and vaccines for animals:
   http://www.oie.int/en/international-standard-setting/
   terrestrial-manual/access-online/

World Health Organization: http://www.who.int/en/

Concise Review of Veterinary Microbiology, Second Edition. P.J. Quinn, B.K. Markey, F.C. Leonard, E.S. FitzPatrick and S. Fanning.
© 2016 John Wiley & Sons, Ltd. Published 2016 by John Wiley & Sons, Ltd.
Companion website: www.wiley.com/go/quinn/concise-veterinary-microbiology

Index

Concise Review of Veterinary Microbiology, Second Edition. P.J. Quinn, B.K. Markey, F.C. Leonard, E.S. FitzPatrick and S. Fanning.
© 2016 John Wiley & Sons, Ltd. Published 2016 by John Wiley & Sons, Ltd.
Companion website: www.wiley.com/go/quinn/concise-veterinary-microbiology